OFFICE ORTHOPEDICS

for

PRIMARY CARE

OFFICE

ORTHOPEDICS

for

PRIMARY

CARE Diagnosis and Treatment

Second Edition

Bruce Carl Anderson, M.D.

Clinical Associate Professor of Medicine
Oregon Health Sciences University
Portland, Oregon

Director, Medical Orthopedic Department
Sunnyside Medical Center
Portland, Oregon

W.B. SAUNDERS COMPANY

A Division of Harcourt Brace & Company

Philadelphia London Toronto Montreal Sydney Tokyo

W.B. SAUNDERS COMPANY
A Division of Harcourt Brace & Company

The Curtis Center
Independence Square West
Philadelphia, Pennsylvania 19106

Library of Congress Cataloging-in-Publication Data

Anderson, Bruce Carl.

Office orthopedics for primary care:diagnosis and treatment / Bruce Carl Anderson.
—2nd ed.

p.   cm.

Includes bibliographical references and index.

ISBN 0–7216–7089–x

1. Orthopedics.   2. Primary care (Medicine)   I. Title.   [DNLM: 1. Musculoskeletal Diseases—diagnosis. 2. Musculoskeletal Diseases—therapy. 3. Fractures—therapy. 4. Family Practice—methods.
WE 141A545o   1999]

RD732.A53   1999   616.7—dc21

DNLM/DLC   98–36303

OFFICE ORTHOPEDICS FOR PRIMARY CARE: Diagnosis and Treatment   ISBN 0–7216–7089–x

Printed in the United States of America.

Last digit is the print number: 9   8   7   6   5   4   3   2   1

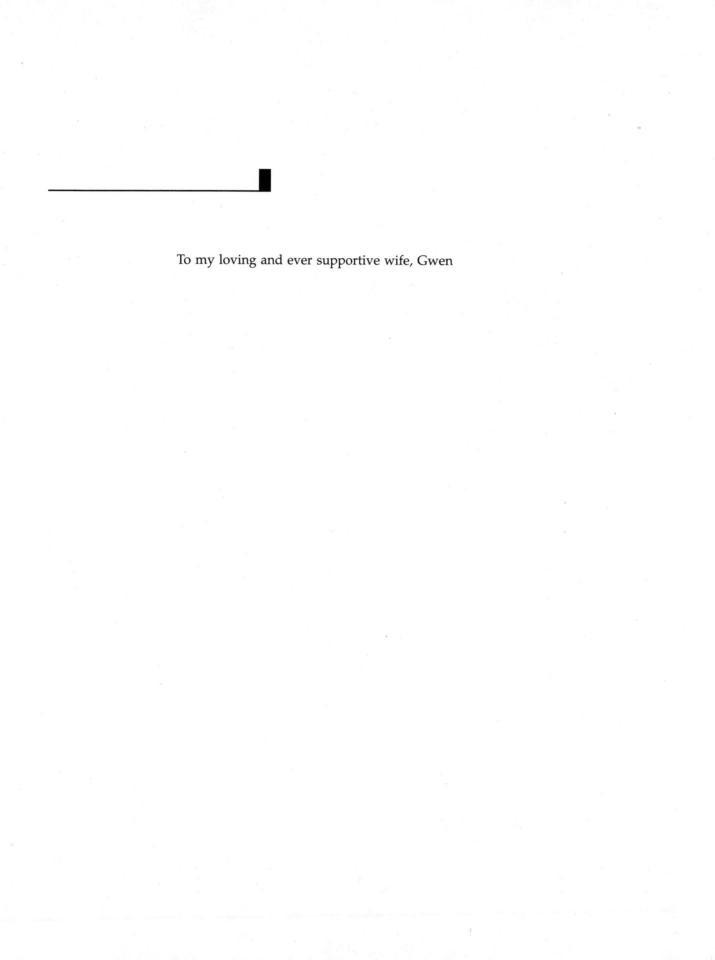

To my loving and ever supportive wife, Gwen

preface

Twenty years ago, in the first year of my internal medicine practice, I was confronted with a most challenging and confounding clinical situation. An extremely muscular, 50-year-old, 250-pound longshoreman presented to my office with an extremely painful right shoulder, demanding a cortisone injection. He said in no uncertain terms, "I'm here for a cortisone shot, and if you won't give me one I want you to find a doctor that will!" I placed his chart down and listened as he went on to say, "I can't stand the pain anymore. It's taken me 5 months to get up the courage to come in. I had the same problem 12 years ago, and my doctor gave me a cortisone injection that cured it! If you won't give me a shot, I'm wasting your time." At that moment, I reflected on my internal medicine teacher's warnings about the hazards and dangers of cortisone injection and was about to pass on to my patient the biases of 20 years of mainstream medical dogma, when he went on to relate, "The shot was the worst pain I ever experienced. All I can remember is the doctor 'digging the needle' on the bone several times before I passed out. My arm was so sore for 3 days that I could hardly move it, but then the pain went away. I have to have another injection so I can get back to work!"

This was not an isolated incident. It was just one of several cases that brought into focus the juxtaposition of the prevailing attitudes of mainsteam internal medicine's teachings regarding injectable corticosteroids—the hazards and dangers of injection, "only as a last resort in treatment," how the treament just covers up the pain, and so forth—and the attitudes and expectations of patients who had received this type of treatment in the past—"an excruciating experience," "cortisone destroys joints," "the only treatment that works." It was this dichotomy that sent this former research chemist on what has turned out to be a lifelong journey of discovery about injectable corticosteroids. Over the next 2 decades, the clinical experiences of hundreds of patients reoriented my attitude and understanding of the utility of local injection of corticosteroids and how this technically demanding part of medicine can be combined with restrictive use, selective immobilization, and physical therapy exercises to successfully and safely manage the conditions that affect the musculoskeletal system.

The cumulative experience and lessons of 20 years of clinical practice, research, and medical residency training are incorporated into this second edition. The book is intended to provide clarity on the treatment of the common outpatient orthopedic problems that are so prevalent in the everyday practice of the primary care physician. Family practitioners, internal medicine specialists, nurse practitioners, and osteopathic and chiropractic physicians will find it a practical guide.

The second edition of this book has expanded. Details of the diagnosis and treatment of 48 common conditions have replaced the first edition's 44. Greater emphasis has been placed on the unique examination skills necessary for diagnosis. The materials included in the appendix have been expanded and updated. However, the format of the book has not been changed. The book is still divided into four sections—the most common conditions, the troublesome fractures, the physical therapy instruction sheets, and the most commonly used supports, braces, and casts—

emphasizing the need to integrate local injection, physical therapy, and immobilization in the complete management of these common conditions.

This book is intended to be comprehensive, providing the practitioner with accurate and easily accessible information on diagnosis and treatment. The "step-care" treatment protocols; the physical therapy exercise instruction sheets; the illustrations of the various braces, casts, and supports; and the detailed descriptions of local injection techniques allow the clinician to "office manage" 90 to 95% of the outpatient medical orthopedic problems. Treatment guidelines provide details on specific restrictions. The length of time for immobilization is both efficacious and practical. The appropriate timing and anatomical details of local injection and the extremely important post-treatment rehabilitation exercises are included. Although local corticosteroid injection has been emphasized, this book was not intended to be simply an "injection manual." Injection of corticosteroids can be exceedingly helpful in arresting the local inflammatory reaction to tissue injury. However, it must not take the place of simpler, less invasive treatments. Local injection of tendons, bursae, ligaments, or joints is indicated when local musculoskeletal inflammation persists despite rest, restriction, appropriate immobilization, and physical therapy.

There are as many ways to accomplish the same treatment goals in the field of musculoskeletal medicine as there are conditions. Differences in technique and approach are widespread in this overlooked part of medicine. This book can serve as a starting point for those interested in expanding their expertise in the treatment of musculoskeletal disease in outpatients. I hope that it bridges the gaps between rheumatology, orthopedics, neurology, and physiatry. In addition, I hope it can serve as a stimulation to greater interest, discussion, and use of local musculoskeletal diagnosis and treatment by internists, family practitioners, osteopathic physicians, and allied health providers. Lastly, I believe it is time to open up the curricula of internal medicine residency programs to a greater emphasis on this very important part of clinical medicine.

acknowledgements

This book represents the outgrowth of 20 years of postresidency education and clinical experience that would not have been possible without the support and encouragement from many sources. I wish to thank all the members of the department of medicine at Sunnyside Medicine Center, especially Dr. Ian MacMillan, for their support in the early years. I also wish to thank my extremely capable physician assistant, Linda Onheiber, and all the medical residents of the graduating classes of 1997 and 1998 at the Oregon Health Sciences University for their constant encouragement, contribution, and critical appraisal of the content of the book, especially Drs. Rick Kadera, Todd Hoechendel, James Chapman, Susan Davids, and Eric Fromme. Thanks to Dr. David N. Gilbert—my internal medicine residency director—for his stimulation to excellence, his encouragement to examine ever deeper into clinical problems, and his support and inspiration in my return to clinical research. Lastly, I wish to thank my loving wife, Gwen, and my three children, Jeremy, Jennifer, and Ryan, for their patience and understanding for the many hours I spent writing, drawing, and editing this work.

contents

Introduction xv

SECTION I
The 48 Most Common Outpatient Orthopedic Conditions 1

Chapter 1
Neck 3
    Cervical Strain 4
    Cervical Radiculopathy 8

Chapter 2
Shoulder 13
    Impingement Syndrome 14
    Rotator Cuff Tendinitis 18
    Frozen Shoulder 23
    Rotator Cuff Tendon Tear 27
    Acromioclavicular Strain-Osteoarthritis 31
    Biceps Tendinitis 35
    Subscapular Bursitis 39
    Glenohumeral Osteoarthritis 41
    Multidirectional Instability of the Shoulder 45

Chapter 3
Elbow 49
    Lateral Epicondylitis 50
    Medial Epicondylitis 54
    Olecranon Bursitis 58
    Radiohumeral Joint Arthrocentesis 61

Chapter 4
Wrist 65
    De Quervain Tenosynovitis 66
    Carpometacarpal Osteoarthritis 69
    Gamekeeper's Thumb 73
    Carpal Tunnel Syndrome 75
    Radiocarpal Joint Arthrocentesis 78
    Dorsal Ganglion 82

Chapter 5
Hand 85
    Trigger Finger 86
    Tendon Cyst 89
    Dupuytren's Contracture 92
    Metacarpophalangeal Joint Arthrocentesis 94
    Osteoarthritis of the Hand 96
    Rheumatoid Arthritis 99

Chapter 6
Chest 103
    Sternochondritis/Costochondritis 104
    Sternoclavicular Joint 107

Chapter 7

Back 111

    Lumbosacral Strain 112

    Lumbar Radiculopathy, Herniated Disk, Sciatica 116

    Sacroiliac Strain 120

Chapter 8

Hip 125

    Trochanteric Bursitis 126

    Gluteus Medius Bursitis/Piriformis Syndrome 130

    Osteoarthritis of the Hip 134

    Meralgia Paresthetica 137

Chapter 9

Knee 139

    Patellofemoral Diseases 140

    Knee Effusion 143

    Dry Tap Injection of the Knee 148

    Osteoarthritis of the Knee 149

    Prepatellar Bursitis 153

    Anserine Bursitis 155

    Baker Cyst 159

    Medial Collateral Ligament Sprain 161

    Meniscal Tear of the Knee 165

Chapter 10

Ankle 169

    Ankle Sprain 170

    Arthrocentesis of the Ankle 174

    Achilles Tendinitis 177

    Pre-Achilles Bursitis 181

    Retrocalcaneal Bursitis 183

    Posterior Tibialis Tenosynovitis 186

    Plantar Fasciitis 188

Chapter 11

Foot 193

    Bunions 194

    Adventitial Bursitis of the First MTP 197

    Gout 200

    Hammer Toes 203

    Morton Neuroma 206

SECTION II

Fractures 209

Chapter 12

Fractures Frequently Encountered in Primary Care 211

    Fractures of the Humerus 217

    Fractures of the Clavicle 218

    Fractures of the Distal Radius 221

    Fractures of the Navicular 222

    Gamekeeper's Thumb, Complete Rupture 224

    Compression Fracture of the Vertebral Body 227

    Rib Fracture 229

    Avascular Necrosis of the Hip 231

    Occult Fracture of the Hip 232

    Tibial Stress Fracture 235

    Gastrocnemius Muscle Tear 236

    Fractures of the Ankle 237

    Heel Pad Syndrome 239

Accessory Bones of the Feet 241
Metatarsal Stress Fractures (March Fracture) 242

SECTION III

Exercise Instruction Sheets 245

Chapter 13

Exercise Instructions for Home Physical Therapy 247
Neck Massage 251
Stretching Exercises for the Neck 252
Home Cervical Traction 253
Pendulum Stretch Exercises for the Shoulder 256
Strengthening Exercises for the Rotator Cuff Tendons 257
Stretching Exercises for a Frozen Shoulder 258
Tennis Elbow Strengthening Exercises 262
Stretching of the Wrist and Hand Tendons 263
Back-Stretching Exercises 266
Advanced Back-Stretching Exercises 267
Back-Strengthening Exercises 268
Stretching Exercises for Arthritis 272
Stretch Exercises for Hip Bursitis 273
Knee-Strengthening Exercises 276
Achilles Tendon Stretching Exercises 279
Ankle Isometric Toning Exercises 280

SECTION IV

Supports, Braces, and Casts 281

Chapter 14

The Most Commonly Used Supports, Braces, and Casts 283
Neck 284
Shoulder 285
Elbow 287
Wrist 288
Hand 293
Lumbosacral Region 295
Knee 297
Ankle 300
Foot 303

Appendix

Fractures, Medications, Lab Values 307
Fractures That Require Referral to a Surgical Orthopedist 307
Nonsteroidal Anti-Inflammatory Drugs 308
Corticosteroids 309
Calcium Supplementation 309
Lab Tests in Rheumatology 310
Synovial Fluid Analysis 311
References 313
Index 321

HEALTH SCIENCES
BOOKSTORE
2109 Aldelbert Road
School of Medicine WB - 10
Cleveland, OH 44106

97 2 11 822

2167089X   7
NDERSON   43.00

              Fee
Postage   3.

              Sub Total   4
      4 - 08 - 7% Tax Total

                       TOTAL

GENERAL CONCEPTS OF LOCAL MUSCULOSKELETAL INJECTION

PRINCIPLES. The successful management of the conditions affecting the musculo-skeletal system requires combining treatment modalities: (1) local injection by *anatomical placement* (as opposed to trigger point injection); (2) *local anesthetic block* to confirm the clinical diagnosis; (3) separate *corticosteroid injection* using a long-acting and concentrated derivative (unmixed); (4) *rest and restricted use* following injection to minimize displacement, lessen inflammatory flare reaction, and optimize anti-inflammatory effect; (5) *adjunctive physical therapy* to recover or enhance lost function; (6) recommendations for *prevention;* and (7) in selected cases, *orthopedic surgical* referral.

MATERIALS. (1) Iodine and alcohol preps; (2) ethyl chloride topical spray; (3) 1% Xylocaine without epinephrine; (4) methylprednisolone (D80) 80 mg/ml (Depo-Medrol), triamcinolone acetonide (K40) 40 mg/ml, tri-iodinated meglumine diatriz-oate radiopaque contrast; (5) 3-, 5-, 10-, and 25-ml disposable syringes; (6) 5/8″ 25-gauge, 1 1/2″ 22-gauge, 3 1/2″ 22-gauge spinal, and 1 1/2″ 18-gauge needles; (7) medium-sized hemostat to facilitate changing syringes; (8) BandAids, 4″ × 4″ gauze, 1″ tape, and elastic wrap.

EXPLANATION AND REASSURANCE. A thorough explanation of the goals of treatment and the details of the procedure engender greater patient confidence and trust. Each patient, especially the anxious one with a previous negative experience with injection, should be counseled in the following: (1) the use of topical anesthesia, (2) the careful use of local anesthesia, (3) the relatively benign side effects of injection, (4) the need to control inflammation to promote healing, (5) the importance of combining treatments, and (6) the expected outcome.

"You don't have to feel the needle go in if we use the cold spray."
"Local anesthetic is always placed first to reduce the irritation of the cortisone."
"There's no question that cortisone causes serious side effects. However, these are generally seen with the cortisone pills taken by mouth, not with injection."
"This is a very small dose of cortisone.... Did you know your body makes 20 to 30 mg of cortisone every day? The cortisone used in injection is only 5 to 10% different from the natural cortisone in your body. The dose is so small and so isolated, it rarely interferes with your body's metabolism!"
"Cortisone given by injection is the single most effective treatment for local inflammation. Would you ignore the inflammation of an infected cut?"
"Cortisone injection is but one tool used in treatment. It dramatically reduces pain and inflammation, allowing you to perform your recovery exercises more effectively."

SKIN PREPARATION. The operator should wear gloves for protection. Iodine followed by alcohol scrub is used to prepare the injection site. Injection is contraindicated in the presence of infected skin, chronically inflamed skin, or systemic infection.

ANESTHETIC INJECTION. A separate anesthetic injection is important for the following reasons: (1) to confirm the diagnosis, especially when two conditions exist simultaneously; (2) to exclude a potential complication (rotator cuff tendinitis vs. tendon tear); and (3) to avoid dilution of the corticosteroid. Anesthesia is placed in several layers, whereas the corticosteroid is injected into a single tissue plane or structure. For example, in the treatment of a dorsal ganglion, anesthetic is injected outside the wall, the viscous fluid is aspirated completely, and the corticosteroid is injected undiluted into the drained cyst.

CORTICOSTEROID INJECTION. The concentrated (mg/ml), long-acting corticosteroid derivatives, when injected *undiluted* into a bursa, joint, or tissue plane, provide the most predictable results. The soluble derivatives do not provide a sufficient suppression of inflammation to be as effective.

INJECTION TECHNIQUE AND VOLUME. Once the point of entry has been chosen, the needle is passed gently through the tissues. The syringe should be held in two or three fingers with the lightest touch, as if holding a dart. As the needle penetrates each tissue, the tissue resistance and pressure required to move through that tissue must be appreciated. Fat has the least tissue resistance and bone the greatest, with muscle, synovial membrane, ligament, and tendon intermediate. If the patient experiences discomfort, the operator should pause, inject anesthetic, partly withdraw the needle, and redirect the needle away from the painful site. All injections of anesthetic or corticosteroid should be performed slowly and with the least possible volume to avoid tissue disruption.

PRECAUTIONS. At the completion of the injection, firm pressure should be immediately applied. The patient must avoid all known aggravations for the first 3 days to protect the injection site and must limit such aggravations for 30 days. In selected cases (Achilles tendinitis, for example), fixed immobilization may be necessary. *Any restrictions the patient has placed upon himself or herself for the past 30 days should be continued for 4 weeks, until the full effect of the medication has been realized.*

SIDE EFFECTS. All patients must be warned about (1) the 30% chance of soreness or pain after the injection (2 to 3 days; ice, Tylenol); (2) the 10% risk of an inflammatory flare reaction (2 to 3 days; ice, narcotics); (3) the 30% chance of fat or skin atrophy (only in the case of superficial injections and with 90% reverting back to normal in 6 to 12 months); (4) the necessity of reevaluation if redness, swelling, and pain persist beyond 3 to 4 days (the chance of infection is 1 in 10,000 or less); and (5) the signs of a more complicated condition.

PHYSICAL THERAPY EXERCISES. The appropriate exercises are usually begun on the fourth day and gradually increased over the next 3 to 4 weeks. All recommended times of rest, restriction of use, and recovery exercises are based on average responses. Individual cases can be treated with specific recommendations based on response and tolerance.

The 48 Most Common Outpatient Orthopedic Conditions

(1) Trigger points are most frequently seen in the middle portion of the upper trapezius muscle, in the long cervical muscles at the base of the neck (at the C6–C7 vertebral level), and in the rhomboid muscles along the medial scapular border. The tenderness may be localized to a small, quarter-sized area or may affect a diffuse area of muscle in chronic cases. (2) The range of motion of the neck may be limited, correlating well with the degree of muscle spasm. As muscle spasm increases, greater loss of ipsilateral neck rotation and of contralateral neck bending is seen. (Normal rotation of the neck is 90 degrees; normal lateral bending is 45 degrees). Flexion and extension of the neck are affected in extreme cases and in cases in which there is underlying arthritis. (3) In an uncomplicated case, the neurologic exam of the upper extremities is normal. (4) Bony structures of the neck, shoulder, and upper back are usually not tender.

X-RAYS.   A cervical spine series (including posteroanterior (PA), lateral, odontoid, and oblique views) is recommended. Mild to moderate cases of cervical strain demonstrate normal x-rays or nonspecific arthritic changes. Changes specific for cervical strain are seen only in moderate to severe cases. The normal cervical lordotic curve can be replaced by a straightened or even a reversed curve. Loss of normal vertebral alignment is best evaluated on the lateral view of the neck. Severe torticollis may cause a lateral deviation of the cervical spine, which is best seen on the PA view of the neck.

SPECIAL TESTING.   Magnetic resonance imaging (MRI) and electromyograms (EMGs) are used for cases complicated by persistent or moderate to severe radicular symptoms (see p. 8).

DIAGNOSIS.   The diagnosis is based on a history and on physical findings of localized upper back and neck tenderness, the characteristic aggravation of symptoms by ipsilateral rotation and contralateral bending of the neck, and the absence of evidence of radiculopathy by history or by exam. Plain x-rays of the cervical spine are used to assess the severity of the condition and to exclude underlying bony pathology. Regional anesthetic block into a trigger point may be helpful in complex cases to differentiate referred pain from cervical radiculopathy or subscapular bursitis.

TREATMENT.   The goals of treatment are to reduce muscle irritability and spasm and to reestablish the normal cervical lordosis. Ice applications, a muscle relaxer at night for 7 to 10 days, and physical therapy exercises are the treatments of choice.

Step 1: Suggest simple changes in lifestyle, including sitting straight with the shoulders held back, sleeping with the head and neck aligned with the body (a small pillow under the neck), driving with the arms slightly shrugged (arm rests), and avoiding straps over the shoulders.

Recommend ice applications to the base of the neck and upper back for temporary relief of pain and muscle spasm in acute cases.

Begin gentle stretching exercises that are to be performed daily, including shoulder rolls, scapular pinch, and neck stretches (p. 252).

Prescribe a muscle relaxer for nighttime use.

Recommend heat and massage for the upper back and the base of the neck (p. 251).

Discuss stress reduction and how stress contributes to symptoms.

Prescribe a nonsteroidal anti-inflammatory drug (NSAID) (e.g., ibuprofen [Advil, Motrin]) and note its secondary role (inflammation is not a prominent part of cervical strain!).

Step 2 (3 to 4 weeks for persistent cases): Order x-rays of the neck.

Prescribe therapeutic ultrasound for persistent strain.

Recommend deep massage for palliative care.

Prescribe gentle cervical traction, beginning at 5 lb for 5 to 10 minutes once a day (p. 253).

Prescribe a soft cervical collar to be worn during the day, especially when involved in physical work (p. 284).

Step 3 (6 to 8 weeks for chronic cases): Perform trigger point injection with a local anesthetic. This can be combined with a long-acting corticosteroid.

Prescribe a tricyclic antidepressant for long-term control of pain.

Consider referral to physical therapy for a transcutaneous electrical nerve stimulator (TENS) unit or to a pain clinic for long-term control of refractory pain.

PHYSICAL THERAPY.   Physical therapy is fundamental in the treatment and prevention of cervical strain.

PHYSICAL THERAPY SUMMARY

1. Ice
2. Heat prior to stretching of the neck and upper back muscles
3. Deep-muscle massage
4. Therapeutic ultrasound
5. Gentle vertical cervical traction, performed manually or with a traction unit

Acute Period.   Heat, massage, and gentle stretching exercises are used to reduce muscular irritation. These exercises should be performed daily at home. *Heat and massage* to the upper back and to the base of the neck provide temporary relief of pain and spasm. These can be combined with a nighttime muscle relaxer for greater effects. *Stretching exercises* are always recommended to regain flexibility and to counteract muscular spasm (p. 250). Heat and a muscle relaxer may enhance the effects of stretching. More advanced or protracted cases may need deep-pressure massage or *ultrasound treatment* from a licensed therapist.

Recovery/Rehabilitation.   Muscular stretching exercises and cervical traction are used to treat persistent or chronic cases. *Stretching exercises* must be continued three times a week to maintain neck flexibility. Chronic cases benefit from gentle *cervical traction,* beginning with a low weight of 5 to 10 lb for 5 minutes once or twice a day (p. 253). Note that severely irritated cervical muscles must be stretched cautiously. Traction can be irritating if applied too long, too frequently, or with too heavy a weight. Assess the patient's tolerance to traction by applying vertical traction in the office, using either manual traction or a cervical traction unit.

INJECTION TECHNIQUE.   Local injection of anesthetic, corticosteroid, or both is used to treat the acute muscle spasms of torticollis and severe cervical strain and to assist in the management of the acute flare-up of fibromyalgia. At best, its use is adjunctive to the physical therapy exercises.

Positioning: The patient is to be sitting up with the shoulders back. The hands are to be placed in the lap.

Surface Anatomy and Point of Entry: The midportion of the superior trapezius is located halfway between the cervical spinous processes and the lateral aspect of the acromion. The paracervical muscles are located 1″ lateral to the spinous processes.

Angle of Entry and Depth: The needle is inserted into the skin at a perpendicular angle. The depth is 1 to 1¼″.

Anesthesia: Ethyl chloride is sprayed on the skin. Local anesthetic is placed at the outer fascial plane (1 ml) and in the belly of the muscle (½ ml with each puncture).

Technique: The success of treatment depends on the accurate injection of the most seriously affected muscle. The point of maximum tenderness is palpated. The thick skin is punctured rapidly. While holding the syringe as lightly as possible, the needle is passed through the subcutaneous layer until the tissue resistance of the outer fascia is met, approximately ¾ to 1″ deep. (Note that the needle will not enter the muscle unless pressure is applied!) One to two ml of local anesthetic is injected just outside the muscle. With light pressure, the needle is passed into the muscle belly, approximately 1 to 1¼″. Often a giving way or popping will be felt as the fascia is penetrated. One to two ml of anesthetic, corticosteroid, or both is injected into an area the size of a quarter with three separate punctures. Restrict treatments to three injections per year to avoid "woody atrophy" of the muscle or the psychologic dependence on injection.

INJECTION AFTERCARE:

1) *Rest* for 3 days, avoiding neck rotation and lateral bending.

2) A soft *Philadelphia collar* should be used in severe cases for 3 to 7 days.

3) *Ice* (15 minutes every 4 to 6 hours) and *Tylenol ES* (1000 mg twice a day) for soreness.

4) *Protection* of the upper back and neck for 30 days by limiting neck rotation and lateral bending and by maintaining good posture.

5) Resume passively performed *rotation stretching exercises* at 2 to 3 weeks.

6) Repeat *injection* at 6 weeks if overall improvement is less than 50%.

7) Obtain *plain x-rays* of the cervical spine to assess for the loss of normal cervical lordosis, the degree of underlying osteoarthritis, and the presence of significant foraminal encroachment disease (greater than 50% narrowing) for refractory cases.

8) Obtain *MRI* to detect an underlying cervical disk in chronic cases (less than 5%).

SURGICAL PROCEDURE.   None.

PROGNOSIS.   Cervical strain is a universal problem. Symptoms frequently recur. Fibromyalgia probably represents a more extensive process that demands a long-term management strategy incorporating all the principles of treatment for cervical strain.

DESCRIPTION: Cervical radiculopathy is an impairment of the upper extremity neurologic function due to an abnormal process in the neck. Cervical arthritis with foraminal encroachment (90%) and a herniated nucleus pulposus (9%) are its two most common causes. Increasing irritation and pressure over the cervical root lead to progressive nerve impairment: sensory loss, loss of deep tendon reflexes, loss of motor strength, tone, or bulk or, in severe cases, long tract symptoms resulting from spinal cord compression.

SYMPTOMS.   Most patients have numbness or tingling in particular fingers. A few patients describe an electric-like pain over the scapula or radiating from the base of

Cervical Radiculopathy

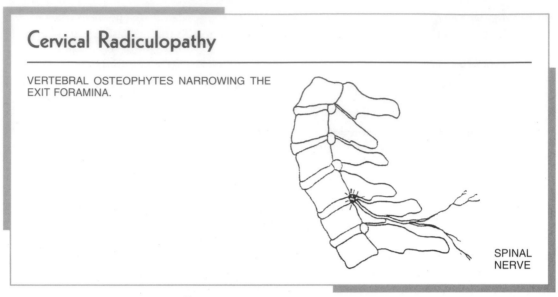

VERTEBRAL OSTEOPHYTES NARROWING THE EXIT FORAMINA.

SPINAL NERVE

Figure 1–2. Cervical radiculopathy

the neck down the arm. Advanced cases may be associated with loss of grip strength (C8) or pushing (C7) or lifting (C6) capacity.

"My fingers feel like they are coming out of Novocain."
"My hand feels numb."
"I think I have a pinched nerve."
*"I have shooting pains down my arm that feel like someone is driving nails into the
    muscles of my arm."*
"It's like your foot goes to sleep—like the nerve is coming out of it."
*"I was working on a ladder, and when I looked straight up, I felt this electric shock
    in the base of my neck."*
"I've been dropping things."

EXAM.   Muscle irritability in the upper back and neck, the range of motion of the neck (particularly in rotation), and the neurology of the upper extremities are examined in each patient.

EXAM SUMMARY

1.   Abnormal upper extremity neurologic exam
2.   Loss of full rotation of the neck and limited extension
3.   A positive Spurling sign
4.   Vertical traction may or may not afford relief
5.   Paracervical tenderness

(1) Findings in the upper extremity neurologic exam are abnormal. Two-point discrimination, light touch, or pinprick sensation may be lost in particular fingers. Deep tendon reflexes may be asymmetric. Grip, triceps, or biceps strength may be impaired in advanced cases. Note that it is important to test strength two or three times to assess the power reserve of the specific muscle groups. (2) The neck often lacks full range of motion, especially in rotation and extension. (Normal rotation of

the neck is 90 degrees.) The loss of rotation correlates directly with the degree of underlying arthritis or the degree of secondary muscular irritation. (3) Nerve root irritation can be brought out by 10 seconds of pressure or by tapping or downward pressure over the top of the cranium (Spurling maneuver) or (4) improved by neck traction applied manually by the examiner. (5) Signs of cervical strain may be present (p. 4).

X-RAYS.   A cervical spine series (including PA, lateral, odontoid, and oblique views) is always recommended. Plain films of the neck may show a loss of the normal cervical lordosis or foraminal encroachment (nearly 90% of cervical radiculopathy is caused by hypertrophic spurs compressing the nerve root at the foraminal level). Because spur formation can occur at multiple levels, the neurologic findings must be correlated with the radiographic abnormalities. For example, symptoms and signs involving the sixth root should correlate with the radiographic changes of foraminal encroachment at vertebral level C5–C6.

SPECIAL TESTING.   An MRI should be obtained when neurologic findings are severe at presentation, when symptoms and signs persist despite reasonable treatment, and when the cervical spine series fails to demonstrate significant (at least 50% narrowing) foraminal encroachment in the oblique views.

DIAGNOSIS.   The diagnosis of cervical radiculopathy is based on a history of radicular pain and paresthesia, neurologic impairment on exam, and correlating abnormalities in x-rays.

TREATMENT.   The goals of treatment are to reduce pressure over the nerve, improve neurologic function, and improve neck flexibility. Ice, a muscle relaxer at night for 7 to 10 days, and rest and protection of the neck are the initial treatments of choice for sensory radiculopathy. Cervical traction, neurosurgical consultation, or both are the treatment recommendations for acute sensorimotor radiculopathy.

Step 1: Perform a complete upper extremity neurologic examination, order neck x-rays or an MRI (depending on the severity), and measure the baseline range of motion of the neck.

Apply ice to the base of the neck and to the upper back to relieve muscle spasm.

Offer a nighttime muscle relaxer (daytime use of a muscle relaxer may aggravate the condition!).

Advise on the proper posture.

Advise on proper nighttime sleeping posture: the patient should sleep with the head and neck aligned with the body (using a small pillow under the neck when lying on the back or several pillows when lying on the side).

Offer a soft cervical collar (p. 284) or a Philadelphia collar for severe muscle irritability (p. 284).

Underscore the importance of stress reduction.

Recommend seat belts and an air bag.

Apply massage and heat to the upper neck and back (p. 251).

Prescribe an NSAID (e.g., ibuprofen [Advil, Motrin]) for pain control.

Step 2 (2 to 3 weeks for persistent cases): Reevaluate neurologic function.

Begin gentle stretching exercises in rotation and lateral bending in sets of 20, performed after heat is applied (p. 252).

Apply vertical cervical traction. A physical therapist can initiate this type of therapy; however, daily traction will have to be performed by the patient at home. A water bag traction unit should be prescribed. Traction is begun at 5 lb for 5 minutes. At intervals of 7 days, the weight and timing are gradually increased to a maximum of 12 to 15 lb for 10 minutes twice a day (p. 253).

Prescribe a stronger muscle relaxant.

Step 3 (4 to 6 weeks for chronic cases): Reevaluate neurologic function.

Maximize vertical cervical traction.

Consult with a neurosurgeon if symptoms persist.

PHYSICAL THERAPY.   Physical therapy plays an integral part in the treatment of cervical radiculopathy and in the prevention of recurrent nerve impingement.

PHYSICAL THERAPY SUMMARY   ● ● ● ● ● ● ● ● ● ● ● ● ● ● ● ●

1. Cautious muscle-stretching exercises, passively performed
2. Cautious stretching plus heat and massage
3. Avoid ultrasound
4. Gradually increase the weight and length of vertical cervical traction

Acute Period.   Ice applications, massage, and gentle muscle-stretching exercises are used to reduce secondary muscular irritation. (All the treatments used for cervical strain can be applied to cervical radiculopathy, but with caution!)

Heat and massage to the upper back and the base of the neck provide temporary relief of pain and muscle spasm. These can be combined with a nighttime muscle relaxer for additional effects.

Stretching exercises to reduce reactive muscular irritation and spasm must be used carefully (p. 252). The extremes of rotation and lateral bending may irritate the nerve roots (especially in foraminal encroachment disease). The tolerance of neck stretching must be assessed in the office prior to home exercise! *Ultrasound* should probably be avoided; it may aggravate nerve impingement.

Recovery/Rehabilitation.   After the acute irritation has subsided, stretching exercises are combined with vertical cervical traction. *Stretching exercises* are continued to maintain neck flexibility and to counteract muscular spasm. *Vertical cervical traction* performed daily will decrease the direct pressure on the cervical roots and nerves. Radiculopathy due to foraminal encroachment uniformly responds to traction (gradually over 4 to 6 weeks). Radiculopathy due to a herniated disk responds less predictably. A poor response to vertical traction suggests severe muscle spasm or herniated disk.

INJECTION TECHNIQUE.   Local injection is not routinely performed. If cervical strain is present, local injection of the trapezius muscle can be performed (p. 4). Facet joint injections should be performed by a neurosurgeon or by an interventional radiologist.

SURGICAL PROCEDURE.   Depending on the cause, foraminotomy or diskectomy are the two most common procedures.

PROGNOSIS.   Cervical radiculopathy is caused by foraminal encroachment in 90% of cases. Only 10% of cases arise from herniated disks (by contrast, 90% of radicular symptoms in the lumbosacral spine arise from herniated disks). Medical therapy is successful in nearly 90% of patients with cervical radiculopathy. However, response to traction may be slow. It is not unusual to require 4 to 6 weeks to resolve sensory or early sensorimotor radiculopathy. Patients with reflex loss or dramatic motor weakness have a poorer response to medical treatment and deserve an early workup with an MRI and an EMG to define the extent of neurologic impairment. Patients failing to respond to conservative therapy over 3 to 4 weeks and those with advanced neurologic symptoms and signs should be evaluated by MRI and should be referred to a neurosurgeon.

chapter 2

Shoulder

Impingement Syndrome

Enter 1½″ below the midpoint of the acromial process; follow the angle of the acromion to the sub-acromial bursa.

Needle: 1½″, 22 gauge

Depth: 1½ to 3½″ (obese patient)

Volume: 2 to 3 ml of anesthetic; 1 ml of D80

Note: NEVER inject under pressure; if bony resistance is encountered, redirect. Restrict use for 3 days and protect the shoulder for 30 days (see p. 18 for details).

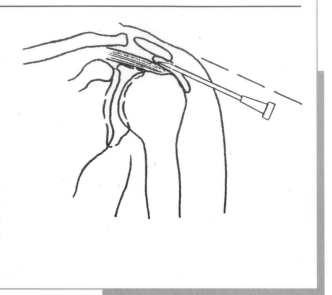

Figure 2–1.   Subacromial bursal injection from the lateral approach

DESCRIPTION.   Impingement syndrome is the term used to describe the symptoms that result from the compression of the rotator cuff tendons and the subacromial bursa between the greater tubercle of the humeral head and the undersurface of the acromial process. It is the mechanical component and principal cause of rotator cuff tendinitis. In the majority of patients, impingement syndrome precedes active rotator cuff tendinitis and subacromial bursitis.

SYMPTOMS.   The patient complains of shoulder pain aggravated by overhead motions or of inability to move the shoulder because of pain. The patient grabs the flesh over the lateral shoulder or rubs the hand up and down the deltoid muscle when describing the pain.

"It's too painful to raise my arm up."
"It feels like a leather strap is holding my shoulder down."
"My shoulder gets so sore after casing mail for an hour."
"If I sleep with my arm above my head, I hurt all the next day."
"It feels like my bones are rubbing together."
"I've had to stop reaching up to the high shelves in the kitchen. I have to stand on the footstool to put my dishes away."

EXAM.   Signs of subacromial impingement and the anatomic position (acromial angle) of the acromial process are assessed in each patient.

EXAM SUMMARY

• • • • • • • • • • • • • • •

1. Pain with the painful arc maneuver—subacromial impingement
2. Focal subacromial tenderness, just below the middle of the acromion
3. *Painless* testing of resisted abduction (supraspinatus), external rotation (infraspinatus), adduction (subscapularis), and elbow flexion (biceps), isometrically performed
4. Normal range of motion of the glenohumeral joint
5. Preserved strength in all directions

(1) The hallmark physical finding of impingement syndrome is pain reproduced by the painful arc maneuver. Passive abduction of the arm at a predictable and reproducible angle causes shoulder pain. This maneuver brings the greater tubercle of the humeral head into contact with the lateral edge of the acromion. When impingement is severe it is often accompanied by muscle spasm and muscle guarding, involuntary contraction of the trapezius muscle. (2) Focal subacromial tenderness is invariably present, although firm to hard pressure with the thumb between the greater tubercle of the humerus and just under the anterior third of the acromial process may be necessary to demonstrate it. This is identical to the local tenderness that occurs with rotator cuff tendinitis. (3) Tendon inflammation signs are not present with pure impingement syndrome. Isometric testing of midarc abduction, adduction, and internal and external rotation is painless! (4) Range of motion of the glenohumeral joint should be normal unless frozen shoulder has developed or underlying glenohumeral arthritis is present. (5) Abduction and external rotation strength should be normal.

X-RAYS.   Routine x-rays of the shoulder (including PA, external rotation, Y-outlet, and axillary views) are optional in patients presenting with a first episode of impingement. Recurrent or persistent cases should undergo radiographic testing. Calcification may be present in the rotator cuff tendons and always underscores the chronicity of the condition. More useful information focuses on the anatomic relationships of the acromion and humeral head. A high-riding humeral head—loss of the normal 1-cm space between the undersurface of the acromion and the top of the humeral head—indicates degenerative thinning of the rotator cuff tendons or a large rotator cuff tendon tear (1%). Long-standing cases of impingement may demonstrate erosive changes at the greater tubercle or bony sclerosis (severe and chronic impingement). Patients with the abnormal down-sloping acromial angle are at higher risk for recurrent or chronic impingement.

SPECIAL TESTING.   Diagnostic ultrasound, arthrography, or MRI are often ordered in the persistent or chronic case to exclude the possibility of rotator cuff tendon tear.

DIAGNOSIS.   The diagnosis of impingement syndrome is based on the history of lateral shoulder pain, the abnormal signs of local subacromial tenderness and a painful arc maneuver on exam, and the absence of signs of active tendinitis.

TREATMENT.   The goals of treatment are to increase the subacromial space, thus reducing the degree of impingement, and to prevent the development of tendinitis and tendon rupture. The pendulum stretching exercise combined with restrictions on overhead reaching and positioning are the treatments of choice.

Step 1: Strongly suggest rest and restriction of overhead positioning and reaching.

Recommend ice applications to control pain.

Demonstrate weighted pendulum stretching exercises using 5 to 10 lb, recommending 5 minutes once or twice a day (p. 256); emphasize the importance of relaxing the shoulder muscles (passive stretching).

Step 2 (2 to 4 weeks for persistent cases): Prescribe an NSAID (e.g., ibuprofen [Advil, Motrin]) given in full dose for 3 to 4 weeks if subtle signs of rotator cuff tendinitis are present.

Discourage the use of a simple arm sling (p. 285). Immobilization in a susceptible patient (often those with a low pain threshold, high stress, or both) may hasten the development of frozen shoulder!

Step 3 (6 to 8 weeks for persistent cases): Reemphasize the pendulum stretching exercise.

If symptoms persist, perform an empiric subacromial injection. Note that impingement syndrome is a mechanical problem with little accompanying inflammation. Local injection with corticosteroids has little therapeutic effect unless tendon inflammation is present.

Recommend general toning exercises in external rotation to enhance muscular support of the glenohumeral joint and to reduce impingement (p. 254).

Suggest a long-term restriction of any repetitious overhead work or positioning for patients with recurrent or persistent impingement.

Step 4 (3 to 6 months for chronic cases): Consider orthopedic consultation for patients with refractory symptoms.

PHYSICAL THERAPY. Physical therapy exercises are the treatments of choice for impingement syndrome.

PHYSICAL THERAPY SUMMARY ● ● ● ● ● ● ● ● ● ● ● ● ● ● ●

1. Ice
2. Weighted pendulum stretching exercises, performed passively with relaxed shoulder muscles
3. Toning exercises for the infraspinatus, performed isometrically
4. Avoidance of simple slings or other shoulder immobilizers

Acute Period. Ice and the weighted pendulum stretching exercises are used to reduce impingement. *Ice* in the form of a bag of frozen corn, blue ice, or a plastic ice bag is used for temporary relief of pain. The *weighted pendulum stretching exercise* is fundamental to stretching the subacromial space. Initially, the exercise is performed with the weight of the arm. With improvement, a hand-held 5- to 10-lb weight is added to increase the stretch (patients with hand and wrist arthritis should use Velcro weights placed just above the wrists). It is exceedingly important to keep the arm vertical and relaxed when performing this exercise. Excessive bending at the waist may aggravate subacromial impingement.

Recovery/Rehabilitation. The weighted pendulum stretching exercises are continued through the recovery period, and the isometric toning exercises are begun 4 to 6 weeks after the acute irritation has resolved. The *weighted pendulum stretching exercise* performed three times a week is effective in preventing the symptoms of recurrent impingement.

Isometric toning exercises of the infraspinatus muscle are used to enhance the stability of the glenohumeral joint and to open the subacromial space (p. 254). Preferential toning of the infraspinatus muscle has the theoretic advantage of increasing the distance between the humeral head and the acromion (vector analysis suggests that preferential toning of the infraspinatus, located between the greater tubercle and the inferior angle of the scapula, leads to a resultant vector in the downward direction and, hence, a downward force on the humeral head).

INJECTION.   Pure impingement syndrome is a mechanical problem and as such does not predictably respond to local injection. However, impingement syndrome can be accompanied by a subclinical degree of rotator cuff tendinitis (see "Rotator Cuff Tendinitis," p. 18). If a subacromial bursal injection of anesthetic (the lidocaine injection test) substantially reduces the patient's pain, improves the overall function of the shoulder, and reduces signs of impingement as noted during a physical exam, then an empiric injection of corticosteroid may be beneficial.

SURGICAL PROCEDURE.   Acromioplasty, performed arthroscopically or by open shoulder exposure, is the surgical procedure of choice for refractory impingement. However, exact indications for this procedure have not been clearly defined. The most common indications for this surgery are: (1) subacromial impingement, with or without rotator cuff tendinitis, in patients who fail to improve after several months of physical therapy (pendulum stretching exercises and external and internal rotation isometric toning exercises) and one or two subacromial corticosteroid injections; (2) symptoms of refractory impingement with high-grade acromial angle (type III acromion, according to Neer's classification); and (3) radiographic changes at the greater tubercle—bony erosions or sclerosis.

PROGNOSIS.   Shoulder impingement is a potential problem for everyone. Who hasn't experienced soreness and pain in the shoulder after unaccustomed work overhead such as painting the ceiling or trying to unscrew the stubborn ceiling light fixture? By contrast, the diagnosis of impingement syndrome is invoked when these same symptoms become persistent and begin to interfere with activities of daily living. Repeated impingement eventually leads to subacromial bursal inflammation, rotator cuff tendinitis, greater tubercle degenerative change and, if left untreated, degenerative thinning or rupture of the rotator cuff tendons.

The overall prognosis for impingement is excellent. Codman weighted pendulum exercises combined with isometrically performed toning exercises will effectively treat the majority of patients. Only a very small percentage of patients experience refractory impingement that would require surgical consultation. Patients with extreme down-sloping acromial processes and patients who have suffered a humeral neck fracture with angulation are at higher risk for chronic impingement.

DESCRIPTION.   Rotator cuff tendinitis is an inflammation of the supraspinatus and infraspinatus tendons lying between the humeral head and the acromial process. Repetitive overhead reaching, pushing, and pulling and lifting with the arms outstretched—repeated abduction, elevation, and torque to the shoulder—lead to compression and irritation of the tendons (subacromial impingement). The subacromial bursa, located just under the inferior surface of the acromion, functions to protect the rotator tendons from the irritation of repeated impingement. If the bursa fails to provide an appropriate amount of lubrication, the rotator cuff tendons become inflamed.

SYMPTOMS.   The patient complains of shoulder pain aggravated by overhead reaching and positioning or inability to move the shoulder because of pain. The patient typically places the hand over the outer deltoid, rubbing the muscle in an up-and-down direction when describing the pain.

"Every time I reach over my head, I get this achy pain in my outer shoulder."
"I can't lift my arm over my head—it hurts so bad."
"I can't sleep on my shoulder! Every time I roll over in bed, my shoulder wakes me up."

Rotator Cuff Tendinitis

Enter 1½" below the midpoint of the acromial process; follow the angle of the acromion to the subacromial bursa.

Needle: 1½", 22 gauge

Depth: 1½ to 3½" (obese patient)

Volume: 2 to 3 ml of anesthetic; 1 ml of D80

Note: NEVER inject under pressure; if bony resistance is encountered, redirect. Restrict use for 3 days and protect the shoulder for 30 days.

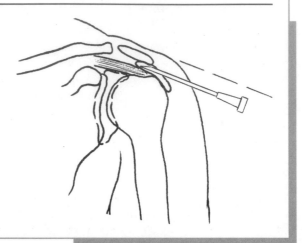

Figure 2–2.   Subacromial bursal injection from the lateral approach

"I can't reach up or back anymore."
"Whenever I move suddenly or reach back, I get this sharp, deep pain in my shoulder."
"The only way I can stop the pain is to hang my arm over the side of the bed."

EXAM.   Signs of subacromial impingement, tendon inflammation, and weakness of the supraspinatus and infraspinatus muscles are looked for in each patient.

EXAM SUMMARY   ● ● ● ● ● ● ● ● ● ● ● ● ● ● ● ● ●

1.   Focal subacromial tenderness
2.   Subacromial impingement, a positive painful arc maneuver
3.   Pain with resisted midarc abduction and external rotation, isometrically performed
4.   Normal range of motion of the glenohumeral joint
5.   Preserved strength of midarc abduction and external rotation (lidocaine injection test)

(1) Subacromial tenderness is located between the greater tubercle of the humerus and the acromial process. Typically, this is a dime-sized area just under the anterior third of the acromion. Diffuse subacromial tenderness usually indicates subacromial bursal inflammation. (2) The impingement sign is always present. Passive abduction of the arm with simultaneous downward pressure on the acromion (the painful arc) reproduces the patient's pain as the swollen tendons and the subacromial bursa are mechanically compressed. (3) The degree of tendon inflammation is assessed by reproducing the patient's pain when resisting midarc abduction and external rotation isometrically. (4) Range of motion of the glenohumeral joint should be normal unless frozen shoulder has developed or underlying glenohumeral arthritis is present. (5) Abduction and external rotation strength should be normal in an uncomplicated case of tendinitis. If the patient's pain interferes with an accurate measurement of strength,

a lidocaine injection test should be performed. The strength of the affected arm should be at least 75% of the strength of the unaffected side, unless a rotator cuff tendon tear is present.

X-RAYS. Routine x-rays of the shoulder (including PA, external rotation, Y-outlet, and axillary views) are optional in patients experiencing their first episode of tendinitis. However, patients with recurrent or chronic tendinitis should be tested to evaluate for high-grade impingement or degenerative change. Tendon calcification—the body's attempt at tendon repair—may be seen in approximately 30% of cases. A high-riding humeral head (loss of the normal 1-cm space between the undersurface of the acromion and the top of the humeral head) indicates either degenerative tendon thinning or rotator cuff tendon tear (1%). Long-standing cases may have arthritic changes at the glenohumeral joint (<1%).

None of these radiographic changes provides conclusive evidence of active tendinitis. The specific diagnosis and the specific treatment recommendations must be based on the clinical exam.

SPECIAL TESTING. Cases accompanied by greater than 50% loss of midarc abduction or external rotation strength and cases with equivocal lidocaine injection tests should be evaluated for rotator cuff tear. Contrast arthrography will demonstrate subtendinous tears, small tendon splits, and large transverse tears. An MRI will demonstrate moderate to large tears and will assess the degree of muscle atrophy and contracture.

Note that patients older than 62 years of age who have suffered a fall onto the outstretched arm or a direct blow to the shoulder are at increased risk for rotator cuff tendon rupture, especially if they have experienced previous episodes of tendinitis. Up to one third of 70-year-old patients with persistent symptoms have either a partial rotator cuff tendon rupture or a full thickness rupture.

DIAGNOSIS. The diagnosis of rotator cuff tendinitis is based on the history of shoulder pain aggravated by reaching, evidence of subacromial impingement, and pain with isometric testing of the supraspinatus, infraspinatus, or subscapularis. The diagnosis is confirmed by regional anesthetic block in the subacromial bursa. Rotator cuff tendon ruptures can accompany rotator cuff tendinitis in 1 to 3% of cases. It is important to perform a lidocaine injection test to exclude an underlying rotator cuff tendon rupture prior to giving a local corticosteroid injection.

TREATMENT. The goals of treatment are to reduce tendon swelling and inflammation, to increase the subacromial space, thus reducing the degree of impingement, and to prevent progressive damage to the tendons (calcification, thinning, and rupture). The pendulum stretching exercise combined with an effective anti-inflammatory treatment is the treatment of choice.

Step 1: Assess the patient's overall shoulder function, order plain x-rays of the shoulder (if the patient is over 60 years of age or has a history of recurrent tendinitis), and estimate the patient's external rotation strength.

Suggest rest and restriction of overhead positioning and reaching.

Recommend ice as the initial anti-inflammatory treatment and as an acute reducer of pain.

Demonstrate weighted pendulum stretching exercises, emphasize the importance of relaxing the shoulder muscles (passive stretching) and begin using a 5- to 10-lb weight for 5 minutes once or twice a day (p. 256).

Step 2 (2 to 4 weeks for persistent cases): Prescribe an NSAID (e.g., ibuprofen [Advil, Motrin]), which is given in full dose for 3 to 4 weeks.

Reemphasize the importance and the proper way of performing the pendulum stretching exercise.

Discourage the use of a simple arm sling (p. 285). Immobilization in a susceptible patient (a diabetic, a patient with a low pain threshold, or a patient with a high degree of stress) may hasten the development of frozen shoulder!

Step 3 (6 to 8 weeks for persistent cases): Perform a lidocaine injection test to exclude the possibility of a tendon tear.

Order an arthrogram or diagnostic ultrasound if the lidocaine injection test result is abnormal (<50% pain relief and <75% of normal strength in abduction or external rotation); or order an MRI if the patient has profound weakness and is a candidate for surgery.

Perform a local injection of D80 if the patient has a normal lidocaine injection test result (>50% pain relief and >75% of normal strength).

Repeat the injection in 4 to 6 weeks if symptoms and signs have improved but linger at or below the 50% improvement level.

Strongly encourage the patient to perform weighted pendulum exercises plus toning exercises in abduction and external rotation to prevent recurrent tendinitis (pp. 254, 256).

Step 4 (3 months or greater for chronic cases): Cautiously perform or limit overhead reaching.

Advise on a long-term restriction of any repetitious overhead work or positioning!

Consider orthopedic consultation if symptoms persist or if tendon rupture is present.

PHYSICAL THERAPY.   Physical therapy plays an active role through the treatment of rotator cuff tendinitis and serves an important role in the prevention of recurrent tendinitis.

PHYSICAL THERAPY SUMMARY   • • • • • • • • • • • • • • •

1. Ice
2. Weighted pendulum stretching exercises, performed passively with relaxed shoulder muscles
3. Toning exercises for the infraspinatus and supraspinatus tendons, isometrically performed
4. Avoidance of simple slings or other shoulder immobilizers

Acute Period.   Ice and the weighted pendulum stretching exercises are used to reduce swelling and impingement. *Ice* in the form of a bag of frozen corn or an ice bag is used for temporary relief of pain and as an initial treatment for inflammation. The *weighted pendulum stretching* exercise is fundamental to stretching the subacromial space, allowing the rotator cuff tendons room to contract and thus helping to prevent frozen shoulder (p. 256). Initially, the subacromial space is stretched by the weight of the arm. With improvement, a 5- to 10-lb weight is used as tolerated. It is exceedingly important to keep the arm vertical and relaxed when performing this exercise. Excessive bending at the waist may aggravate subacromial impingement. Active use of the shoulder muscles (as opposed to relaxing them and allowing them to stretch) may aggravate the underlying tendon inflammation!

TABLE 2–1. CLINICAL OUTCOMES OF ROTATOR CUFF TENDINITIS AFTER SUBACROMIAL INJECTION OF DEPO-MEDROL 80 mg/ml

Complete resolution		
One injection		48
Two injections 6 weeks apart		8
Total		56 (62%)
Recurrence (averaged 5 to 6 months)		
Reinjected once	14	
Reinjected twice	7	
Multiple injections	3	
Total		24 (27%)
Failed to respond; chronic tendinitis		7 (8%)
Rotator cuff tendon rupture (developed in the follow-up period)		3 (3%)
Lost to follow-up		9
TOTAL		99

Note: Diagnosis confirmed with local anesthetic block; 1 ml of D80; home physical therapy; pendulum stretching exercises plus isometric toning exercises; 18-month prospective follow-up of 91% of patients enrolled.
Data collected at the Medical Orthopedic Clinic, Sunnyside Medical Center, Portland, OR.

Recovery/Rehabilitation. The *weighted pendulum stretching exercise* is continued through the recovery period. Continuing this exercise should be strongly encouraged in patients with high-grade impingement and in those who have suffered more than one episode of tendinitis. Maintenance exercises three times a week will reduce the chance of recurrent tendon compression.

Isometric toning exercises of the infraspinatus and supraspinatus muscles are used to strengthen the weakened tendons, to stabilize the glenohumeral joint, and to open the subacromial space (p. 254). These exercises are begun 4 to 6 weeks after the acute pain and swelling have resolved. (Toning exercises begun too soon can reignite tendon inflammation!) Preferential toning of the infraspinatus muscle has the theoretical advantage of increasing the distance between the humeral head and the acromion.

INJECTION. Local injection of anesthetic and corticosteroid is used (1) to confirm the diagnosis of an uncomplicated rotator cuff tendinitis, (2) to treat active rotator cuff tendinitis that has persisted for 6 to 8 weeks or that has failed to improve with steps 1 through 4 above, (3) to treat rotator cuff tendinitis that accompanies frozen shoulder, and (4) to palliate the symptoms that accompany rotator cuff tendon tear in patients who are incapable of undergoing surgery (see Tables 2–1 and 2–2).

Positioning: The patient is to be sitting up, with the hands placed in the lap. The patient is asked to relax the shoulder and neck muscles. Traction applied to the flexed elbow may be necessary to open the subacromial space!

Surface Anatomy and Point of Entry: The lateral edge of the acromion is located and its midpoint marked. The point of entry is 1 to 1½" below the midpoint.

TABLE 2–2. ADVERSE REACTIONS TO A SUBACROMIAL INJECTION OF DEPO-MEDROL 80 mg/ml

None	48 (49%)
Pain	32 (33%)
Inflammatory flare reaction (pain, heat, swelling)	7 (7%)
Vasovagal reaction	4 (4%)
Bruise	4
Stiffness	2
Swelling; itching; nausea; flushing	1 each
Postinjection infection	0
Postinjection tendon rupture (within 6 weeks of injection)	1

Data collected at the Medical Orthopedic Clinic, Sunnyside Medical Center, Portland, OR.

Angle of Entry and Depth: The angle of entry should *parallel* the patient's own acromial angle (averaging 50 to 65 degrees). The depth will vary according the patient's weight and muscle development (1½" in an asthenic patient and up to 3½" in an obese patient 30% over ideal body weight). Note that the depth and angle of injection can be measured directly off the PA shoulder x-ray with a metal marker placed at the point of entry. This is particularly helpful in an obese patient or a patient with a well-developed deltoid muscle.

Anesthesia: Ethyl chloride is sprayed on the skin. Local anesthetic is placed in the deltoid muscle (1 ml), the deep deltoid fascia (½ ml), and the subacromial bursa (1 to 2 ml). Note that the subacromial bursa will accept only 2 to 3 ml of total volume before rupturing!

Technique: Successful treatment depends on the accurate injection of the subacromial bursa. The lateral approach is the most accessible and safest to perform (injection into the rotator cuff tendons is nearly impossible with this technique). The needle is advanced through the subcutaneous tissue and the deltoid muscle until the subtle resistance of the deep deltoid fascia is encountered. If firm or hard tissue resistance is encountered (deltoid tendon or periosteum, often painful), then the needle is withdrawn ½" and the angle is redirected 5 to 10 degrees up or down. A "giving way" or "popping" sensation is often appreciated when the subacromial bursa is entered. Following 1 to 2 ml of anesthesia (the needle can be left in place), the patient's strength is retested. If pain is reduced by 50% and the strength of abduction and external rotation is 75 to 80% of the unaffected side, then 1 ml of D80 is injected. Note: never inject under moderate to high pressure (tension generated by an anxious patient or placement outside the bursa!).

INJECTION AFTERCARE

1) *Rest* for 3 days, avoiding reaching, overhead positioning, lifting, pushing, and pulling.

2) *Ice* (15 minutes every 4 to 6 hours and *Tylenol ES* (1000 mg twice a day) for soreness.

3) *Protect* the shoulder for 30 days by limiting reaching, overhead positioning, lifting, pushing, and pulling.

4) Resume passively performed *pendulum stretching exercises* on day 4.

5) Begin *isometric toning exercises* of abduction and external rotation at 3 to 4 weeks, after the acute pain and inflammation have resolved.

6) Repeat *injection* at 6 weeks if overall improvement is less than 50%.

7) Delay *regular activities, work, and sports* until the majority of lost muscular tone has been recovered.

8) Obtain *plain x-rays* or a *shoulder arthrogram* in all patients who fail to experience at least 2 months of relief; evaluate for rotator cuff tear, AC joint disease with inferior-directed osteophytes, and high-grade impingement.

SURGICAL PROCEDURE.   Surgery is indicated for chronic or persistent rotator cuff tendinitis complicated by high degrees of subacromial impingement or tendon tear. The various procedures attempt (1) to reduce impingement (subacromial decompression and acromioplasty devised by Dr. C. S. Neer), (2) to remove devitalized tissue (excision of calcific deposits or necrotic tendons), and (3) to repair torn tissue (primary tendon repair). Unfortunately, surgical treatment is successful only about 70 to 75% of the time. The procedure often reduces pain but fails to return the patient to his or her original level of function. The patient must be advised that the success of surgery depends, as a rule, on the degree of irreparable tendon damage and degeneration.

PROGNOSIS.   Uncomplicated rotator cuff tendinitis treated with one or two injections 6 weeks apart does extremely well; 85 to 90% of patients will respond completely, with approximately one in three requiring retreatment in the next few years. The prognosis is governed by the accuracy of injection, the use of a concentrated, long-acting corticosteroid, the degree of subacromial impingement, the degree of chronic tendon degeneration (the number of recurrences and the width of the subacromial space), and the compliance of the patient (exercises and restrictions).

Frozen Shoulder

Frozen shoulder can be injected at the subacromial bursa (see p. 18 for details) or intra-articularly. The intra-articular injection enters just below the coracoid and is directed outward (fluoroscopy is strongly recommended when performing dilation).

Needle: 1½ to 3½" spinal needle, 22 gauge

Depth: 1½ to 2½"

Volume: 4 ml of anesthetic; 10 to 15 ml of saline for dilation; and 1 ml of K40

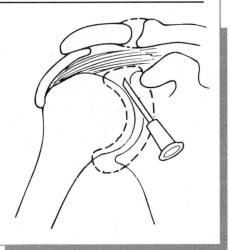

Figure 2–3.   Intra-articular injection for frozen shoulder

DESCRIPTION.   Frozen shoulder is a descriptive term that refers to a stiff shoulder joint—a glenohumeral joint that has lost significant range of motion. Pathologically, the glenohumeral joint capsule has lost its normal distensibility. In long-standing cases, adhesions may form between the joint capsule and the humeral head (adhesive capsulitis). Rotator cuff tendinitis, acute subacromial bursitis, fractures about the humeral head and neck, and paralytic stroke are common causes. Protracted cases with severe restriction of motion may be complicated by hand swelling, finger discoloration, Sudeck atrophy of bone, and an unusual pattern of pain that radiates up and down the arm (reflex sympathetic dystrophy (RSD)).

SYMPTOMS.   The patient complains of a gradual loss of shoulder function and motion. The patient often rubs the outer shoulder and demonstrates the inability to move it in certain directions when describing the condition.

"My shoulder is stiffening up."
"I can't reach up over my head."
"I can't reach back to fasten my bra. I have to fasten it in front and rotate it around."
"It's getting harder and harder to put on my coat."
"I can't shave under my armpit anymore."
"My shoulder used to be quite sore and tender. The pain has gotten a lot better, but I can't move it now."

EXAM.   The range of motion of the glenohumeral joint is measured, and a specific cause of local pain or inflammation (rotator cuff tendinitis, fracture, dislocation, and so forth) is identified in each patient.

EXAM SUMMARY   • • • • • • • • • • • • • • • •

1.   An abnormal Apley scratch test (inability to scratch the lower back)
2.   Restricted abduction and external rotation, measured passively
3.   No radiographic evidence of glenohumeral arthritis
4.   Hand swelling, finger discoloration, synovitis (complicating RSD)

(1) General function of the shoulder is assessed by asking patients to raise their arms overhead and to scratch the lower back, the Apley scratch test. These simple maneuvers are used to assess glenohumeral motion rapidly. Patients with normal glenohumeral motion should be able to raise their arms straight overhead and scratch the midback at the T8 to T10 vertebral level. Patients with frozen shoulder lack full overhead reaching and are unable to scratch even the lower back at the L4 or L5 level. (2) Next, individual motions are measured. In many patients, abduction and external rotation are reduced and should be estimated or measured with a goniometer (measurements are made passively). The glenohumeral joint normally rotates externally to 90 degrees and abducts to 90 to 110 degrees. Note that in order to measure abduction accurately, shrugging must be prevented by placing downward pressure over the acromion. (3) Frozen shoulder must be distinguished from advanced glenohumeral arthritis; upon examination, glenohumeral arthritis appears similar to frozen shoulder. However, arthritis will often show loss of motion in all directions and will have characteristic changes on plain x-rays of the shoulder. (4) Severe frozen shoulder (months in duration) may be associated with diffuse hand pain and swelling, finger discoloration, abnormal patterns of sweating, or unilateral joint synovitis (RSD).

X-RAYS.   X-rays are not required in order to diagnose or stage frozen shoulder. However, routine views (including PA, external rotation, Y-outlet, and axillary views) are often obtained because of the protracted nature of the condition and to satisfy the patient's expectations. Most plain films are nondiagnostic, although rotator cuff tendon calcification is found in 30% of cases.

SPECIAL TESTING.   No special studies are required or used routinely. Shoulder arthrography, often ordered to rule out subtle glenohumeral arthritic change or rotator cuff tendon tear, may show the characteristic changes of a contracted glenohumeral capsule. Normally the glenohumeral joint easily fills with 8 to 10 ml of radiopaque contrast. An advanced case of frozen shoulder may accept only 4 to 5 ml of contrast.

DIAGNOSIS.   The diagnosis of frozen shoulder requires demonstrating a loss of range of motion of the glenohumeral joint, a loss that is not attributable to glenohumeral arthritis or to a painful periarticular process, such as tendinitis or fracture. X-rays of the shoulder are required to rule out arthritis of the glenohumeral joint. A lidocaine injection test is used to reduce the dramatic levels of pain and muscle spasm that can interfere with an accurate measurement of the range of motion of the joint.

TREATMENT.   The goals of treatment are to treat any underlying periarticular or bony process, gradually stretch out the glenohumeral joint lining, and restore normal range of motion to the shoulder. Weighted pendulum stretching exercise combined with passively performed glenohumeral stretches in abduction and external rotation is the treatment of choice.

Step 1: Determine the general function of the shoulder, rule out glenohumeral osteoarthritis with plain x-rays, and perform a lidocaine injection test to obtain accurate measurements of abduction and external rotation.

Educate the patient about the slow recovery time, especially in diabetic and stroke patients: "It may take 6 to 18 months to recover."

Advise on the application of heat to the anterior shoulder prior to stretching.

Begin twice-a-day pendulum stretching exercises (p. 255).

Recommend an individualized program of passively performed stretching exercises in the directions of motion with the greatest loss, commonly abduction and external rotation (p. 258).

Suggest elimination of over-the-shoulder work in patients with signs of tendinitis.

Prescribe an NSAID (e.g., ibuprofen [Advil, Motrin]) for pain control, noting that inflammation is not prominent in pure frozen shoulder.

Step 2 (6 to 8 weeks for routine follow-up): Reevaluate the range of motion.

Reinforce the specific passive stretching exercises.

Consider a subacromial or intra-articular injection of corticosteroid, especially if an underlying tendinitis is present.

Step 3 (3 months with persistent loss of range of motion): Reevaluate the range of motion.

Encourage the patient.

Consider intra-articular dilation with lidocaine and saline.

Step 4 (6 to 12 months for chronic cases): Gradually resume normal activities as motion improves.

Suggest pendulum stretching exercises to prevent a recurrence.

Consider arthroscopic dilation of the joint.

Resort to shoulder manipulation under general anesthesia if symptoms fail to improve.

PHYSICAL THERAPY. The principal treatment for frozen shoulder involves an individualized program of shoulder-stretching exercises.

PHYSICAL THERAPY SUMMARY ● ● ● ● ● ● ● ● ● ● ● ● ● ● ● ●

1. Heating of the shoulder
2. Weighted pendulum stretching exercise twice a day, performed passively with relaxed shoulder muscles
3. Daily stretching exercises in the directions most affected, performed passively
4. Rotator cuff muscle toning after motion has been significantly restored, performed isometrically

Acute Period/Recovery. Heat, the weighted pendulum stretching exercises, and passive stretching exercises are used to restore glenohumeral flexibility. The shoulder is *heated* for 10 to 15 minutes with moist heat or in a bathtub or shower.

Weighted pendulum stretching exercises are performed for 5 minutes (p. 256). The arm is kept vertical while the patient bends slightly at the waist. The patient should be instructed on relaxing the shoulder muscles when performing this exercise: "This is a pure stretching exercise; don't swing the weight more than 1 foot in distance or diameter; let the weight do the work." *Passive stretching exercises* are performed after the pendulum stretching exercises. Individualize your recommendations. Emphasize stretching exercises that focus on the directions in which the patient has suffered the greatest loss, usually abduction and external rotation (p. 258). Limit the abduction stretching to no higher than shoulder level, especially if the frozen shoulder resulted from rotator cuff tendinitis. Emphasize the need to stretch to the point of tension, but not pain. Multiple repetitions performed twice a day will gradually stretch the glenohumeral capsule.

General *rotator cuff tendon toning exercises* may play a minor role in recovery, especially if rotator cuff tendinitis preceded the frozen shoulder (p. 254).

INJECTION.   A subacromial injection of corticosteroid is indicated when concurrent rotator cuff or bicepital tendinitis is present (see "Rotator Cuff Tendinitis," p. 18). A glenohumeral intra-articular injection combined with saline dilation is indicated when >50% of range of motion has been lost despite an adequate trial of physical therapy, subacromial injection, or both.

Positioning: The patient is to be recumbent with the head raised to 30 degrees.

Surface Anatomy and Point of Entry: The coracoid process is located and marked. The point of entry is ½ to ¾" caudal to the coracoid.

Angle of Entry and Depth: The angle of entry is perpendicular to the skin and slightly outward. The depth is 1½ to 2½". Fluoroscopy is strongly advised if dilation is performed.

Anesthesia: Ethyl chloride is sprayed on the skin. Local anesthetic is placed at the pectoralis major fascia (1 ml), at the subscapularis fascia (1 ml), and at the periosteum of the glenoid or humeral head (1 to 2 ml).

Technique: Successful dilation requires fluoroscopy to assure an accurate intra-articular injection. Following anesthesia, 2 to 3 ml of radiopaque contrast is injected through the same needle to confirm the intra-articular position. Subsequently, 10 to 15 ml of normal saline is slowly but gradually injected. The volume will be determined by the increasing pressure to injection and the patient's aware-ness of a sense of tightening. At the completion of dilation, 1 ml of K40 is injected.

INJECTION AFTERCARE

1) *Rest* for 3 days, avoiding reaching, overhead positioning, lifting, pushing, and pulling.

2) *Ice* (15 minutes every 4 to 6 hours) and *Tylenol ES* (1000 mg twice a day) for soreness.

3) *Protect* the shoulder for 30 days by limiting reaching, overhead positioning, lifting, pushing, and pulling.

4) Resume passively performed *pendulum stretching exercises* as well as passively performed *stretching exercises* of abduction and external rotation on day 4.

5) Begin *isometric toning exercises* of abduction and external rotation after 75% of normal range of motin has been restored.

6) Repeat *injection* at 2 to 3 months if overall improvement is less than 50%.

7) Delay *regular activities, work, and sports* until the majority of the shoulder's range of motion has been recovered and at least 75% of muscular tone has been restored.

8) Request a *consultation* with a surgical orthopedist if the range of motion fails to increase by an average of 10 to 15% per month.

SURGICAL PROCEDURE.   Arthroscopic dilation of the glenohumeral joint or ma-nipulation under general anesthesia (<2%).

PROGNOSIS. Frozen shoulder is a reversible condition. It slowly improves over several months, with 90 to 95% of patients recovering completely. However, a loss of 50% or more external rotation or abduction may be associated with incomplete recovery and permanent stiffness, especially in the diabetic patient. The British method of intra-articular dilation (*Br Med J* 1991; 302:1498–1501) is very successful and should be considered when physical therapy stretching fails to improve range of motion over 2 months or when the patient presents with a dramatic loss of motion. Arthroscopic dilation—a replacement for the archaic manipulation under general anesthesia—is indicated for the refractory case of adhesive capsulitis.

ROTATOR CUFF TENDON TEAR

Transverse or longitudinal tendon tears at the musculotendinous juncture

"Milwaukee shoulder": a combination of a large tendon tear, a large joint effusion, and radiographic evidence of glenohumoral joint osteoarthritis

Diagnostic testing: plant x-rays, shoulder arthrography diagnostic ultrasound, or MRI

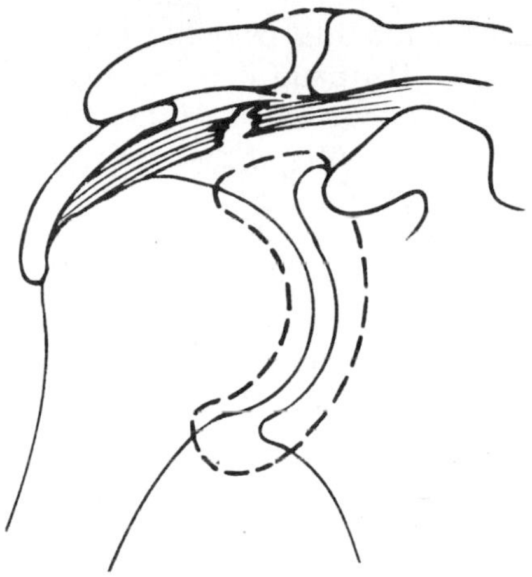

Figure 2–4. Rotator cuff tendon tear

DESCRIPTION. Rotator cuff tendon tears, loss of the normal integrity of the infraspinatus or supraspinatus tendons or both, occur as the end result of chronic subacromial impingement and progressive tendon degeneration or from traumatic injury or both. Chronic subacromial impingement over many years causes chronic tendon inflammation which, in turn, leads to progressive mucinoid degeneration, tendon thinning and, ultimately, tendon rupture. Injuries that are most commonly associated with rotator cuff tendon tears include falls onto the outstretched arm, falls directly onto the outer shoulder, vigorous pulling on a lawn mower cable, and unusual heavy pushing and pulling. Tears are classified anatomically as tendon splits or transverse ruptures and functionally as partial or complete.

Rotator cuff tendon tears are common, although many elude clinical detection. Cadaver studies show an incidence of 15% of tendon disruption.

SYMPTOMS. The patient complains of weakness of the shoulder, localized pain over the upper back, or a popping sensation whenever the shoulder is moved. The patient often tries to reach over the shoulder attempting to touch the affected area of the upper back when describing the condition or asks the examiner to listen to the popping sound.

"Every time I roll my shoulder, it pops."
"I can't sleep on my back anymore. There's this spot of pain over my shoulder blade."
"I can't sit against a hard-backed chair."
"Doc, what makes my shoulder pop all the time?"

"I work at an assembly table. I have to reach back and forth. The back of my shoulder began to hurt when I took this new job."

"That cortisone shot for my bursitis really took the pain away. I could finally get back to my gardening; however, when I was rototilling, my arm was jerked forward. It felt like a .22 shell went off in my shoulder. Now the pain is worse than ever and I can't lift my arm."

EXAM. General function of the shoulder, specific weakness of glenohumeral external rotation and abduction, and signs of active rotator cuff tendinitis are examined in each patient.

EXAM SUMMARY   • • • • • • • • • • • • • • • •

1. Loss of smooth overhead motion
2. *Weakness* and pain with isometric testing of midarc abduction, external rotation, or both
3. The painful arc maneuver is usually positive (p. 15)
4. Subacromial tenderness
5. Atrophy of the infraspinatus and/or supraspinatus muscles noted over the scapula

(1) The general function of the shoulder is assessed first. Large tears dramatically affect shoulder mobility and strength, interfering with the ability to reach overhead (large tear), to lift a 2- to 5-lb weight overhead (moderate), to lift an object with an outstretched arm (moderate), or to smoothly raise the arm overhead (small). (2) Next, the integrity of the specific tendons is assessed by strength testing. Weakness of external rotation (the function of the infraspinatus tendon) or midarc abduction (the function of the supraspinatus tendon) is the hallmark sign of rotator cuff tendon tear. Since pain often accompanies weakness (concurrent rotator cuff tendinitis), a lidocaine injection test is often necessary to isolate true weakness from weakness due to pain or poor effort. (3) As with active rotator cuff tendinitis, the painful arc maneuver is positive and (4) tenderness is present in the subacromial area. (5) Moderate to large tears that have been present for several weeks to months are associated with atrophy of the infraspinatus and supraspinatus muscles in their respective scapular fossae. Lastly, some cases demonstrate crepitation or popping with passive circumduction of the shoulder.

X-RAYS. Plain x-rays of the shoulder (including PA, external rotation, Y-outlet, and axillary views) are always recommended if a rotator cuff tendon tear is suspected. A subacromial space measurement less than 1 cm—the distance between the undersurface of the acromion and the head of the humerus—is highly suggestive of degenerative thinning, tear, or both. Calcification will be present in 30% of cases but does not correlate directly with the presence of tendon disruption.

SPECIAL TESTING. Cases accompanied by greater than 50% loss of midarc abduction or external rotation strength after a lidocaine injection test (and those with an equivocal lidocaine injection test) deserve either an arthrogram or an MRI of the shoulder to evaluate for rotator cuff tear. All those patients who have three of the major risk factors for tear should undergo further testing with shoulder arthrography, diagnostic ultrasound, if available, or MRI.

Note that patients older than 62 years of age who have suffered a fall onto the outstretched arm or a direct blow to the shoulder are at increased risk for rotator cuff tendon rupture. Up to one third of 70-year-olds with persistent symptoms have either a partial rotator cuff tendon rupture or a full thickness rupture.

DIAGNOSIS.   A presumptive diagnosis of tendon tear can be made in the setting of rotator cuff tendinitis with persistent weakness after a lidocaine injection test. If the patient is elderly, suffers serious medical comorbidities, or elects to avoid an operation, then further testing is not necessary. However, a definitive diagnosis of tendon tear requires special testing. Shoulder arthrography will demonstrate subtendinous tears, small splits, and large tendon tears. An MRI will demonstrate large tears. Unfortunately, an MRI cannot distinguish a small tear from active tendinitis.

TREATMENT.   The goals of treatment are to recover and improve lost strength in external rotation and abduction, to improve the global function of the shoulder, and to treat any concurrent rotator cuff tendinitis. The treatment of choice is immediate surgical consultation in the 50- to 62-year-old patient with a large, dominant shoulder tear. For the elderly patient with major medical problems, for patients with medium-sized tears (especially on the nondominant side), and for patients with small tears, physical therapy toning exercises of external rotation and abduction are the nonsurgical treatments of choice.

Step 1: Assess the patient's overall shoulder function, order plain x-rays of the shoulder, and evaluate the patient's strength of external rotation.

> Immediately order a diagnostic arthrogram or MRI for the 50- to 62-year-old male who demonstrates clinical findings of a large tear of the dominant shoulder (profound weakness, inability to raise the arm above shoulder level and so forth) and refer to an orthopedic surgeon with experience in shoulder surgery.

> Suggest a restriction of overhead positioning and reaching.

> Apply ice over the deltoid muscle to acutely reduce pain and inflammation.

> Perform weighted pendulum stretching exercises passively, using a 5- to 10-lb weight for 5 minutes once or twice a day (p. 256).

> Begin isometric toning exercises at a level that does not cause pain or soreness during the exercise, hours later, or the next day.

Step 2 (2 to 4 weeks for persistent cases): Prescribe an NSAID (e.g., ibuprofen [Advil, Motrin]) in full dose for 3 to 4 weeks.

> Perform a local corticosteroid injection if the signs of tendinitis predominate, the patient has mild to moderate weakness, and the subacromial space is greater than 6 to 7 mm in diameter (mild degenerative change only).

> Reemphasize the pendulum stretching exercises, passively performed.

> Continue isometric toning exercises at a level that does not cause pain or soreness during the exercise, hours later, or the next day.

> Discourage the use of a simple arm sling (p. 285). Immobilization in a susceptible patient (often with a low pain threshold or with stress) may hasten the development of frozen shoulder!

Step 3 (6 to 8 weeks for persistent cases): Order an arthrogram or diagnostic ultrasound if symptoms and signs fail to improve with steps 1 and 2 and if surgery is contemplated.

> Consider orthopedic surgical referral for primary repair of the small to medium-sized tears if symptoms persist.

Step 4 (3 months or longer for chronic cases): Prescribe weighted pendulum stretching exercises and toning exercises in abduction and external rotation to prevent a recurrence (pp. 254, 256).

Restrict or avoid any repetitive overhead work or positioning in a patient with chronic symptoms arising from medium-sized to large tears.

Consider orthopedic surgical consultation for total joint replacement if symptoms persist, function is dramatically interfered with, and the patient is willing to undergo the risks of surgery.

PHYSICAL THERAPY.   Physical therapy plays an essential role in the active treatment and rehabilitation of small to medium-sized rotator cuff tendon tears and a significant role in the postoperative recovery of surgically repaired medium-sized to large tears.

PHYSICAL THERAPY SUMMARY   ● ● ● ● ● ● ● ● ● ● ● ● ● ● ●

1. Ice to control the acute pain or swelling
2. Weighted pendulum stretching exercises, performed passively with relaxed shoulder muscles
3. Isometrically performed toning exercises in external rotation and abduction
4. Active exercises as tolerated

Acute Period/Recovery.   Exercises to stretch the glenohumeral space are combined with toning exercises and restricted use. Daily *isometric toning exercises* of glenohumeral abduction and external rotation are essential to the rehabilitation of small to medium-sized rotator cuff tendon tears (p. 254). These exercises are performed with low tension and high repetition, using a TheraBand, large rubber bands, a spring-tension chest expander, or similar aid. Enough tension is used to stress the rotator cuff tendon muscles but not enough to aggravate an underlying tendinitis! The toning is enhanced if it is preceded by the heating of the shoulder for 10 to 15 minutes and by the stretching of the subacromial space with *weighted pendulum stretching exercises* (p. 256). These exercises are also very important to the overall success of the surgical repair of complete rotator cuff tendon tears.

Rehabilitation.   General care of the shoulder coupled with a long-term restriction of overhead work are necessary to prevent further tendon degeneration. Emphasis is placed on prevention, using the *weighted pendulum stretching exercises* and *isometric toning exercises.*

INJECTION.   A subacromial injection of anesthetic is used to confirm the diagnosis of rotator cuff tendinitis complicated by tear. Patients with medium-sized to large tears, persistent pain, and persistent loss of shoulder function should be treated surgically. Patients with small to medium-sized tears can be treated cautiously with physical therapy and medication. Corticosteroid injection is used to treat concomitant tendinitis and to palliate symptoms in the nonsurgical candidate (see "Rotator Cuff Tendinitis," p. 18).

Note that in order to prevent tension across the healing tendons, injection should be combined with immobilization. An abduction pillow immobilizer or a simple shoulder immobilizer (p. 286) should be used concurrently for 30 days, the duration of action of the long-acting injectable corticosteroid.

SURGICAL PROCEDURE.   Primary tendon repair can be combined with a procedure to reduce impingement such as acromioplasty.

PROGNOSIS.   Rotator cuff tendon tears vary in cause (degenerative vs. traumatic tears), size (small, medium-sized, or large), location (infraspinatus vs. supraspinatus), pathology (splits vs. transverse tears), functional loss (minor weakness vs. inability to

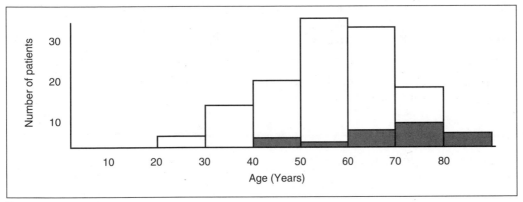

Figure 2–5.   The results of Hypaque 60 subacromial bursography in 124 consecutive patients presenting with signs and symptoms of rotator cuff tendinitis (RCT). Of 124 cases, 104 patients were diagnosed as uncomplicated RCT (average age, 57 years) and 20 had RCT complicated by tendon tears (average age, 67 years). N = 124: uncomplicated RCT = 104; RCT Tears = 20 (shaded areas). (These data were collected at the Medical Orthopedic Clinic, Sunnyside Medical Center, Portland, OR.)

raise the arm over the head), and symptoms. A general prognosis cannot be given for all cases.

Small to medium-sized tears with loss of 25 to 50% of strength and function can be treated medically. At least half of these smaller tears will respond to treatment that includes restrictions in use, physical therapy exercises and, in selected cases, a subacromial injection of corticosteroid. The duration of treatment often exceeds 6 months. Patients who do not respond to 4 weeks of conservative care should be promptly referred to the orthopedic surgeon.

Medium-sized to large tears, especially in a working male between 50 and 62 years of age, should be referred to the orthopedic surgeon immediately. Unnecessary delays in referral may lead to muscle atrophy, making surgical recovery more difficult and prolonged.

Risk factors that should alert the clinician to rotator cuff tendon tear include (1) age over 62 years (Figure 2–5), a fall onto the outstretched arm or a direct blow to the shoulder, a history of recurrent shoulder tendinitis, weakness on examination that cannot be accounted for by pain or poor effort (the lidocaine injection test), and a narrowed subacromial space measurement on plain x-rays of the shoulder. The common denominator in all these risk factors consists of the underlying degenerative changes of tendon attrition. If the patient has two or three of these five risk factors, special studies should be strongly considered.

DESCRIPTION.   The acromioclavicular (AC) joint and its supporting ligaments are susceptible to injury from repetitive reaching (especially across the chest and over the head) and from trauma. The AC, the coracoclavicular, and the coracoacromial ligaments, binding the acromion, clavicle, and coracoid process together, can be strained, partially torn, or completely disrupted (first-degree, second-degree, or third-degree separation, respectively). Repeated strain or injury to the supporting ligaments may progress to osteoarthritis of the AC joint many years later.

SYMPTOMS.   The patient complains of shoulder pain or swelling at the AC joint. The symptoms are often so localized that when describing the condition, the patient points to the end of the collar bone with the index finger.

"Whenever I reach up or across my shoulder, I get a pain right here (pointing to the AC joint)."
"I fell off my mountain bike and landed right on my shoulder. Ever since then I have had achy pain and swelling right here (pointing to the AC joint)."
"If I reach up, I feel a grinding in my shoulder."

Acromioclavicular Strain/Osteoarthritis

Enter just over the end of the clavicle (1½″ medially to the lateral edge of the acromion).

Needle: ⅝″, 25 gauge

Depth: ⅜ to ⅝″, down to the periosteum

Volume: 1 ml of anesthetic + ½ ml of K40

Note: The needle does not enter the joint directly. The injection is placed under the synovial membrane.

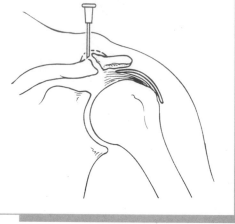

Figure 2–6.   Injection of the acromioclavicular joint

"The bones seem to be rubbing against one another."
"I can't lie on my shoulder. Sharp pain will wake me up."

EXAM.   Each patient is examined for joint inflammation, arthritic change, and disruption of the ligaments that support the joint.

EXAM SUMMARY   ● ● ● ● ● ● ● ● ● ● ● ● ● ● ●

1.   AC joint enlargement or deformity
2.   AC joint tenderness (with or without swelling)
3.   Pain aggravated by downward traction or forced adduction, performed passively
4.   AC joint widening with downward traction on the arm

(1) Simple inspection may reveal that the AC joint is distorted by tissue swelling, bony osteophytes, or elevation of the clavicle (third-degree separation). (2) Local tenderness (the most common sign) is located at the top of the joint, approximately 1½″ medial to the lateral edge of the acromion. (3) Pain is consistently aggravated by passively adducting the arm across the chest, thereby forcing the ends of the articulating surfaces together. (4) Pain may be aggravated by placing downward traction on the arm. In second-degree and third-degree separations, this may be accompanied by a widening of the gap between the clavicle and the acromion (palpable or visible in asthenic individuals and in those with high-grade separations). (5) The diagnosis is supported by a local anesthetic block placed just over the joint.

X-RAYS.   X-rays of the shoulder (including PA, external rotation, Y-outlet, and weighted views of the AC joint) are recommended. Plain films of the shoulder may show degenerative change, such as narrowing, sclerosis, "squaring-off" of the bones of the clavicle or proximal acromion, or osteophytic spurring. Weighted views of the shoulder (with and without hand-held weights) may show excessive widening between the end of the clavicle and the acromial process (>5 mm).

Note that severe osteophytic enlargement of the AC joints can contribute to subacromial impingement. Large, inferiorly directed osteophytes (4 to 5 mm in length) can irritate the subacromial bursa or the rotator cuff tendons!

Osteolysis of the clavicle—resorption of the distal end of the clavicle—is a rare complication of injury to the joint.

SPECIAL TESTING.   Weighted views of the AC joint are used to determine the severity of AC separation.

DIAGNOSIS.   The diagnosis of AC joint disease is easily made by physical examination. The degree of osteoarthritis or the extent of AC separation is determined by x-rays.

TREATMENT.   The goal of treatment is to reduce direct pressure and traction at the AC joint in order to allow the ligaments to reattach to their respective bony insertions. Restriction of reaching and direct pressure over the outer shoulder, combined with immobilization, are the treatments of choice.

Step 1: Examine the joint, order weighted views of the AC joints, and determine the stage of the injury (first, second, or third degree) and the degree of osteoarthritic change.

Advise the patient to avoid sleeping on either side.

Recommend restriction of reaching over the head and across the chest.

Limit lifting to 10 to 20 lb held close to the body.

Recommend applications of ice to control swelling and pain.

Prescribe a shoulder immobilizer for 3 to 4 weeks (p. 286).

Educate the patient: "If the ligaments aren't allowed to reattach to the bone, symptoms may recur over and over."

Step 2 (2 to 4 weeks for persistent cases): Reemphasize the restrictions.

Perform a local injection of K40, especially if swelling is prominent.

Perform a second injection 4 to 6 weeks after the first injection and combine it with a Velcro shoulder immobilizer to protect the injection and the joint.

Step 3 (8 to 10 weeks for chronic cases): Consider an orthopedic referral for palliative surgery.

PHYSICAL THERAPY.   Physical therapy plays a minor role in the treatment of AC strain and degenerative arthritis of the AC joint. Ice over the AC joint can provide temporary symptomatic relief. Unfortunately, there are no effective isometric toning exercises or stretching exercises that will provide direct support to the joint. General shoulder conditioning is recommended for the athlete.

PHYSICAL THERAPY SUMMARY   • • • • • • • • • • • • • •

1.   Ice
2.   General shoulder conditioning

INJECTION.   Local injection of anesthetic is used to confirm the diagnosis (to differentiate it from concurrent rotator cuff disease, for example). Corticosteroid injection is used to control the symptoms of a persistent sprain or the acute arthritic flare-up.

Positioning: The patient is to be sitting up with the shoulders held back and the hands in the lap.

Surface Anatomy and Point of Entry: The acromion and clavicle are identified. The AC joint is located as a ¼" depression at the distal end of the clavicle or 1½" medial to the lateral edge of the acromion. The point of entry is over the anterosuperior portion of the distal clavicle.

Angle of Entry and Depth: The 25-gauge needle is inserted at a perpendicular angle. The depth is ⅜ to ⅝".

Anesthesia: Ethyl chloride is sprayed on the skin. Local anesthetic is placed in the subcutaneous tissue (½ ml) and ¼" above the periosteum of the distal clavicle (½ ml). Note that all anesthesia is injected ¼" above the joint, thereby providing the highest concentration of corticosteroid to the joint.

Technique: The success of treatment depends on an undiluted injection of corticosteroid atop the joint or just under the synovial lining that attaches to the adjacent bone. After anesthesia is injected just outside the synovium, the 25-gauge needle is gently advanced down to the firm resistance of the periosteum of the clavicle. Using a separate syringe, ½ ml of K40 is injected flush against the bone. Note that the joint will not accommodate much medication. If the patient experiences increasing pressure, the needle should be withdrawn ⅛" and the remaining steroid injected just outside of the joint.

INJECTION AFTERCARE

1) *Rest* for 3 days, avoiding overhead reaching, reaching across the chest, lifting, leaning on the elbows, and sleeping directly on the shoulder.

2) Use a *shoulder immobilizer* with the injection to maximize protection of the joint (optional).

3) *Ice* (15 minutes every 4 to 6 hours) and *Tylenol ES* (1000 mg twice a day) for soreness.

4) *Protect* the shoulder for 30 days by limiting the movements referred to in (1).

5) Begin *general shoulder conditioning* 3 to 4 weeks after most of the pain and inflammation have resolved.

6) Repeat the *injection* and combine it with 3 to 4 weeks of immobilization at 6 weeks if overall improvement is less than 50%.

7) Delay *regular activities, work, and sports* until the pain has resolved.

8) Request *consultation* with a surgical orthopedist if two injections are unsuccessful.

SURGICAL PROCEDURE.   Several procedures are performed to stabilize the second- or third-degree separations. The most definitive surgical procedure involves distal clavicle resection.

PROGNOSIS.   Success of medical treatment is determined by adequate and anatomic healing of the injured ligaments. The emphasis of treatment must be on immobilization rather than on the anti-inflammatory action of injection. Unfortunately, since proper reattachment of the ligaments does not always occur, recurrent injury is seen frequently. Surgical consultation can be considered in recurrent cases, although distal clavicle resection or internal fixation is performed infrequently.

DESCRIPTION.   Biceps tendinitis is an inflammation of the long head tendon as it passes through the bicipital groove of the anterior humerus. Repeated irritation leads to microtearing and degenerative change. Vigorous or unusual lifting can lead to the

Biceps Tendinitis

Enter 1 to 1¼" below the anterolateral corner of the acromion, directly over the bicipital groove.

Needle: 1½", 25 gauge

Depth: ½ to ¾" to either tubercle and ¾ to 1" to the bottom of the bicipital groove

Volume: 1 to 2 ml of anesthetic and/or 1 ml of D80

Note: Gently locate the periosteum of the tubercle, anesthetize the bone, and carefully "walk down" the bone to the bottom of the groove.

CAUTION: Maintain the bevel of the needle parallel to the fibers of the tendon!

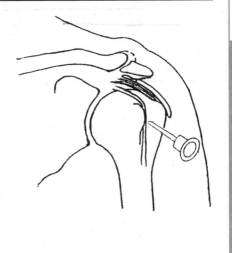

Figure 2–7.   Bicipital groove injection for bicipital tendinitis

spontaneous rupture of a chronically inflamed tendon. The risk of rupture approaches 10 to 12%, which is the highest spontaneous rupture rate of any tendon in the body.

SYMPTOMS.   The patient has shoulder pain aggravated by lifting or overhead reaching. The patient often takes one finger and points directly to the bicipital groove when describing the condition.

"The front of my shoulder hurts every time I lift my mail tray."
"I get this pain right here (pointing to a vertical line of pain running up the upper arm) whenever I move my shoulder."
"My shoulder has been sore for a long time. Yesterday, I tried to place my trailer on the trailer hitch when I felt and heard this loud pop!"
"My shoulder used to hurt a lot every day. Two days ago, it stopped hurting. Now I have this big bruise near my elbow, and the muscle seems bigger."

EXAM.   Each patient is examined for swelling and inflammation of the long head of the biceps in the bicipital groove for signs of subacromial impingement and for tendon rupture.

EXAM SUMMARY   • • • • • • • • • • • •

1. Local tenderness in the bicipital groove
2. Pain aggravated by flexion of the elbow, isometrically performed
3. A painful arc maneuver is often positive (p. 15)
4. A bulge in the antecubital fossa, signifying long head tendon rupture

(1) Local tenderness is present in the bicipital goove approximately 1" below the anterolateral tip of the acromion. The bicipital groove can be identified by palpating the anterior humeral head while passively internally and externally rotating the arm.

(2) Pain is aggravated by resisting elbow flexion isometrically. The patient describes a line of pain along the anterior humerus. (3) Pain may be aggravated by passively abducting the arm (the painful arc maneuver), as the long head tendon traverses between the humeral head and the undersurface of the acromion on its way to attach to the glenoid process. (4) Rupture of the tendon is usually manifested by a bulge several inches above the antecubital fossa and a large ecchymosis present along the inner aspect of the distal arm. Strength of elbow flexion is usually preserved because the short head and the brachioradialis tendons combine to make up 80% of the strength of elbow flexion.

X-RAYS. X-rays of the shoulder (including PA, external rotation, Y-outlet, and axillary views) are not always necessary. Plain films may demonstrate calcification in the bicipital groove. However, treatment decisions are based on the clinical findings of the exam rather than on the presence or absence of calcification.

Note that if bicipital rupture is present and the painful arc maneuver is dramatically positive, plain x-rays of the shoulder should be obtained to evaluate for concurrent rotator cuff tendon inflammation or rotator cuff tendon tear.

SPECIAL TESTING. Arthrography or MRI is indicated if concurrent rotator cuff tendon tear is suggested by examination.

DIAGNOSIS. The diagnosis is suggested by a history of anterior humeral pain and by an exam showing local tenderness in the bicipital groove that is aggravated by resisted elbow flexion. A regional anesthetic block in the bicipital groove may be necessary to differentiate biceps tendinitis from referred pain from the rotator cuff tendons or pain arising from the glenohumeral joint.

TREATMENT. The goals of treatment are to reduce the inflammation and swelling in the tendon, to strengthen the biceps muscle and tendon, and to prevent rupture. Restriction of lifting and reaching combined with an effective anti-inflammatory regimen is the treatment of choice.

Step 1: Eliminate lifting.

> Restrict over-the-shoulder positions and reaching.

> Apply ice over the anterolateral shoulder.

> Suggest an NSAID (e.g., ibuprofen [Advil, Motrin]) for 3 to 4 weeks.

> Educate the patient: "If restrictions aren't followed, there is a 5 to 10% risk of rupture."

Step 2 (2 to 4 weeks for persistent cases): Perform a local injection of D80 in the bicipital groove for patients younger than 50 or in the subacromial bursa for patients more than 50 years old.

> Repeat the injection in 4 to 6 weeks if symptoms have not decreased by at least 50%.

> Combine the injection with a simple sling or shoulder immobilizer to provide maximum protection against rupture (see pp. 285 to 286).

Step 3 (2 to 3 months for chronic cases): Consider an orthopedic consultation for persistent symptoms or if rupture has occurred. Note that surgery is rarely indicated.

PHYSICAL THERAPY. Physical therapy plays a minor role in the treatment of bicipital tendinitis and bicipital tendon rupture.

PHYSICAL THERAPY SUMMARY   • • • • • • • • • • • • •

1. Ice
2. Phonophoresis
3. Weighted pendulum stretching exercises, performed passively with relaxed shoulder muscles
4. Toning exercises for the short head biceps and brachioradialis tendons (with rupture)

Acute Period.   Ice, phonophoresis, and the weighted pendulum stretching exercises are used in the early treatment of bicipital tendinitis. *Ice* placed over the anterior humeral head provides temporary relief of pain. *Phonophoresis* over the anterior humeral head may provide relief of pain and swelling in thin patients. For an uncomplicated case of bicipital tendinitis, *weighted pendulum stretching exercises* are to be performed daily (p. 256). Increasing the subacromial space can provide the long head tendon more freedom of motion.

Recovery/Rehabilitation.   Weighted pendulum stretching exercises are combined with isometric toning of the elbow flexors.

Weighted pendulum stretching exercises are continued through the recovery period. When these exercises are performed three times a week, the chance of recurrent tendinitis is reduced.

Isometric toning exercises of elbow flexion are begun 3 to 4 weeks after the acute pain has resolved. These should be performed at 45 degrees of passive abduction of the shoulder to minimize the amount of friction in the bicipital groove. Daily toning exercises are particularly important when bicipital tendon rupture has occurred. Strengthening the short head of the biceps and brachioradialis just 15 to 20% will counteract the loss of strength from the rupture of the long head of the biceps.

INJECTION.   Local injection of anesthetic is used to confirm the diagnosis and corticosteroid to treat the chronic tendon inflammation. A subacromial or intra-articular injection is preferred after age 50 because the risk of tendon rupture is greater in this patient group and because these methods avoid direct needle penetration of the tendon. Bicipital groove injection—the most precise anatomic injection—is recommended in patients under age 50.

Positioning: The patient is to be sitting up, and the hands are placed in the lap. The patient is asked to relax the shoulder and neck muscles.

Surface Anatomy and Point of Entry: The humeral head and the lateral edge of the acromion are located and marked. The point of entry is directly over the bicipital groove, which is located 1 to 1¼" caudal to the anterolateral edge of the acromion. When the examiner's fingers are over the anterolateral humeral head, the groove is palpable when the arm is passively rotated internally and externally.

Angle of Entry and Depth: The angle of entry is perpendicular to the skin. The depth is ½ to ¾" to either bony prominence and ¾ to 1" to the bottom of the groove.

Anesthesia: Ethyl chloride is sprayed on the skin. Local anesthetic is placed at the firm tissue resistance of the lesser or greater tubercle (¼ to ½ ml) and at the bottom of the bicipital groove (½ ml).

Technique: The success of treatment depends on the accurate injection of the bicipital groove. In addition, in order to protect the tendon from damage, the bevel of the 25-gauge needle must be kept *parallel* to the fibers of the tendon during the entire procedure! The needle is gently advanced down to the firm tissue resistance of the periosteum of either the lesser or the greater tubercle, anesthetizing one or both. Having identified the adjacent bone, the needle is withdrawn ¼ to ⅜" and redirected into the groove (¼" deeper) until the rubbery, firm resistance of the tendon or the hard resistance of the humerus is felt. Inject only under light pressure! High pressure to injection suggests either an intratendonous or periosteal injection. If reexamination shows less local tenderness and less pain from isometric testing of arm flexion (>50%), then 1 ml of D80 is injected.

INJECTION AFTERCARE

1) *Rest* for 3 days, avoiding all lifting.

2) *Ice* (15 minutes every 4 to 6 hours) and *Tylenol ES* (1000 mg twice a day) for soreness.

3) *Protect* the tendon for 30 days by avoiding or at least limiting lifting (held close to the body, with low weight) and overhead reaching and positioning (the biceps tendon is located under the acromion).

4) Resume passively performed *pendulum stretching exercises* on day 4.

5) Begin isometric *elbow flexion exercises* after the pain has resolved (several weeks).

6) Repeat *injection* at 6 weeks if overall improvement is less than 50% (accompanied by a discussion of the risk factors for tendon rupture: age over 50, recurrent tendinitis, a previous tendon rupture, poor general shoulder conditioning, and rheumatoid arthritis).

7) Delay *regular activities, work, and sports* until the lost tone has been fully recovered.

SURGICAL PROCEDURE.   Bicipital tendon ruptures are rarely repaired (the short head of the biceps and the brachioradialis provide 80% of flexion strength).

PROGNOSIS.   A significant number of patients develop degenerative changes in the tendon. Spontaneous rupture occurs in 10% of cases. Surprisingly, little functional disability results because the short head of the biceps and the brachioradialis provide 80% of the strength of elbow flexion. Rupture often cures the problem but leads to a minor deformity. For these reasons, surgical repair is performed infrequently. Heavy laborers, violinists, and other patients who demand the utmost from their upper extremities should be referred for surgical consultation.

DESCRIPTION.   Constant friction (to-and-fro motions of the arm) and direct pressure (lying on hard surfaces) cause irritation and inflammation to develop between the scapula and the underlying rib. This focal inflammation just under the superomedial angle of the scapula is referred to as subscapular bursitis or as scapulothoracic syndrome (the difference in nomenclature reflects the confusion over the exact nature of the structure; it is neither a true bursa nor a true articulation, simply a friction point of the body). The condition must be distinguished from the more common rhomboid or levator scapular muscle irritation (posture, stress, whiplash) and the referred pain of the lower cervical roots.

SYMPTOMS.   The patient complains of localized pain over the upper back or a popping sound whenever the shoulder is shrugged. The patient often tries to reach over the shoulder in an attempt to touch the affected area of the upper back when describing the condition.

"Every time I roll my shoulder, it pops."
"I can't sit against a hard-backed chair."
"I work at an assembly table. I have to reach back and forth. The back of my shoulder began to hurt when I took this new job."
"I can't sleep on my back anymore. There's this spot of pain over my shoulder blade."

Subscapular Bursitis

Enter directly over the second or third rib, which-ever is closer to the superomedial angle of the scapula.

Needle: 1½", 22 gauge

Depth: ¾ to 1¼" down to the periosteum of the rib

Volume: 1 to 2 ml of anesthetic plus 1 ml of K40

Note: Place one finger above and one finger be-low the rib in the intercostal spaces and enter between the two; never advance more than 1¼" (too deep, pleura!).

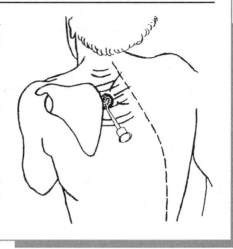

Figure 2–8.   Subscapular bursa injection

EXAM.   The patient is examined for localized tenderness under the superomedial angle of the scapula atop the second or third ribs.

EXAM SUMMARY

• • • • • • • • • • • • • • • •

1. Local tenderness under the superomedial angle of the scapula, directly over the rib
2. Full range of motion of the shoulder
3. No evidence of cervical root irritation or rhomboid or trapezius muscle strain
4. Confirmation with local anesthetic block

(1) Local tenderness is present in a half-dollar sized area just under the supero-medial angle of the scapula. The tenderness is palpated along the second or the third rib, whichever is closer to the angle. Palpation of the exact site of irritation requires that the patient's arm be fully adducted. Have the patient place the hand on the contralateral shoulder and then relax the shoulder muscles. (2) The condition does not affect the range of motion of the glenohumeral joint. (3) Because cervical radicu-lopathy can refer pain in the identical area of the upper back, the neck must be examined in each case. In an uncomplicated case of bursitis, the range of motion of the neck should be unaffected (a normal 90 degrees of painless rotation) and the upper extremity neurologic examination should be normal. (4) Local anesthetic block plays an integral part in the diagnosis. One or two ml of lidocaine placed at the level of the periosteum of the closest rib should totally eliminate the patient's pain and local tenderness.

X-RAYS.   X-rays of the shoulder are not necessary in an uncomplicated case.

SPECIAL TESTING.   None.

DIAGNOSIS.   Focal tenderness just under the superomedial angle of the scapula is highly suggestive of subscapular bursitis. However, in order to distinguish this local inflammatory condition from referred pain from the cervical roots or the muscular irritation of upper back strain, the diagnosis must be confirmed by local anesthetic block at the level of the adjacent rib.

TREATMENT. The goals of treatment are to reduce the acute inflammation and to prevent further episodes by improvement in posture and in shoulder muscle tone. Local corticosteroid injection with K40 is the treatment of choice.

Step 1: Perform a neck and upper back exam, and if symptoms are localized to the superomedial angle of the scapula, confirm the diagnosis with local anesthesia.

If the diagnosis is confirmed, perform an injection of 1 ml of K40.

Emphasize the importance of correct posture.

Advise on avoiding direct pressure over the scapula.

Recommend limitations of to-and-fro motions and overhead reaching of the affected arm.

Step 2 (4 to 6 weeks for persistent cases): Repeat the K40 injection if the symptoms and signs have not improved by at least 50%.

Reemphasize correct posture.

Begin isometric toning exercises of internal and external rotation.

Perform therapeutic ultrasound for refractory cases.

PHYSICAL THERAPY. Physical therapy plays a minor role in the treatment of subscapular bursitis. General shoulder conditioning can be combined with enhancement of the subscapularis muscle tone. Increases in the tone and bulk of the shoulder's principal internal rotator has the theoretical advantage of providing a natural padding between the ribs and the undersurface of the scapula. This exercise must be combined with improvements in sitting posture to be effective.

INJECTIONS. Local injection of anesthetic is used to confirm the diagnosis and corticosteroid is used to treat the active inflammation. The NSAIDs are not effective for this condition.

Positioning: The patient is to be sitting up, and the shoulder on the affected side is to be fully adducted. The patient is asked to place his or her hand on the contralateral shoulder.

Surface Anatomy and Point of Entry: The superomedial angle of the scapula is identified. With the shoulder fully adducted, the second and third ribs are identified and marked. With one finger in the intercostal space above and one finger in the intercostal space below, insert the needle directly over the rib.

Angle of Entry and Depth: The angle of entry is perpendicular to the skin. The depth is ¾″ in thin patients and up to 1¼″ in heavier patients. *Caution:* never advance deeper than 1¼″ (pleura)! If periosteum has not been encountered at 1¼″, withdraw the needle and redirect!

Anesthesia: Ethyl chloride is sprayed on the skin. Local anesthetic is placed at the firm tissue resistance of the periosteum of the rib (1 to 2 ml). Avoid putting anesthesia into the muscular layer above the rib so as to differentiate the degree of bursitis from any associated involvement of the overlying rhomboid muscles.

Technique: The successful injection of the bursa depends on the proper positioning of the patient and the accurate placement of medication just atop the periosteum of the rib. The needle is advanced through the trapezius muscle and the rhomboid muscle to the hard resistance of the periosteum of the rib. Both the anesthetic and the corticosteroid are injected at this site.

INJECTION AFTERCARE

1) *Rest* for 3 days, avoiding all direct pressure and to-and-fro shoulder motions.

2) *Ice* (15 minutes every 4 to 6 hours) and *Tylenol ES* (1000 mg twice a day) for soreness.

3) *Protect* the shoulder for 30 days by limiting direct pressure and the extremes of shoulder motion.

4) Reemphasize the need for good *posture.*

5) Begin *isometric toning exercises* of internal rotation and adduction at 3 weeks. If the bulk and tone of the subscapularis muscle can be increased, the scapula will be less likely to rub against the underlying ribs.

6) Repeat the *injection* at 6 weeks if overall improvement is less than 50%.

7) Delay *regular activities, work, and sports* until the pain and inflammation have resolved and improvement in adduction and internal rotation strength is substantial.

SURGICAL PROCEDURE. None.

PROGNOSIS. Local injection of anesthesia followed by corticosteroid is highly effective in treating the acute inflammation of subscapular bursitis. Prevention of recurrent bursitis depends on correcting posture, reducing muscular stress, and enhancing the tone and bulk of the subscapularis muscle. Long-term complications do not occur.

Glenohumeral Osteoarthritis

Intra-articular injection enters ½″ below the coracoid process and is directed outward toward the medial portion of the humeral head (see p. 23 for details).

Needle: 1½ to 3½″ spinal needle, 22 gauge

Depth: 1½ to 2½″, down to humeral periosteum

Volume: 3 to 4 ml of anesthetic plus 1 ml of K40

Note: Fluoroscopy is strongly recommended in obese patients.

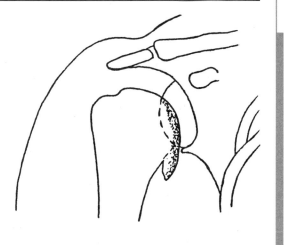

Figure 2–9. Glenohumeral osteoarthritis

DESCRIPTION. Osteoarthritis of the glenohumeral joint—wear and tear of the articular cartilage of the glenoid labrum and humeral head—is an uncommon problem. In most cases, trauma precedes the condition, although the injury may have occurred years earlier. Injuries that are associated with the development of osteoarthritis include previous dislocation, humeral head or neck fracture, large rotator cuff tendon tears, and rheumatoid arthritis. X-rays are diagnostic and demonstrate osteophyte formation at the inferior humeral head, flattening and sclerosis of the humeral head, and narrowing of the inferior portion of the articular cartilage, which has a normal width of 3 to 4 mm.

SYMPTOMS. The patient complains of the gradual development of shoulder pain and stiffness over a period of months to years. The patient often rubs the front of the shoulder when describing the symptoms.

"My shoulder is stiff."
"I can't reach back to put my coat on."
"I dislocated my shoulder in football. The coach said I would get arthritis in my shoulder. Now I'm 58 years old and my shoulder is gradually losing its motion . . . it's getting stiffer and stiffer."
"My shoulder makes this terrible clunking noise, like the front of my car when the steering went out."

EXAM. The patient is examined for local glenohumeral joint line tenderness and swelling, loss of range of motion of external rotation and abduction, and crepitation.

EXAM SUMMARY

1. Local tenderness located anteriorly, just under the coracoid process
2. Restricted abduction and external rotation, measured passively
3. Crepitation with circumduction or clunking on release of isometric tension
4. Swelling of the infraclavicular fossa or general fullness to the shoulder

(1) Tenderness is located anteriorly, just under the thumb-shaped projection of the coracoid process. Firm outward and slightly upward pressure is necessary to assess the irritation along the anterior glenohumeral joint line. (2) Endpoint stiffness and restricted range of motion are the hallmark physical signs of arthritis of the shoulder. The global function of the shoulder is reduced. Overhead reaching and reaching to the lower lumbosacral spine (the Apley scratch test) are impaired. Loss of glenohumeral abduction and external rotation predominate and are used to gauge the severity of the condition. (3) Noise arising from the joint is common. Crepitation or a clunking sound is palpable anteriorly and in moderate to severe cases can be audible. This is reproduced best by resisting abduction in midarc and feeling for the crepitation as tension is released (the humeral head rapidly moves across the irregular glenoid cartilage, causing the noise). (4) Dramatic involvement of the glenohumeral joint is associated with a joint effusion. Small effusions are usually too subtle to detect. Moderate to large effusions present with infraclavicular swelling or general fullness to the shoulder. General fullness is best assessed by looking down on the joint from above and comparing the PA dimension with the unaffected side.

X-RAYS. Plain x-rays of the shoulder (including PA, external rotation, Y-outlet, and axillary views) are strongly recommended. The earliest changes include narrowing of the articular cartilage and irregularities at the inferior glenoid fossa. As the disease progresses, the distance between the inferior glenoid and the humeral head gradually decreases, and spurring off the inferior portion of the humeral head gradually increases. Advanced arthritis presents with a large humeral head spur, a flattening of the humeral head, and obliteration of the articular cartilage at the inferior glenoid.

SPECIAL TESTING. Special testing is not necessary in the moderate to advanced case with well-established changes on plain x-rays. However, to detect early disease, computerized tomography (CT) arthrography can be ordered. Iodine contrast arthrography with CT is indicated to detect subtle irregularities of the inferior glenoid labral cartilage or early thinning of the articular cartilage in the young, active patient who has suffered trauma to the shoulder. These patients tend to complain of deep anterior shoulder pain, loss of smooth motion, and crepitation with movement, and they demonstrate hypermobility on examination.

DIAGNOSIS.   A diagnosis of osteoarthritis is suggested by a history of progressive loss of range of motion, crepitation or crunching with circumduction, and documentation of a loss of external rotation and abduction. Since the findings on physical examination of frozen shoulder are nearly identical to the findings of glenohumeral osteoarthritis, the diagnosis must be confirmed by plain x-rays. Note that early presentations of osteoarthritis may require CT arthrography to show clearly the early thinning of the inferior glenoid articular cartilage.

TREATMENT.   The goals of treatment combine exercises to improve range of motion and muscular support with ice applications and medication to reduce the inflammation. Weighted pendulum stretching exercises performed daily and isometric toning exercises of external rotation and abduction are the initial treatments of choice.

Step 1: Determine the severity of the condition by assessing the patient's reaching overhead and reaching to the lower back (the Apley scratch test), by measuring the loss of abduction and external rotation, and by estimating the strength of external rotation.

Obtain baseline x-rays of the shoulder.

Educate the patient about the slowly progressive nature of the condition: "This is a wear-and-tear type of arthritis that progresses very slowly."

Recommend heat applications to the anterior shoulder prior to stretching.

Prescribe weighted pendulum stretching exercises with the shoulder muscles relaxed, once a day (p. 256).

Prescribe passive stretching exercises in the directions of motion with the greatest loss, commonly abduction and external rotation (p. 258).

Suggest an elimination of heavy work, overhead reaching, and forceful pushing and pulling.

Prescribe an NSAID (e.g., ibuprofen [Advil, Motrin]) in full dose for 3 to 4 weeks and then substitute it with *ES Tylenol, 1000 mg* twice a day.

Step 2 (6 to 8 weeks for routine follow-up): Reevaluate the range of motion.

Reinforce the specific passive stretching exercises.

Perform an intra-articular injection of corticosteroid or refer patient to a radiologist to perform this under fluoroscopic control.

Evaluate and treat any concurrent rotator cuff tendinitis.

Begin isometric toning exercises of external rotation to improve the stability of the joint.

Step 3 (3 months for follow-up): Reevaluate the range of motion.

Encourage the patient.

Perform repeat x-rays if the patient has lost significant range of motion and symptoms have been relentlessly progressive.

Step 4 (6 to 12 months for chronic cases): Gradually increase activities of daily living, as tolerated. Consider referral to an orthopedic surgeon with experience in shoulder replacement.

PHYSICAL THERAPY. Physical therapy plays a significant role in the rehabilitation of the acute osteoarthritic flare and a vital role in the prevention of future episodes.

PHYSICAL THERAPY SUMMARY ● ● ● ● ● ● ● ● ● ● ● ● ● ● ●

1. Ice placed over the anterior shoulder
2. Range-of-motion exercises to restore or enhance lost external rotation and abduction
3. Gentle pendulum stretching exercises, as tolerated
4. Isometrically performed toning exercises in rotation and abduction, followed by more active exercises

---

Acute Period/Recovery. Heat, the weighted pendulum stretching exercises, and passive stretching exercises are used to improve glenohumeral flexibility. The shoulder is *heated* for 10 to 15 minutes with moist heat or in a bathtub or shower. *Weighted pendulum stretching exercises* are performed for 5 minutes (p. 256). The arm is kept vertical, and the patient bends slightly at the waist. The patient should be instructed on relaxing the shoulder muscles when performing this exercise: "This is a pure stretching exercise; don't swing the weight in a diameter greater than 1 foot; let the weight do the work." *Passive stretching exercises* are performed after the pendulum stretching exercises. Individualize your recommendations. Emphasize stretching exercises that address the directions in which the patient has suffered the greatest loss, usually abduction and external rotation (p. 258). Limit the abduction stretch to no higher than shoulder level, especially if rotator cuff tendinitis accompanies arthritis. Emphasize the need to stretch to the point of tension but not pain. Multiple repetitions performed daily will gradually stretch the glenohumeral capsule.

General *rotator cuff tendon toning exercises* may play a major role in recovery, especially if arthritis is complicated by rotator cuff tendinitis (p. 254). Gradually increasing the tone of the infraspinatus tendon (external rotation) and the subscapularis tendon (internal rotation) will enhance stability, provide greater support, and reduce arthritic flare-ups. Activities of daily living should be postponed until muscle tone in external and internal roation are restored.

INJECTION. Local injection of anesthetic is used to confirm the diagnosis (to separate it from concurrent rotator cuff disease, for example). Corticosteroid injection is used to control the symptoms of the acute arthritic flare (see "Frozen Shoulder," p. 23).

SURGICAL PROCEDURE. Shoulder replacement (arthroplasty) for intractable symptoms or loss of 50% range of motion is the procedure of choice.

PROGNOSIS. Osteoarthritis of the glenohumeral joint is a slowly progressing process. Physical therapy exercises combined with intra-articular injection are effective in controlling the acute inflammatory flare. Maintenance toning exercises in external and internal rotation are fundamental to providing stability, improved motion, and fewer recurrent arthritic flares. Total shoulder replacement is indicated when overall function is impaired, activities of daily living are significantly impacted, and pain is intractable.

DESCRIPTION. Multidirectional instability of the shoulder is synonymous with "subluxation," "loose" shoulder, or partial dislocation. It is more common in young women with poor muscular support of the shoulder, in patients with large rotator cuff tendon tears (loss of support as exemplified in the patient with Milwaukee shoulder), and in athletic patients under the age of 40 (especially swimmers and

MULTIDIRECTIONAL INSTABILITY OF THE SHOULDER

The treatment of choice is isometric toning exercises involving internal and external rotation, with the shoulder kept in neutral position; resistance is accomplished by using a TheraBand, bungy cord, inner tube, or similar aid.

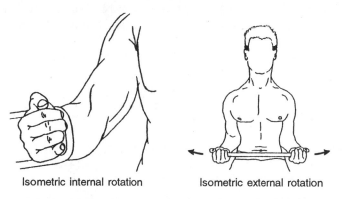

Isometric internal rotation   Isometric external rotation

Figure 2–10. Multidirectional instability of the shoulder

throwers). It is an uncommon problem after age 40 because of the natural stiffening of the tissues around the shoulder.

SYMPTOMS. The patient complains of looseness of the shoulder, a noisy shoulder, or anterolateral shoulder pain typical of rotator cuff tendinitis. The patient often grabs hold of the deltoid muscle, securing it in place, or rubs over it when describing the condition.

"It feels like my shoulder is going to pop out."
"Every time I try to lift something heavy, my shoulder seems to slip."
"My shoulder seems weak."
"My shoulder makes this crunching sound."
"I'm afraid to rock-climb because I can't trust my shoulder."

EXAM. Each patient is examined for the degree of instability (subluxation), for the presence of subacromial impingement and tendon inflammation, and for early signs of glenohumeral osteoarthritis.

EXAM SUMMARY ● ● ● ● ● ● ● ● ● ● ● ● ● ● ● ●

1. Downward traction on the arm causing the sulcus sign
2. Increased anteroposterior mobility of the humeral head (relative to the glenoid fossa)
3. The painful arc maneuver may be positive (p. 15).
4. A positive apprehension sign when the arm is placed at 70 to 80 degrees of abduction and passively rotated externally

(1) The hallmark sign of hypermobility is the sulcus sign, an objective measurement of the looseness of the glenohumeral joint. By placing downward traction on

the arm (pressure applied to the antecubital fossa when the elbow is flexed to 90 degrees) the humerus can be observed to pull away from the acromion. A gap of ½ to ¾" that forms between the humeral head and the undersurface of the acromion indicates severe hypermobility. By contrast, it is impossible to create a subacromial gap in patients with fibromyalgia, stress, or highly toned muscles. (2) Hypermobility can be confirmed by applying pressure to the humeral head in the anteroposterior direction while simultanteously holding the acromion in a fixed position. The humeral head can be felt to move in the glenoid with moderate to severe hypermobility. Sharp pain or a grinding crunch may indicate osteoarthritic change or a tear of the glenoid labrum. (3) Rotator cuff tendinitis can accompany hypermobility. The painful arc may be positive and anterolateral shoulder pain may be reproduced by isometric testing of midarc abduction (supraspinatus) and external roation (infraspinatus). (4) An apprehension sign can be demonstrated in patients with true dislocation. With the arm passively abducted to 70 to 80 degrees, tolerance of forced passive external rotation is assessed.

X-RAYS.   Plain x-rays of the shoulder (including PA, external rotation, Y-outlet, and axillary views) are highly recommended for patients with persistent pain, loss of range of motion, or persistent signs of rotator cuff tendinitis.

SPECIAL TESTING.   CT arthrography is the test of choice to assess the integrity of the glenoid labral cartilage (thinning or tears) and to determine the degree of early osteoarthritis of the glenohumeral joint (early inferior glenoid osteophyte formation or loss of glenoid articular cartilage). The most common indication for this test is poor response to isometric toning exercises, persistent lack of full range of motion, or persistent clicking or crepitation with circumduction of the shoulder.

DIAGNOSIS.   The diagnosis of hypermobility is made by clinical exam.

TREATMENT.   The goals of treatment are similar to the recommendations for rotator cuff tendinitis. Emphasis is placed on performing isometric toning exercises to improve the stability of the glenohumeral joint and thus reduce the risk of osteoarthritis. Isometric toning exercises in external and internal rotation are the treatment of choice.

Step 1: Assess the patient's degree of hypermobility, estimate the range of motion, and order x-rays of the shoulder.

Advise rest and restriction of overhead positioning, reaching, pushing, pulling, and lifting.

Recommend ice for concurrent rotator cuff tendinitis.

Prescribe isometric toning exercises in external and internal rotation, beginning at low tension.

Step 2 (2 to 4 weeks for persistent cases): Prescribe an NSAID (e.g., ibuprofen [Advil, Motrin]) in full dose for 3 to 4 weeks or perform a subacromial injection of D80.

Reemphasize the isometric toning exercises in external and internal rotation.

Step 3 (6 to 8 weeks for persistent cases): Order a CT arthrogram to exclude a glenoid labral tear if symptoms fail to respond to exercises and an empiric injection of D80.

Repeat the injection in 4 to 6 weeks if symptoms and signs have improved but linger at or below the 50% improvement level.

Step 4 (3 months or longer for chronic cases): Emphasize the need to continue the toning exercises to maintain stability.

Recommend cautious performance of or limitations of overhead reaching.

Tell a patient with recurrent or persistent symptoms to avoid all repetitive overhead work or positioning!

Refer the patient to an orthopedic surgeon with experience in shoulder surgery for a stabilization procedure.

PHYSICAL THERAPY. Isometric toning exercises in external and internal rotation combined with general shoulder conditioning are the mainstays of treatment for hypermobility of the shoulder.

PHYSICAL THERAPY SUMMARY ● ● ● ● ● ● ● ● ● ● ● ● ● ● ●

1. Ice if concurrent rotator cuff tendinitis is present
2. Isometrically performed toning exercises in external and internal rotation
3. General shoulder conditioning with emphasis on rotation and deltoid muscle toning

---

Acute Period. *Ice* can provide temporary relief of pain and swelling if rotator cuff tendinitis is present.

Recovery/Rehabilitation. *Isometric toning exercises* of the external rotation (infraspinatus muscle) and internal rotation (subscapularis muscle) are combined to enhance the stability of the glenohumeral joint and to counteract the hypermobility (p. 254). Ideally, the strength of external rotation should equal the strength of internal rotation which, in turn, should be close to the strength of the biceps muscle. Once rotation is enhanced, *general shoulder conditioning* can be started. These exercises should be performed daily until tone is enhanced and then three times a week indefinitely.

INJECTION. Local anesthetic injection can be used to identify the presence or degree of subclinical or overt rotator cuff or bicipital tendinitis (see details, p. 18). If subacromial or bicipital groove anesthetic block improves pain and function significantly, empiric corticosteroid injection can be performed.

SURGICAL PROCEDURE. Variations of the Putti-Platt procedure to remove redundant capsule and to reinforce the anterior joint capsule with the subscapularis tendon is the procedure of choice.

PROGNOSIS. A patient with recurrent dislocation should be evaluated by an orthopedic surgeon for consideration of a stabilization procedure. Recurrent dislocation must be managed properly to avoid glenohumeral osteoarthritis later in life.

A patient with recurrent subluxation and episodic rotator or bicipital tendinitis should be managed with long-term physical therapy toning exercises. Surgical consultation is dependent on the overall impairment of shoulder function and the number of episodes and frequency of shoulder tendinitis. By contrast, surgical consultation should not be entertained in every case. The natural history of the condition is to improve slowly as the body gradually stiffens during the 40- to 50-year age range.

chapter 3

Elbow

Lateral Epicondylitis

Enter directly over the prominence of the lateral epicondyle; use skin traction to identify the interface of the subcutaneous fat and the extensor carpi radialis tendon.

Needle: ⅝″, 25 gauge

Depth: ¼ to ½″, just above the tendon

Volume: 1 to 2 ml of anesthetic plus ½ ml of D80

Note: Never inject under forced pressure or if the patient experiences sharp pain (too deep and likely intratendinous).

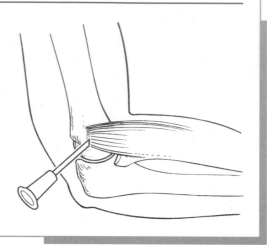

Figure 3–1.   Injection for lateral epicondylitis

DESCRIPTION.   Lateral epicondylitis (tennis elbow) is an injury of the common extensor tendon at the lateral epicondyle of the humerus. Unaccustomed or repetitive lifting, tooling, or hammering and sports activities involving tight gripping and repetitive impact cause microtearing or microavulsion of the origin of the extensor carpi radialis tendon. Secondary inflammation develops at the epicondyle after this mechanical injury. Symptoms persist because of constant traction that occurs as a result of everyday use of the wrist and hand. The radiohumeral joint range of motion and function are unaffected in this classic periarticular condition.

SYMPTOMS.   The patient has elbow pain and weakness of the forearm. The patient points to the lateral epicondyle or rubs the outer aspect of the lower humerus with the fingertips when describing the condition.

"The pain in my elbow has gotten so bad that I can't even lift my coffee cup."
"After a couple of hours of using my screwdriver, my elbow starts to ache really badly."
"I was pounding nails over the weekend, and ever since then my elbow has been aching."
"Anytime I try to use my torque wrench, I get this sharp pain on the outside of my elbow."
"You've got to do something, doc. I can't spike the volleyball anymore."

EXAM.   Each patient is examined for local irritation at the lateral epicondyle, for the strength and integrity of the common extensor tendon mechanism, and for weakness of grip.

(1) Local tenderness is the most common sign and is located over a dime-sized area at the lateral epicondyle. A few patients will have local tenderness between the radial head and the lateral epicondyle (the radial humeral bursa, an extension of the joint lining of the elbow). (2) This lateral elbow pain is aggravated by resisting wrist extension and radial deviation performed isometrically with the wrist held in neutral position. (The tendon most commonly involved in tennis elbow is the extensor carpi radialis brevis whose function is to extend and radially deviate the wrist.) (3) Pain is aggravated by strong gripping. In severe cases, weakness of grip occurs from disuse but also from the mechanical disruption of the injury. Objective measurement of grip strength and endurance with a dynamometer can be used to document severe

involvement. (4) The range of motion of the elbow is preserved. Loss of extension or flexion is almost always indicative of a primary elbow joint process.

EXAM SUMMARY   ● ● ● ● ● ● ● ● ● ● ● ● ● ● ●

1. Local epicondylar tenderness
2. Pain aggravated by resisting wrist extension and radial deviation, isometrically performed
3. Decreased grip strength
4. Full range of motion of the elbow joint

X-RAYS. X-rays of the elbow are not necessary. Routine films of the elbow are normal in nearly all cases.

SPECIAL TESTING. None.

DIAGNOSIS. The diagnosis is based on a history of pain over the lateral epicondyle and on an examination demonstrating local epicondylar tenderness and lateral elbow pain aggravated by isometric wrist extension or radial deviation. Regional anesthetic block at the epicondyle can be used to confirm the diagnosis and differentiate it from the referred pain of carpal tunnel syndrome, cervical radiculopathy, or rotator cuff tendinitis.

TREATMENT. The goals of treatment are to allow the microtorn common extensor tendon to reapproximate or reattach to the lateral epicondylar process, to reduce the secondary inflammation, and to restore forearm muscle strength. Ice to reduce inflammation at the lateral epicondyle combined with immobilization of the wrist to prevent traction and tension is the treatment of choice.

Step 1: Evaluate flexion and extension of the elbow, estimate the strength of gripping, and obtain baseline measurements of the patient's strength of wrist extension.

Recommend limitations on lifting, hammering, repetitive wrist motion, and fine hand work.

Apply ice over the epicondyle.

Prescribe a Velcro wrist splint (p. 288).

Empirically prescribe an NSAID (e.g., ibuprofen [Advil, Motrin]) for 3 to 4 weeks. Note that oral medication may not concentrate sufficiently in this relatively avascular tendon site.

Educate the patient: "You may feel the pain at the elbow, but it is the wrist and hand motions that aggravate it the most."

Step 2 (3 to 4 weeks for persistent cases): Order a short-arm cast (p. 288).

Suggest a long-arm cast if supination and pronation of the forearm prominently affect the pain at the elbow.

Discontinue the NSAID at 4 weeks if symptoms have not responded dramatically.

Continue with applications of ice.

Step 3 (6 to 8 weeks for persistent cases): Perform a local injection of D80 if a 3-week period of fixed immobilization with casting has failed.

Repeat the injection in 4 to 6 weeks if symptoms have not been reduced by at least 50%.

Step 4 (6 to 10 weeks for chronic cases): Begin toning exercise (p. 262) after the pain has subsided.

Use a tennis elbow band (p. 287) to prevent a recurrence.

Advise patient to gradually resume activities.

Demonstrate palms-up lifting and explain how this avoids putting direct tension on the elbow.

Consider an orthopedic referral for persistent symptoms, especially for laborers and carpenters.

PHYSICAL THERAPY. Physical therapy plays a minor role in the active treatment of lateral epicondylitis and a vital role in its rehabilitation and prevention.

PHYSICAL THERAPY SUMMARY

1. Ice
2. Phonophoresis with a hydrocortisone gel
3. Gripping exercises, isometrically performed
4. Toning exercises of wrist extension, isometrically performed

Acute Period. *Ice* and *phonophoresis* using a hydrocortisone gel provide temporary relief of pain and swelling. Ice is routinely recommended and is particularly helpful for inflammatory flare reactions after local corticosteroid injection. Phonophoresis is an alternative treatment that is used when inflammatory changes are prominent and have failed to respond to ice. Both must be combined with immobilization to be effective.

Recovery/Rehabilitation. Isometric exercises are used to restore the strength and tone of the extensor muscles. Between 3 and 4 weeks after the symptoms and signs have resolved, *isometric toning exercises* are begun (p. 262). Initially, *grip exercises* using grip putty, a small compressible rubber ball, or an old tennis ball are performed daily in sets of 20, with each hold lasting 5 seconds. The strength and endurance of the forearm flexor and extensor muscles are gradually built up. (When actively flexing the forearm muscles by gripping, the extensor muscles are activated as well.) These exercises are followed by *isometric toning exercises of wrist extension*, which are essential to restoring full strength to the forearm and to preventing future recurrences. Each episode of epicondylitis appears to weaken the common extensor mechanism. To overcome the loss of tensile strength, toning exercises must continue to be done three times a week and should be combined with an ongoing limitation on lifting, torquing, and heavy gripping. For recurrent disease, these exercises should be continued for up to 6 to 12 months.

INJECTION. Local injection with corticosteroid is indicated when initial management with immobilization fails to reduce symptoms sufficiently to allow participation in the physical therapy recovery exercises.

Positioning: The patient is to be in the supine position, the elbow is flexed to 90 degrees, and the hand is placed under the ipsilateral buttock (for maximum exposure of the epicondyle).

Surface Anatomy and Point of Entry: The lateral epicondyle is easily palpated with the elbow flexed to 90 degrees. It is located ½" proximal to the radial head (the radial head should rotate smoothly under the examiner's fingers when passively supinating and pronating the forearm). The point of entry is directly over the center of the epicondyle.

Angle of Entry and Depth: The angle of entry is perpendicular to the skin. The depth is ¼ to ⅜" down to the extensor tendon (*not* down to the periosteum!). If the patient is thin, pinch up the skin, enter from an angle, and use 1 ml of anesthesia to dilate the subcutaneous tissue, thereby creating a space for the injection of corticosteroid.

Anesthesia: Ethyl chloride is sprayed on the skin. Local anesthetic is placed in the subcutaneous tissue only (½ ml). If the patient is thin, use 1 ml of anesthetic to distend the tissues over the epicondyle, thereby creating more space for the corticosteroid.

Technique: Successful treatment combines the protection of immobilization with the accurate placement of injection followed by isometrically performed recovery exercises. The depth of injection can be accurately determined by gradually advancing the needle until the patient feels mild discomfort (the subcutaneous tissue is usually pain-free) or until the rubbery resistance of the tendon is felt. Note: a painful reaction to injection or firm resistance during injecting suggests that the needle is too deep and is within the body of the tendon (withdraw ⅛"!). In addition, the proper depth can be confirmed by applying traction to the overlying skin. The needle should move freely with skin traction if the tip is above the tendon. Conversely, the needle will stick in place if the tip is within the body of the tendon. The corticosteroid should always be injected at the tissue plane between the subcutaneous fat and the tendon!

INJECTION AFTERCARE

1) *Rest* for 3 days, avoiding all lifting, typing, writing, turning of the forearms, tooling, and hammering.

2) *Ice* (15 minutes every 4 to 6 hours) and *Tylenol ES* (1000 mg twice a day) for soreness.

3) *Protect* the elbow for 3 to 4 weeks by the continuous wearing of the Velcro brace or a short-arm cast. Instruct the patient to restrict the turning of the forearm (the only motion wrist immobilization cannot restrict).

4) Emphasize the need to perform lifting palms-up, to use a wrist bar when typing, and to use thick, padded grips on tools.

5) Begin *gripping exercises* at half tension after the brace or cast is discontinued. The patient should start with a half grip and gradually build up over 1 to 2 weeks.

6) With restoration of normal grip strength, *isometric toning exercises of wrist extension* are begun at low tension and slowly increased. The patient should exercise only to the edge of discomfort; patients experiencing forearm muscle soreness are probably exercising too aggressively. Exercises must be interrupted if the lateral epicondyle becomes progressively more irritated.

7) Repeat *injection* at 6 weeks if recovery exercises are poorly tolerated or improvement is less than 50%.

8) Delay *regular activities, work, and sports* until the pain and inflammation have resolved and grip and wrist extension strength have increased substantially.

9) Obtain *plain x-rays* of the elbow and a *consultation* with a surgical orthopedist for chronic symptoms.

SURGICAL PROCEDURE.   Tendon excision or débridement, tendon lengthening, or tenotomy is performed uncommonly (approximately 3 to 5% of cases). Surgery can

be considered when two courses of immobilization combined with local ice applications and at least one local corticosteroid injection have failed to resolve the acute symptoms.

PROGNOSIS.   Of these patients, 95% should respond to immobilization combined with corticosteroid injection. The remaining 5% may respond to long-term physical therapy toning exercises with severe restrictions of forearm use. Patients failing to improve (those with chronic tendinitis or mucinoid degeneration of the tendon, or both) can be considered for surgical exploration and primary tendon repair.

Medial Epicondylitis

Enter ⅜ to ½" distal to the prominence of the medial epicondyle; use skin traction to identify the interface between the subcutaneous fat and the tendon.

Needle: ⅝", 25 gauge

Depth: ¼ to ⅜", just above the tendon

Volume: 1 to 2 ml of anesthetic plus ½ ml of D80

Note: Never inject under forced pressure or if the patient experiences sharp pain (too deep, within the tendon).

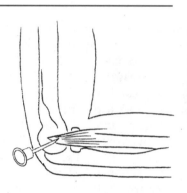

Figure 3–2.   Injection for medial epicondylitis

DESCRIPTION.   Medial epicondylitis (golfer's elbow) is an injury of the common flexor tendon at the medial epicondyle of the humerus. Unaccustomed or repetitive lifting, tooling, or hammering and sports activities involving tight gripping and repetitive impact cause microtearing or microavulsion of the origin of the flexor carpi radialis tendon. Secondary inflammation develops at the epicondyle after this mechanical injury. Symptoms persist because of the constant tension and traction that occur during everyday use of the wrist and hand. The radiohumeral joint's range of motion and function are unaffected in this periarticular condition.

SYMPTOMS.   The patient has elbow pain and weakness of the forearm. The patient points to the medial epicondyle or rubs the inner aspect of the lower humerus when describing the condition.

"I have constant pain in my neck, shoulder, and arms because of my fibromyalgia. However, I have this very severe pain along the inside of my elbow."
"After a couple of hours of using my computer, my elbow starts to ache really badly."
"Everytime I brush my elbow against my side, I get this sharp pain."
"I'm losing the strength of my grip . . . my elbow hurts so bad."
"I can't believe there's no swelling. My elbow (pointing to the inner aspect of the joint) hurts so badly I would think there would be something showing."

EXAM.   Each patient is examined for local irritation at the medial epicondyle, for the strength and integrity of the common flexor tendon mechanism, and for weakness of grip.

EXAM SUMMARY

> 1. Local epicondylar tenderness
> 2. Pain aggravated by resisting wrist flexion and radial deviation, isometrically performed
> 3. Decreased grip strength
> 4. Full range of motion of the elbow joint

(1) Local tenderness is the most common sign and is located over a dime-sized area just distal to the medial epicondyle. This is in contrast to the local tenderness of lateral epicondylitis, which occurs directly over the bone. (2) This medial elbow pain is aggravated by resisting wrist flexion and radial deviation performed isometrically (the flexor carpi radialis is the tendon most commonly involved, and its function is to flex and radially deviate the wrist). (3) Pain is aggravated by strong gripping. In severe cases, weakness of grip occurs from disuse but also from the mechanical disruption of the tendon. Objective measurement of grip strength and endurance with a dynamometer can be used to document severe involvement. (4) The range of motion of the elbow is preserved. Loss of flexion or extension is almost always indicative of a primary elbow joint process.

X-RAYS. X-rays of the elbow are not necessary. Routine films of the elbow are normal in most cases.

SPECIAL TESTING. None.

DIAGNOSIS. The diagnosis is based on a history of medial epicondylar pain and on an examination demonstrating local tenderness and pain aggravated by isometric wrist flexion, radial deviation, or both. Regional anesthetic block at the epicondyle confirms the diagnosis and differentiates it from the pain of cubital tunnel syndrome, cervical radiculopathy, or the referred pain of rotator cuff tendinitis.

TREATMENT. The goals of treatment are to allow the microtorn common flexor tendon to reapproximate or reattach to the medial epicondylar process, to reduce the inflammation at the epicondyle, and to restore forearm muscle strength by performing isometric toning exercises of gripping and wrist flexion. Ice to reduce inflammation at the medial epicondyle combined with immobilization of the wrist to prevent traction and tension at the elbow is the treatment of choice.

Step 1: Evaluate flexion and extension of the elbow, estimate the strength of gripping, and obtain baseline measurements of patient's strength of wrist extension.

Limit lifting, hammering, and repetitious wrist and hand work.

Apply ice over the epicondyle.

Prescribe a Velcro wrist splint (p. 288).

Empirically prescribe an NSAID (e.g., ibuprofen [Advil, Motrin]) for 3 to 4 weeks; note that oral medication may not concentrate sufficiently in this relatively avascular tendon site.

Educate the patient: "You may feel the pain at the elbow, but it is the wrist and hand motions that aggravate the tendon."

Step 2 (3 to 4 weeks for persistent cases): Prescribe a short-arm cast (p. 288) to replace the splint.

Prescribe a long-arm cast if supination and pronation of the forearm prominently affect the pain at the elbow.

Discontinue the NSAID if the pain at the elbow has not responded at 3 to 4 weeks.

Continue with applications of ice.

Step 3 (6 to 8 weeks for persistent cases): Perform a local injection of D80 if 3 weeks of fixed immobilization with casting has failed.

Repeat the injection in 4 to 6 weeks if symptoms have not been reduced by at least 50%.

Step 4 (6 to 10 weeks for chronic cases): Begin toning exercises (p. 262) after the pain has subsided.

Use a tennis elbow band (p. 287) to prevent a recurrence.

Advise the patient to gradually resume activities.

Demonstrate palms-down lifting and explain how this protects the elbow against traction from the wrist.

Consider an orthopedic referral for persistent symptoms, especially for laborers and carpenters.

PHYSICAL THERAPY.   Physical therapy plays a minor role in the active treatment of the tendinitis of the common flexor origin but a vital role in its rehabilitation and prevention.

PHYSICAL THERAPY SUMMARY   ● ● ● ● ● ● ● ● ● ● ● ● ● ● ● ●

1.   Ice
2.   Phonophoresis with a hydrocortisone gel
3.   Isometrically performed toning of gripping
4.   Isometrically performed toning of wrist flexion

Acute Period.   *Ice* and *phonophoresis* using a hydrocortisone gel provide temporary relief of pain and swelling. Ice is routinely recommended and is particularly helpful for inflammatory flare reactions after local corticosteroid injection. Phonophoresis is an alternative treatment used when inflammatory changes are prominent and have failed to respond to ice. Both must be combined with immobilization to be effective.
Recovery/Rehabilitation.   Isometric exercises are used to restore the strength and tone of the flexor muscles. Between 3 and 4 weeks after the symptoms and signs have resolved, *isometric toning exercises* are begun (p. 261). Initially, *gripping exercises* using grip putty, a small compressible rubber ball, or an old tennis ball are performed daily in sets of 20, with each grip being held for 5 seconds. The strength and endurance of the forearm flexor muscles are gradually built up. These exercises are followed by *isometric toning exercises of wrist flexion* which are essential to restore full strength to the forearm and to prevent recurrences. Each episode of epicondylitis appears to weaken the common flexor mechanism. In order to overcome the loss of tensile strength, toning exercises must continue to be performed three times a week and combined with an ongoing limitation on lifting, torquing, and heavy gripping. For recurrent disease, these exercises should be continued for up to 6 to 12 months.

INJECTION.   Local injection with corticosteroid is indicated when initial management with immobilization fails to reduce symptoms sufficiently to allow participation in the physical therapy recovery exercises.

Positioning: The patient is to be in a supine position, the elbow is flexed to 90 degrees, and the arm is rotated externally as far as is comfortable.

Surface Anatomy and Point of Entry: The medial epicondyle is easily palpated with the elbow flexed to 90 degrees. The point of entry is ½" distal to the center of the epicondyle.

Angle of Entry and Depth: The angle of entry is perpendicular to the skin. The depth is ¼ to ⅝" down to the flexor tendon. If the patient is thin, pinch up the skin and enter from an angle. Use 1 ml of anesthesia to create a space for the corticosteroid.

Anesthesia: Ethyl chloride is sprayed on the skin. Local anesthetic is placed in the subcutaneous tissue only (½ ml or up to 1 ml to create a greater space for the steroid).

Technique: Successful treatment combines the protection of immobilization with the accurate placement of injection, followed by isometrically performed recovery exercises. The depth of injection can be determined by gradually advancing the needle until the patient feels mild discomfort (the subcutaneous tissue is usually pain-free) or until the rubbery resistance of the tendon is felt. Note: A painful reaction to injection or firm resistance when injecting suggests the needle is too deep and is within the body of the tendon (withdraw ⅛"!). In addition, the proper depth can be confirmed by applying traction to the overlying skin. The needle should move freely with skin traction if the tip is above the tendon but will stick in place if the tip is within the body of the tendon. The corticosteroid should always be injected just atop the tendon!

INJECTION AFTERCARE

1) *Rest* for 3 days, avoiding lifting, typing, turning of the forearms, tooling, and hammering.
2) *Ice* (15 minutes every 4 to 6 hours) and *Tylenol ES* (1000 mg twice a day) for soreness.
3) *Protect* the elbow for 3 to 4 weeks by the continuous wearing of the Velcro brace or a short-arm cast emphasizing the restriction of turning of the forearm.
4) Begin *gripping exercises* at half tension after the brace or cast is discontinued.
5) With restoration of normal grip strength, *isometric toning exercises of wrist flexion* are begun at low tension and slowly increased.
6) Repeat *injection* at 6 weeks if recovery exercises are poorly tolerated or improvement is less than 50%.
7) Delay *regular activities, work, and sports* until the pain and inflammation have resolved and grip and wrist extension strength have increased substantially.
8) Obtain *plain x-rays* and an orthopedic *consultation* for chronic symptoms.

SURGICAL PROCEDURE.   Tendon excision or débridement and tendon lengthening or tenotomy are performed uncommonly (approximately 3 to 5% of cases). Surgery can be considered when two courses of immobilization combined with local ice applications and at least one local corticosteroid injection have failed to resolve the symptoms.

PROGNOSIS.   Up to 95% of patients should respond to immobilization combined with corticosteroid injection. The remaining 5% may respond to long-term physical therapy toning exercises with severe restrictions of forearm use. Patients failing to improve (those with chronic tendinitis or mucinoid degeneration of the tendon, or both) can be considered for surgical exploration and primary tendon repair.

Olecranon Bursitis

Enter at the base of the bursa, paralleling the ulna; rotate the bevel so that it faces the bone; aspirate completely with the syringe or with manual pressure; send for studies.

Needle: 1½", 18 gauge

Depth: ¼ to ⅜"

Volume: ½ ml of anesthetic (only in the subcutaneous tissues) plus ½ ml of K40 for nonseptic effusions

Note: Apply a compression dressing for 24 hours.

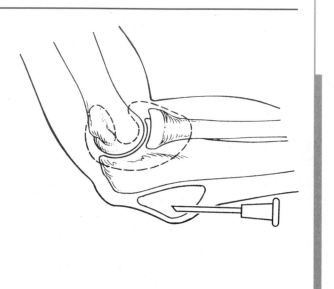

Figure 3–3.   Olecranon bursa aspiration and injection

DESCRIPTION.   Olecranon bursitis is an inflammation of the bursal sac located between the olecranon process of the ulna and the overlying skin. It is a low-pressure bursa that is susceptible to external pressure. Most cases are caused by repetitive trauma in the form of pressure, referred to as draftsman's elbow. It is one of two bursal sacs that are uniquely susceptible to infection (5% are caused by *Staphylococcus aureus* infection) and gout (5%).

SYMPTOMS.   The patient has pain and swelling just behind the elbow. The patient will rub over the olecranon process or elevate the flexed elbow to demonstrate the swelling when describing the symptoms.

"Within 5 hours, I had this golf ball show up at the end of my elbow."
"I am a mapmaker. I slowly developed this swelling over my elbow."
"When I rub the skin over my elbow, I feel a bunch of little marbles."
"I've got this sack of fluid hanging off my elbow."
"All of a sudden I developed this red, hot, swollen area over my elbow."

EXAM.   Bursal sac swelling, inflammation, and thickening are examined in each patient.

EXAM SUMMARY   • • • • • • • • • • • • • • • •

1.   Swelling, redness, and heat over the olecranon process
2.   Full range of motion of the elbow joint
3.   A characteristic aspirate

(1) Cystic swelling, redness, heat, or all three are present over the proximal 1 to 2" of the olecranon process. (2) The range of motion of the elbow joint should be unaffected. (3) The diagnosis is confirmed by aspiration of fluid from the bursal sac. Note that if redness extends beyond the immediate area of the bursa and is accompanied by induration, septic bursitis with accompanying cellulitis should be suspected.

X-RAYS. X-rays of the elbow are not necessary. Routine films of the elbow demonstrate soft-tissue swelling over the olecranon. An olecranon spur may be present in approximately 20% of cases. Treatment is rarely influenced by radiographic studies.

SPECIAL TESTING. Bursal fluid analysis.

DIAGNOSIS. The diagnosis is based on the laboratory evaluation of the bursal aspirate. The cell count, Gram stain, and crystal analysis will help to differentiate acute traumatic bursitis from the inflammatory reaction of gout and infection. All bursae should be aspirated. It is not possible to distinguish clinically inflamed traumatic bursitis from septic bursitis without bursal fluid analysis!

TREATMENT. The goals of treatment are to determine the cause of the swelling, to reduce swelling and inflammation, to encourage the walls of the bursa to reapproximate, and to prevent chronic bursitis. The treatment of choice is aspiration, drainage, and lab analysis.

Step 1: Aspirate the bursa for diagnostic studies: Gram stain and culture, uric acid crystals, and hematocrit.

Apply a simple compression dressing for 24 to 36 hours (gauze and Elastoplast).

Avoid direct pressure.

Prescribe a neoprene pull-on elbow sleeve (p. 287).

Step 2 (1 to 2 days after lab analysis): Prescribe an antibiotic for the infection (*S. aureus*), evaluate and treat for gout, or perform an intrabursal injection of K40 for traumatic bursitis.

Continue with the neoprene pull-on sleeve.

Step 3 (4 to 6 weeks for persistent cases): Repeat the aspiration and local injection with K40 if there is persistent swelling and pain.

Educate the patient: "In 10 to 20% of cases there is persistence of swollen or thickened sacs."

Step 4 (3 months for chronic cases): Consider consultation with an orthopedist if thickening has developed and it is interfering with the patient's activities of daily living.

PHYSICAL THERAPY. Physical therapy does not play a significant role in the treatment or rehabilitation of olecranon bursitis.

INJECTION. Local injection with corticosteroid is indicated when initial management with simple aspiration and compression dressing fails to control swelling or thickening, or both.

Positioning: The patient is to be placed in the supine position, the elbow is flexed to 90 degrees, and the arm is placed over the chest.

Surface Anatomy and Point of Entry: The bursal swelling is located directly over the olecranon process. The point of entry is at the base of the bursa along the ulna.

Angle of Entry and Depth: The angle of entry is parallel to the ulna. The depth is ¼ to ⅜" from the surface.

Anesthesia: Ethyl chloride is sprayed on the skin. Local anesthetic is placed in the subcutaneous tissue only (½ ml), adjacent to the bursal wall.

Technique: The successful treatment combines complete aspiration of the fluid with compression of the bursal sac. After the subcutaneous tissue has been anesthetized, an 18-gauge needle is passed, bevel outward, into the center of the bursal sac. The bevel is then rotated 180 degrees toward the ulna. Aspiration of the contents of the bursal sac is accomplished with the syringe and is assisted by manual compression from either side. For aseptic bursitis—sepsis excluded by clinical criteria, a negative Gram stain, or clear, noncellular-appearing serous fluid—the needle is left in place and the bursa is injected with ½ ml of K40.

INJECTION AFTERCARE

1) *Rest* for 3 days with the bulky compression dressing worn for the first 24 to 36 hours and avoidance of all direct pressure and extremes of range of motion of the elbow.

2) *Ice* (15 minutes every 4 to 6 hours) and *Tylenol ES* (1000 mg twice a day) for soreness.

3) *Protect* the elbow for 3 to 4 weeks with a pull-on neoprene elbow sleeve, worn continuously.

4) Prescribe daily passive flexion or extension *stretching exercises* over the next several weeks if range of motion has been affected (the range of motion of the elbow is rarely affected except in the case of septic bursitis accompanied by cellulitis).

5) Septic bursitis may need to be *reaspirated* at 7 to 10 days.

6) Repeat the *injection* at 6 weeks if swelling persists or chronic thickening develops (*"It feels like I have gravel under my skin"*).

7) Avoid direct pressure for the next 6 to 12 months.

8) Obtain a *consultation* with a surgical orthopedist if the bursal sac does not diminish naturally over the course of 6 months.

SURGICAL PROCEDURE.   Bursectomy can be considered for persistent swelling or chronic bursal thickening that fails to improve with the combined treatment (aspiration, drainage, and injection of K40 on two successive attempts).

PROGNOSIS.   Between 80 and 85% of cases resolve with aspiration alone or with aspiration combined with corticosteroid injection. Approximately 15% develop some degree of chronic bursal thickening. Less than 5% of cases will require surgical removal.

DESCRIPTION.   Aspiration of the radiohumeral joint and fluid analysis will distinguish between inflammatory, noninflammatory, and septic elbow effusions (see the synovial fluid table, p. 311). Rheumatoid arthritis, osteoarthritis due to trauma, and spondyloarthropathy are the conditions most likely to cause elbow effusions.

SYMPTOMS.   The patient complains of an inability to move the elbow through a full range of motion or of a pressure-like pain in the antecubital fossa or both. When describing the condition, the patient actively flexes and extends the arm, demonstrates the lack of full extension or flexion of the joint, or tries to reproduce the recurrent popping sound.

"I can't straighten my arm."
"I feel a pressure buildup in my elbow."
"My elbow doesn't move smoothly anymore. It's like a rachet that catches as I try to straighten it."
"I can't throw any more. My elbow hurts too much and it's getting weaker."

Radiohumeral Joint Arthrocentesis

Enter laterally in the center of the triangle formed by the lateral epicondyle, the radial head, and the olecranon process, paralleling the radial head (the center of lateral bulge); the elbow should be flexed at 90 degrees.

Needle: 1″, 21–22 gauge

Depth: ⅝ to ¾″ down to and through the radial collateral ligament

Volume: 1 to 2 ml of anesthetic plus ½ ml of K40

Note: Redirect the needle if bone is encountered at ⅜″.

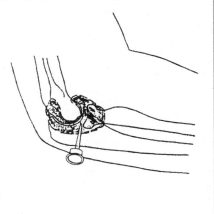

Figure 3—4.   Aspiration and injection of the elbow

EXAM. An examination of the range of motion, the smoothness of motion, and endpoint stiffness is performed in flexion, extension, supination, and pronation. Joint line tenderness and signs of effusion should be assessed in the center of the triangle formed by the lateral epicondyle, the radial head, and the olecranon process.

EXAM SUMMARY

1. Loss of full flexion, extension, supination, or pronation
2. Lack of smooth motion or catching (loose body or osteochondritis dissecans)
3. Lateral joint line tenderness and swelling (the bulge sign)
4. Endpoint stiffness or pain with forced passive flexion or extension

(1) The hallmark finding of radiohumeral joint disease is a loss of full range of motion. The earliest sign of an elbow effusion is a loss of full extension. As the condition advances, full flexion may become limited. If the radial head is involved with osteochondritis dissecans or osteoarthritis from previous injury, supination and pronation will be affected as well. In either case there will be endpoint stiffness at the extremes of range of motion. (2) Lack of smooth motion or locking with passive flexion and extension is suggestive of an intra-articular loose body. Osteochondritis dissecans is the most common cause of this unique sign. (3) The characteristic swelling of the elbow joint is best observed laterally. With the elbow flexed to 90 degrees, a bulge sign should be observable or palpable in the triangle formed by the radial head, the lateral epicondyle, and the olecranon process.

X-RAYS. X-rays of the elbow (including lateral and PA views) are always indicated when the elbow joint is involved. Osteoarthritic narrowing between the radius and the humerus or the olecranon and the humerus may be seen. Evidence of an old fracture may be present. However, plain films may not show evidence of osteochondritis dissecans with accompanying loose body.

SPECIAL TESTING.   If elbow signs persist and true locking of the joint has been demonstrated, an MRI is advisable to evaluate for osteochondritis dissecans or intra-articular loose body.

DIAGNOSIS.   The diagnosis of radiohumeral joint disease is strongly suggested by the loss of full range of motion of the joint. The diagnosis is confirmed by aspiration of joint fluid or improvement in pain and range of motion after intra-articular injection of lidocaine or both.

TREATMENT.   Although passive range-of-motion exercises are fundamental in restoring the normal range of motion of the joint, aspiration and synovial fluid analysis is the treatment of choice. Fluid analysis will differentiate the three most common causes of joint effusion, namely, traumatic hemarthrosis, rheumatoid arthritis, and posttraumatic osteoarthritis. Septic arthritis is rare.

Step 1: Aspirate the joint for diagnostic studies: Gram stain and culture, uric acid crystal analysis, and cell count and differential.

Recommend avoidance of repetitious bending and extension.

Prescribe a neoprene pull-on elbow brace (p. 287) to protect and support the joint.

Step 2 (1 to 3 days after lab analysis): After excluding infection, perform an intra-articular injection of K40 for the rheumatoid or osteoarthritic effusion.

Continue the neoprene pull-on.

Begin range-of-motion exercises to restore full flexion and extension.

Step 3 (3 to 4 weeks for persistent cases): Repeat the joint aspiration and local injection with K40 if there is persistent swelling and pain.

Continue range-of-motion exercises to restore full flexion and extension.

Step 4 (3 months for chronic cases): If locking or effusion persists, consider an orthopedic consultation for joint débridement.

PHYSICAL THERAPY.   *Ice* placed over the outer elbow will provide temporary control of pain and swelling. *Passive range-of-motion exercises* are vital in restoring full range of motion to the joint. These are best performed after the acute symptoms of pain and swelling have subsided. After restoring the normal range of motion of the joint, *isometric toning exercises* are performed to restore the strength of the biceps, brachioradialis, and triceps muscles.

PHYSICAL THERAPY SUMMARY   • • • • • • • • • • • • • •

1. Ice placed over the outer elbow
2. Range-of-motion exercises in flexion and extension, passively performed
3. Isometrically performed toning of flexion and extension after the range of motion has been restored

INJECTION.   Aspiration and drainage should be considered for tense, painful hemarthrosis. Corticosteroid injection is indicated for any inflammatory condition (rheumatoid arthritis or the acute osteoarthritic flare) accompanied by a loss of 15 to 20 degrees of extension and flexion.

Positioning: The patient is to be in the supine position, the elbow is flexed to 90 degrees, and the arm is placed over the chest.

Surface Anatomy and Point of Entry: Joint swelling is most readily seen between the lateral epicondyle, the olecranon process, and the radial head when the elbow is flexed to 90 degrees (the bulge sign of an elbow effusion). The point of entry is at the center of the triangle formed by these three bony prominences.

Angle of Entry and Depth: The angle of entry is perpendicular to the skin, paralleling the radial head. The synovial cavity depth is ¾".

Anesthesia: Ethyl chloride is sprayed on the skin. Local anesthetic is placed in the subcutaneous tissue (¼ ml), in the hard resistance of any bony prominence encountered at a superficial depth (¼ ml), and at the firm resistance of the deep ligaments (¼ ml).

Technique: Successful aspiration and drainage requires accurate localization of the point of entry and careful redirection of the needle if bone is encountered at a superficial depth. A *lateral approach* provides the best access. A 21- or 22-gauge needle is gently advanced down to the firm resistance of the radial collateral ligament, paralleling the radial head. Note that if bone is encountered at a superficial level (⅜"), local anesthesia is injected, and the needle is withdrawn ¼" and redirected. After placing anesthesia just outside the radial collateral ligament, the needle is advanced ¼" through the firm resistance of the ligament and joint capsule. Aspiration is attempted at this depth. If fluid is not obtained, turn the bevel of the needle 180 degrees and repeat the aspiration. For the aseptic effusion, the needle is left in place and the joint is injected with ½ ml of K40.

INJECTION AFTERCARE

1) *Rest* for 3 days, avoiding repetitious motion and tension at the elbow.

2) *Ice* (15 minutes every 4 to 6 hours) and *Tylenol ES* (1000 mg twice a day) for soreness.

3) *Protect* the elbow for 3 to 4 weeks with a pull-on neoprene elbow sleeve, worn continuously.

4) Begin daily passive flexion or extension *stretching exercises* as soon as the pain and swelling have abated.

5) Septic arthritis may need to be *reaspirated* at 7 to 10 days.

6) Repeat *injection* at 6 weeks if swelling persists or chronic synovial thickening develops.

7) Obtain an *MRI* and *consultation* with a surgical orthopedist if full, smooth range of motion is not restored (osteochondritis dissecans or loose body).

SURGICAL PROCEDURE.   Arthroscopy is indicated to remove loose bodies, to evaluate and treat osteochondritis dissecans, or to débride the osteoarthritic joint.

PROGNOSIS.   Local injection is very effective in providing temporary improvement in the symptoms and signs of radiohumeral joint effusions. Persistent low-grade inflammatory effusions may be an indication of osteochondritis dissecans or loose body, or both.

chapter 4

Wrist

De Quervain Tenosynovitis

Enter ⅜" proximal to the tip of the radial styloid, angling at 45 degrees to the bone (approach the bone very carefully because of its sensitivity).

Needle: ⅝", 25 gauge

Depth: ⅜ to ½", flush against the periosteum of the radial styloid

Volume: 2 to 3 ml of anesthetic (for dilation) plus ½ ml of D80

Note: The tenosynovial sac should form a palpable "bubble" 1½" long.

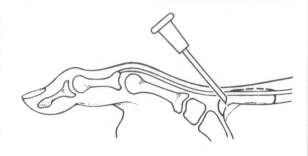

Figure 4–1.   Injection and dilation of de Quervain's tenosynovitis

DESCRIPTION.   De Quervain tenosynovitis is an inflammation of the extensor and flexor tendons of the thumb. Repetitive or unaccustomed use of the thumb (gripping and grasping) leads to friction and irritation of the snuffbox tendons as they course over the distal radial styloid. If left untreated, this friction-induced tenosynovitis can progress to fibrosis and to loss of flexibility of the thumb in flexion. The latter condition is referred to as stenosing tenosynovitis.

SYMPTOMS.   The patient has wrist pain and difficulties with gripping. The patient often rubs over the distal styloid when describing the condition.

"I can't grip anymore."
"Every time I try to pick up my baby, I get this sharp pain in my wrist."
"I have had this sharp pain over my wrist (pointing to the end of the radius) ever since I had a needle stuck into my vein."
"It's very sore right here (pointing to the end of the radius), and it has begun to swell."
"My bone is getting bigger (pointing to the radial styloid)."

EXAM.   Each patient is examined for tenderness and swelling at the radial styloid process, for the degree of inflammation of the extensor pollicis longus, extensor pollicis brevis, and abductor pollicis longus tendons, and for the range of motion of the thumb.

EXAM SUMMARY   • • • • • • • • • • • • • •

1. Local tenderness at the tip of the radial styloid
2. Pain aggravated by resisting thumb extension or abduction, isometrically performed
3. A positive Finklestein test (pain aggravated by passive stretching the thumb in flexion)
4. A distensible tenosynovial sac

(1) Local tenderness is present over the distal portion of the radial styloid, adjacent to the abductor pollicis longus tendon. (2) Pain is aggravated by resisting thumb extension and abduction isometrically (thumb abduction is moving the thumb perpendicular to the palm). (3) Pain is aggravated by passively stretching the thumb tendons over the radial styloid in thumb flexion (the Finklestein maneuver). This maneuver is so painful that the patient often responds by lifting the shoulder to prevent the examiner from stretching the tendons! (4) Tendon fibrosis is assessed by evaluating flexion and circumduction of the thumb and by assessing the distensibility of the tissues over the radial styloid. Normally, the soft tissues over the radial styloid should distend readily with 2 to 3 ml of local anesthetic, forming a bubble 1½" long.

X-RAYS. X-rays of the wrist and thumb are not necessary. Plain films of the wrist and thumb are normal; calcification of these tendons does not occur.

SPECIAL TESTING. None.

DIAGNOSIS. The diagnosis is suggested by a history of radial-side wrist pain and an exam showing local radial styloid tenderness and pain aggravated by resisting thumb extension. The diagnosis is confirmed by regional anesthetic block placed directly over the radial styloid. Effective relief of signs and symptoms excludes carpometacarpal arthritis and radiocarpal arthritis. A distensible tenosynovial sac essentially excludes stenosing tenosynovitis.

TREATMENT. The goals of treatment are to reduce the inflammation in the tenosynovial sac, to prevent adhesions from forming, and to prevent recurrent tendinitis (by tendon stretching exercises and by altering lifting and grasping). Corticosteroid injection placed at the radial styloid is the treatment of choice.

Step 1: Confirm the diagnosis and assess for stenosing tenosynovitis.

> Suggest rest and restriction of thumb gripping and grasping.

> Apply ice at the radial styloid.

> Prescribe buddy-taping of the thumb to the base of the first finger (p. 293), a dorsal hood splint (p. 289), or a Velcro thumb spica splint (p. 291).

Step 2 (3 to 4 weeks for more severe or persistent cases): Perform a local injection of D80.

> Repeat the injection at 4 to 6 weeks if the symptoms are not reduced by 50%.

> Severe cases that require a second injection can be treated concurrently with either a dorsal hood splint or a short-arm cast with a thumb spica (p. 288).

Step 3 (6 to 8 weeks for chronic cases): Apply gentle stretching exercises of the thumb in flexion if the symptoms have improved (p. 263).

> Consider a surgical consultation for persistent symptoms.

PHYSICAL THERAPY. Physical therapy does not play a prominent role in the treatment of de Quervain tenosynovitis.

PHYSICAL THERAPY SUMMARY ● ● ● ● ● ● ● ● ● ● ● ● ● ● ●

1. Ice
2. Phonophoresis with a hydrocortisone gel
3. Gentle stretching exercises in flexion, passively performed (prevention)

Acute Period.   Ice and phonophoresis are used in the treatment of active tenosynovitis. *Ice* applied to the radial styloid can effectively reduce local pain and swelling. *Phonophoresis* with a hydrocortisone gel may be helpful in minor cases but cannot take the place of a local corticosteroid injection in persistent or chronic cases.

Recovery/Rehabilitation.   Stretching exercises are used to prevent recurrent tenosynovitis. After the signs and symptoms of active tenosynovitis have resolved (3 to 4 weeks), gentle *passive stretching exercises* of the extensor and abductor tendons into the palm are performed. Sets of 20 stretches, each held 5 seconds, are performed daily (p. 262).

INJECTION.   Corticosteroid injection is the treatment of choice for patients experiencing symptoms longer than 6 weeks.

Positioning: The wrist is to be kept in neutral position and turned on its side, radial side up.

Surface Anatomy and Point of Entry: The radial styloid is identified and marked. The point of entry is halfway between the abductor pollicis longus and the extensor pollicis longus tendons at the radial styloid.

Angle of Entry and Depth: The needle is carefully advanced at a 45-degree angle down to the hard resistance of the radial styloid periosteum (pain). If the bone is not encountered at ⅜ to ½" (the typical depth), the point of entry may have been too distal.

Anesthesia: Ethyl chloride is sprayed on the skin. Local anesthetic is placed at the radius.

Technique: Successful treatment involves a single passage of the needle down to the periosteum of the radius, slow dilation of the tissues with anesthesia, and injection with D80, all in one step. After freezing the skin with ethyl chloride spray, a 25-gauge needle is gently advanced down to the radial styloid and 2 to 2½ ml of anesthesia is injected to dilate the soft tissues around the tendons (a bubble should appear). Moderate pressure to injection, a poorly distensible sac, or both may indicate a chronic stenosis of the tendons, that is, adhesions. With the needle left in place (avoid multiple punctures!), the syringe containing the anesthetic is removed and replaced with the syringe containing ½ ml of D80. The treatment is completed by injecting the corticosteroid.

INJECTION AFTERCARE

1) *Rest* for 3 days, by avoiding all gripping and grasping.
2) *Ice* (15 minutes every 4 to 6 hours) and *Tylenol ES* (1000 mg twice a day) for soreness.
3) *Protect* the wrist for 3 to 4 weeks with a dorsal hood splint, a thumb spica splint, or a Velcro wrist immobilizer worn during the day (optional).
4) Begin passive *stretching exercises* of the thumb in flexion at 3 weeks.
5) Repeat *injection* at 6 weeks if symptoms have not improved by 50% (warning: skin and subcutaneous fat atrophy may be greater or permanent with a second injection in 30% of patients).
6) Reemphasize the need to avoid grasping and lifting with the wrist ulnar deviated.
7) Obtain a *consultation* with a surgical orthopedist if two injections in 1 year fail to resolve the condition.

SURGICAL PROCEDURE.   Surgical release of the first dorsal compartment is recommended if two injections within a year fail to resolve the condition.

TABLE 4-1. CLINICAL OUTCOMES OF 55 CASES OF DE QUERVAIN TENOSYNOVITIS TREATED WITH DEPO-MEDROL 80*

Complete resolution (single injection)	30 (58%)
Recurrence (reinjected; average 11.9 months to recurrence)	17 (32%)
Failed to respond; chronic tendinitis	5 (10%)
Total	52

*Prospective follow-up of 95% of patients enrolled: 4.2 years.
These data were published in *Arthritis Rheum* 1991;34:793–798.

PROGNOSIS. Patients who receive treatment within 6 months of developing de Quervain tenosynovitis have an excellent prognosis. Local injection combined with dilation of the soft tissues over the radial styloid should be effective in 95% of cases. Patients who have had symptoms for longer than 6 months are at risk for fibrosis (stenosing tenosynovitis). Local injection and dilation can be used in these patients but the results of treatment are not as predictably successful (Table 4–1).

Carpometacarpal Osteoarthritis

Enter ⅜" proximal to the base of the metacarpal bone, in the "anatomic snuffbox" adjacent to the abductor pollicis longus tendon

Needle: ⅝", 25 gauge

Depth: ½ to ⅝", flush against the trapezium bone

Volume: ½ ml of anesthetic injected at ⅜" depth plus ½ ml of K40 injected flush against the trapezium

Note: Moderate pressure may be needed.

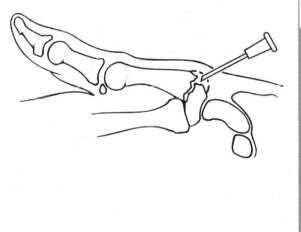

Figure 4–2.   Carpometacarpal joint injection

DESCRIPTION. Carpometacarpal (CMC) joint arthritis is a very common form of osteoarthritis. Repetitive gripping and grasping and excessive exposure to vibration in susceptible patients (those with a positive family history) lead to wear and tear of the articular cartilage at the base of the thumb. Over many years, bony enlargement, loss of range of motion, and progressive subluxation occur. Although this is a common form of osteoarthritis, it does not herald the onset of systemic forms of osteoarthritis.

SYMPTOMS. The patient has pain, swelling, or enlargement at the base of the thumb. The patient frequently rubs over the radial side of the wrist and the base of the thumb when describing the condition. Note that not every patient with bony enlargement becomes symptomatic.

"I've had to stop crocheting and knitting because of the constant pain in my thumbs."
"My thumbs are starting to look like the arthritis my grandmother had."
"Every time I lift my coffee cup, I get this terribly sharp pain in the base of my thumb."
"It looks like the bones in my thumb are getting bigger."
"The only way I can do my housework is if I put pressure over the thumb and hold it in place."

When asking an 85-year-old Russian woman, a former potato harvester from Odessa, whether she needed treatment for her severely subluxed and arthritic CMC joint she replied, "No doctor, it's past the pain part."

EXAM.   Each patient is examined for swelling and inflammation at the base of the thumb, the degree of subluxation of the metacarpal bone, and loss of range of motion of the joint.

EXAM SUMMARY   • • • • • • • • • • • • • • • •

1. Compression tenderness across the joint
2. Crepitation of the joint in circumduction
3. Pain aggravated at the extremes of thumb motion
4. Bony deformity, subluxation, or both (the shelf sign)
5. Atrophy of the thenar muscles

(1) Tenderness and swelling are present over the base of the thumb. Sensitivity is best demonstrated by compressing the joint in the anteroposterior plane. Pressure applied from the snuffbox is usually much less painful. Swelling is best seen with the wrist turned radial side up. An accurate assessment of the enlargement of the base of the thumb is best appreciated in this position. (2) Crepitation is palpable when the metacarpal is forcibly rotated against the trapezium (the mortar and pestle sign). (3) Pain is often aggravated when the joint is passively stretched to the extremes of extension and flexion. (4) As the condition progresses, greater degrees of bony deformity and metacarpal subluxation contribute to the enlargement of the base. Progressive subluxation creates an abnormality referred to as the shelf sign. The smooth contours of the distal radius and thumb are replaced by a bony protuberance of the metacarpal. (5) End-stage disease often shows atrophy of the thenar muscles.

X-RAYS.   X-rays of the wrist (including PA and lateral views) are often sufficient to determine the degree of osteoarthritic wear and tear in the thumb. Nearly all symptomatic cases will have abnormal x-rays. Variable degrees of bony sclerosis, asymmetric joint narrowing, spur formation, and radial-side subluxation can be seen at the trapezial-metacarpal articulation. Note that the early changes on plain x-rays are not always appreciated or commented on by the radiologist (these x-rays should be viewed by the examining provider).

SPECIAL TESTING.   None.

DIAGNOSIS.   The diagnosis is based on the clinical findings of local joint tenderness, joint crepitation, and painful motion of the joint coupled with the characteristic abnormalities on plain films at the trapezial-metacarpal articulation. X-rays are often used to gauge the severity of the condition and to predict the need for surgery. A regional anesthetic block is occasionally necessary to differentiate de Quervain tenosynovitis and radiocarpal arthritis from symptomatic carpometacarpal arthritis.

TREATMENT.   The goals of treatment are to relieve swelling and inflammation, to reduce subluxation (allowing the joint to articulate more freely), and to assess the need for surgery. Overlap-taping along with restrictions on heavy gripping and exposure to vibration are the treatments of choice for early disease. Local corticosteroid injection placed in the depths of the anatomic snuffbox is the treatment of choice for the more advanced or persistent cases.

Step 1: Assess the joint for soft-tissue swelling, bony enlargement, and subluxation; obtain plain x-rays of the wrist (including PA and lateral views).

Suggest rest and restriction of gripping and grasping.

Recommend oversized tools, grips, and other occupational adjustments.

Demonstrate overlap-taping of the joint (p. 291) or prescribe a dorsal hood splint (p. 289) or a Velcro thumb spica splint (p. 291).

Prescribe a 3- to 4-week course of an NSAID (e.g., ibuprofen [Advil, Motrin]).

Step 2 (3 to 4 weeks for persistent cases): Perform a local injection of K40.

Repeat the injection at 4 to 6 weeks if symptoms have not decreased by 50%.

Step 3 (6 to 8 weeks for resistant cases): Combine fixed immobilization using a thumb spica cast (p. 288) with a local corticosteroid injection.

Step 4 (2 to 3 months for chronic cases): Perform isometric toning exercises of the thumb flexors and extensors (if the patient has improved sufficiently to tolerate them).

Consult with a hand surgeon for implant arthroplasty or tendon graft interposition.

PHYSICAL THERAPY. Physical therapy does not play a significant role in the treatment of CMC osteoarthritis. Instead, the focus of therapy is on restricted use, immobilization/taping, and anti-inflammatory treatments. If significant loss of muscle tone has occurred, isometric toning of flexion, extension, abduction, and adduction is recommended. Preferential toning of extension (almost always weaker than flexion) may reduce the tendency of the joint to sublux to the radial direction.

INJECTION. Local anesthetic injection is used to differentiate CMC arthritis from de Quervain tenosynovitis or radiocarpal joint conditions. Corticosteroid injection is the anti-inflammatory treatment of choice for symptoms persisting beyond 6 to 8 weeks.

Positioning: The wrist is to be kept in neutral position and turned on its side, radial side up.

Surface Anatomy and Point of Entry: The proximal end of the metacarpal bone is identified and marked. The point of entry is ⅜″ proximal to the metacarpal and adjacent to the abductor pollicis longus tendon.

Angle of Entry and Depth: The needle is carefully advanced at a 45-degree angle down to the hard resistance of the trapezium (typical depth is ½ to ⅝″).

Anesthesia: Ethyl chloride is sprayed on the skin. Local anesthetic is placed in the subcutaneous fat (½ ml) and ¼″ above the trapezium (½ ml).

Technique: The successful injection must be placed against the trapezium at the proper depth! After anesthesia, the needle is gently advanced at a 45-degree angle down to the trapezium bone (½ to ⅝″). If the hard resistance of bone is encountered at a superficial depth (⅜″), withdraw and redirect the needle. In this case, the point of entry may have been too distal—a common error. Note: Be sure to inject the anesthesia above the bone and the corticosteroid at the periosteum. Firm but not hard pressure may be required when injecting at the deeper site. If the radial artery is encountered (10% chance), withdraw, hold pressure for 5 minutes, and redirect the injection.

INJECTION AFTERCARE

1) *Rest* for 3 days, avoiding all grasping, pinching, and exposure to vibration.
2) *Ice* (15 minutes every 4 to 6 hours) and *Tylenol ES* (1000 mg twice a day) for soreness.

3) *Protect* the thumb for 3 to 4 weeks by limiting grasping, pinching, and exposure to vibration and by overlap-taping the joint or using a dorsal hood splint or a thumb spica splint.

4) Reemphasize light gripping of pens, padding of hand tools, antivibration types of gloves, and oversized grips for golf clubs, rackets, and so forth.

5) Begin passive *stretching exercises* of the thumb in flexion and extension at 3 weeks.

6) Repeat *injection* at 6 weeks if symptoms have not improved by 50%.

7) Obtain a *consultation* with a surgical orthopedist if two injections fail to provide at least 3 to 4 months of symptomatic relief.

SURGICAL PROCEDURE.   Surgery is often necessary in working or active patients who present with symptoms and are in the 45- to 55-year age range. Surgery is indicated when symptoms become refractory to treatment or when restrictions, immobilization, and two consecutive injections fail to provide months of symptom-free use. Tendon interpositional arthroplasty—interposition of the flexor carpi radialis tendon between the bones of the joints—is recommended for patients under the age of 62, and trapezial arthroplasty—replacement of the trapezium bone—is performed in patients over 62. Both procedures are well tolerated.

PROGNOSIS.   Local injection is highly successful in the temporary relief of symptoms in most patients. A single injection can provide control of symptoms and improvement in function, especially when swelling predominates over bony enlargement. Two or three treatments over the course of several years can serve as a bridge from the symptomatic phase of the condition to the "burnt-out" phase of the condition. Since symptoms usually fade over several years in the majority of patients, referral to surgery will be necessary infrequently (5 to 10% of cases) (Table 4–2).

DESCRIPTION.   The gamekeeper of a royal court was likely to injure the ulnar collateral ligament of the metacarpophalangeal (MP) joint when twisting the necks of the fowl hunted for the king. Today, ski pole injuries are the most common cause of this condition. Whether by injury or repetitive use, the disrupted ligament leads to instability of the MP joint, poor pinching and opposition function and, in later years, degenerative arthritic change.

SYMPTOMS.   In the acute phase, the patient complains of pain and swelling along the ulnar side of the MP joint. In the chronic phase, the patient complains of pain, weakness, or loss of stability. The patient often takes the thumb and first finger and rubs over the MP joint when describing the condition.

"I took a bad fall while skiing. My thumb got caught in my pole straps."
"It's hard for me to sew. My thumb (pointing to the MP joint) hurts when I try to thread the needle."
"My thumb hurts whenever I try to use a hammer."
"I think I dislocated my thumb when I fell down."

TABLE 4-2. CLINICAL OUTCOMES OF 50 CASES OF CMC OSTEOARTHRITIS TREATED WITH KENALOG-40

Epidemiology: average age, 50 years (range, 34 to 83); ratio of women to men, 7 to 1; right side and left side were equally affected
Injection results: 46 or 50 (92%) responded to single or multiple treatment, averaging 10 months of relief (range, 3 to 19 months)
Surgery: 4 patients failed to respond and underwent surgery

These data were generated between 1990 and 1996 at the Sunnyside Medical Orthopedic Clinic, Portland, OR.

Gamekeeper's Thumb

Enter ¼″ distal to the prominence of the distal metacarpal head on the ulnar side of the joint; use anesthesia to differentiate this soft tissue injury from involvement of the joint.

Needle: ⅝″, 25 gauge

Depth: between ⅛ and ¼″, just under the skin and above the ulnar collateral ligament

Volume: ¼ ml of anesthetic (corticosteroid is not used for this condition).

Note: In order to locate the proper depth of injection, advance the needle to the hard resistance of the bone and then withdraw ⅛″.

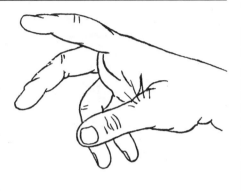

Figure 4–3.   Gamekeeper's thumb: ulnar collateral ligament injury of the metacarpal joint

EXAM.   The metacarpophalangeal joint of the thumb is examined for local tenderness, swelling, and instability.

EXAM SUMMARY   • • • • • • • • • • • • • • •

1.   Local tenderness and swelling along the ulnar side of the MP joint
2.   Pain or excessive motion with valgus stress testing of the ulnar collateral ligament
3.   Inability to fully flex the joint (when acute or swollen)
4.   Decreased pinching strength due to instability or acute pain

(1) MP joint tenderness is localized to the ulnar side of the joint. The entire joint may be swollen or the swelling may be restricted to the ulnar side. (2) The MP joint is unstable to stress testing. With the examiner's thumb at the MP joint and index finger at the interphalangeal joint, valgus stability and valgus-induced pain are assessed. A comparison should be made to the stability of the contralateral thumb. (3) The MP joint may not fully flex to 90 degrees. (4) The strength or holding power of thumb and first finger may be compromised.

X-RAYS.   Plain x-rays of the hand are usually normal. Late-onset degenerative changes may be present years after the initial injury. No special testing is used at this small joint.

DIAGNOSIS.   The diagnosis is based on the history of injury to the thumb coupled with the local signs of inflammation and instability. Occasionally, local anesthetic block placed along the ulnar side of the joint is necessary to differentiate symptoms arising from the CMC joint or referred from the carpal tunnel.

TREATMENT.   The treatment of choice is immobilization for the acute injury. Local corticosteroid injection is reserved for the case complicated by osteoarthritis.

Step 1: Obtain x-rays of the thumb (including PA and lateral views).

Apply ice over the MP joint.

Immobilize with overlap-taping (p. 291), a dorsal hood splint (p. 289), or a thumb spica splint (p. 291).

Educate the patient: "The thumb must be protected and completely rested over several weeks to allow the ligaments to reattach in their proper positions."

Step 2 (3 to 6 weeks for recovery): After immobilization, perform gentle, passive range-of-motion exercises of the thumb.

Begin isometric toning of thumb flexion (gripping).

Avoid heavy gripping or grasping until grip has been restored isometrically.

Avoid exposure to vibration.

Step 3 (6 to 10 weeks for chronic cases): Consider orthopedic consultation if the thumb remains unstable, and gripping and grasping are interfered with.

Step 4 (years): Consider intra-articular injection for secondary osteoarthritic changes.

PHYSICAL THERAPY.   *Ice* will provide temporary relief of pain and swelling in the acute stage of this injury. Following immobilization, gentle, passive *range-of-motion exercises* in flexion and extension are performed for several days to restore full mobility to the thumb. Subsequently, *isometric toning exercises* of thumb flexion (gripping) are begun and followed by more active exercises after range of motion and baseline grip strength are restored.

PHYSICAL THERAPY SUMMARY   ● ● ● ● ● ● ● ● ● ● ● ● ● ● ●

1.   Ice over the MP joint
2.   Passive range of motion exercises in flexion and extension
3.   Toning exercises of gripping, isometrically performed

INJECTION.   The indication for injection at the MP joint is limited. Local anesthetic block may be necessary to distinguish ligament injuries from involvement of the joint. Local corticosteroid injection is used to treat the secondary osteoarthritis.

SURGICAL PROCEDURE.   Reattachment of the torn distal ligament, tendon graft repair, or arthrodesis (fusion) are indicated when the stability of the joint has been severely compromised.

PROGNOSIS.   The outcome of treatment is directly related to the severity of the initial injury. For example, the prognosis is excellent for a patient with a microtorn ligament and mild secondary swelling. The prognosis is poor for a patient with a macrotorn ligament, regardless of the amount of secondary inflammatory response. Most patients have pathology that falls between these two extremes. To ensure the optimal results, immobilization must be combined with a sufficient amount of anti-inflammatory treatment.

DESCRIPTION.   Carpal tunnel syndrome (CTS) is a compression neuropathy of the median nerve. Compression occurs under the transverse carpal ligament at the wrist, at the pronator teres muscle in the proximal forearm or, rarely, in the distal forearm following penetrating trauma. Traditionally and anatomically, the term CTS is used to refer to the compression at the wrist. "Compression neuropathy of the medial

Carpal Tunnel Syndrome

Enter ½ to ¾" proximal to the palmar prominence of the wrist, at the distal volar crease and on the ulnar side of the palmaris longus tendon (there is more room on the ulnar side of the tendon).

Needle: ⅝", 25 gauge

Depth: ½ to ⅝"

Volume: 1 to 2 ml of the anesthetic plus ½ ml of K40

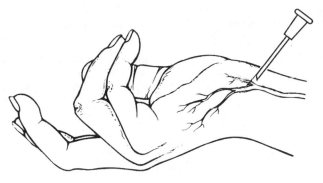

Figure 4–4.   Carpal tunnel injection

nerve" is a more general term that encompasses all causes of median nerve symptoms. The stage of the condition (from sensory loss to motor loss with atrophy) correlates directly with the degree of compression and the chronicity of the symptoms. Most cases present at an early stage with intermittent sensory symptoms only.

SYMPTOMS.   The patient complains of a loss of sensation in the tips of the first three fingers, pain traveling through the forearm and wrist, weakness of grip, or all three. The variability in symptoms reflects the stage of the condition, the amount of nerve compression, the length of time symptoms have been present, and so forth. The patient often rubs the fingers across the wrist, palm, and first three fingers when describing the condition.

"My thumb and first two fingers go to sleep at night."
"After I've typed all day, I get these shooting pains up and down my arm."
"My hand keeps going numb."
"After long bike rides, my fingers go to sleep."
"My hand feels dead. I've started to drop things."

EXAM.   The degree of median nerve dysfunction is assessed by examining the sensation of the first three fingers, the degree of nerve irritability with provocative testing, and the integrity of the thumb muscles by inspection and by function-testing of thumb opposition. If median nerve symptoms do not appear to be arising from the wrist, then examination is performed at the pronator teres muscle and then at the distal forearm.

EXAM SUMMARY   • • • • • • • • • • • • • • •

1. Sensory loss in the first three fingers
2. Loss of thumb opposition
3. Positive Tinel sign, Phalen sign, or both
4. Pressure over the pronator teres in the proximal forearm
5. Median nerve block confirming the diagnosis

Depending on the time of day, the amount of use, and the daily variation of symptoms, the examination of the median nerve may reveal total normality despite a clinically significant problem. (1) Two-point discrimination, light touch, and pain sensation may be decreased at the fingertips of the first three digits. (2) The strength of thumb opposition may be decreased. This is best tested by asking the patient to hold the thumb and fifth finger together. (3) Tests for Tinel sign and Phalen sign are performed at the wrist to test nerve irritability. The test for the Tinel sign should be performed using vigorous tapping over the transverse carpal ligament, with the wrist held in extension. The test for the Phalen sign—holding both wrists in extreme volarflexion—should be held for 30 to 60 seconds. (4) If these results are negative, then compression in the forearm should be performed. Pressure is applied 1 to 2″ distal to the antecubital fossa. This can be enhanced by resisting forearm pronation. (5) Further confirmation of the diagnosis can be made by median nerve block at the wrist or short-term response to corticosteroid injection.

Note that median nerve distribution varies from one patient to another. Most patients experience paresthesia in the first three fingers; however, a few patients may experience symptoms in the second and third fingers, with little involvement of the thumb. Occasionally, a median nerve will involve the radial side of the fourth finger.

SPECIAL TESTING.   No characteristic changes in x-rays occur with CTS. X-rays of the wrist are not necessary unless there is clinical evidence of an underlying carpal or radiocarpal arthritis. Nerve conduction velocity (NCV) testing is the test of choice. The result of an NCV test will be positive in approximately 70% of cases. Note that a negative result on an NCV test does *not* totally exclude the presence of median nerve compression.

DIAGNOSIS.   In advanced cases, such as those involving prolonged symptoms or motor involvement, the NCV test is the diagnostic test of choice, and it has high predictive value; however, patients with intermittent symptoms or mild sensory symptoms present a diagnostic dilemma. The result of the NCV test is often normal in these patients. When the diagnosis is suspected on clinical grounds (for example, a characteristic pain pattern, the Tinel sign, or the Phalen sign), a regional anesthetic block plus a corticosteroid injection should be considered. Almost 90% of patients experience relief from this procedure, helping to confirm the clinical suspicion of CTS.

TREATMENT.   The goals of treatment are to reduce compression of the nerve, to treat concurrent flexor tenosynovitis, and to prevent a recurrence of CTS through improved ergonomics. Adjustments at the work station as well as wrist splinting are the treatments of choice for early disease. Advanced disease with motor involvement should be treated with surgery.

Step 1: Evaluate the stage of the condition and the underlying cause by clinical or NCV testing. Treat the underlying cause using diuretics (if fluid retention is found), anti-inflammatory medication (if there is rheumatoid arthritis), or levothyroxine (for the obvious case of myxedema), and so forth.

Reduce repetitive wrist motion.

Use antivibration padded gloves (Sorbothane orthotic devices).

Reposition the wrist at the keyboard, assembly line, and so forth.

Use a Velcro wrist splint at night (p. 288).

Step 2 (2 to 4 weeks for persistent cases): Reevaluate the stage of the condition.

Order an NCV test in patients with persistent symptoms or significant motor symptoms.

Order x-rays of the wrist (including PA, lateral, and carpal tunnel views) to exclude primary arthritis of the wrist and a lunate dislocation.

Perform a local injection of K40 (for sensory symptoms only).

Prescribe a Velcro wrist splint to be used during the day and at night.

Repeat the injection in 4 to 6 weeks if symptoms have not been reduced by 50%.

Step 3 (6 to 8 weeks for chronic symptoms): Begin stretching exercises for the flexor tendons if symptoms have improved (p. 263).

Reemphasize ergonomics and proper use.

Request a surgical consultation if motor symptoms have developed or symptoms have failed to improve.

PHYSICAL THERAPY.   Although surgical release is still the mainstay of treatment, more and more emphasis has been placed on the role of physical therapy in the management of CTS. Ergonomic adjustments can have a tremendous impact on the response to treatment and on the rehabilitation of the condition. Proper hand and wrist placement according to normal anatomic position cannot be overemphasized. In addition, stretching exercises of the nine flexor tendons of the hand may reduce the overall recurrence rate (p. 263). These stretching exercises are especially helpful when combined with local corticosteroid injection.

INJECTION.   Injection with corticosteroids can be used for definitive treatment of mild to moderate sensory CTS, or it can be used empirically to diagnose mild CTS with normal NCV testing. Of patients with CTS, 90% will respond to corticosteroid injection. By contrast, the results of NCV testing are diagnostic in only 70% of patients.

Positioning: The wrist is placed palm up, dorsiflexed to 30 degrees (see Fig. 4–4).

Surface Anatomy and Point of Entry: The pisiform bone and the palmaris longus tendons are located and marked. The point of entry is at the intersection of the distal volar crease and the ulnar side of the palmaris longus.

Angle of Entry and Depth: The needle is carefully advanced at a 45-degree angle down to and through the transverse carpal ligament (typical depth is ⅜ to ½"). This angle coupled with the short ⅝" needle make it nearly impossible to enter the nerve.

Anesthesia: Ethyl chloride is sprayed on the skin. Local anesthetic is placed in the subcutaneous fat (½ ml), in the firm resistance of the transverse carpal ligament (½ ml), and in the carpal tunnel (½ to 1 ml). A median nerve block confirms the accurate placement.

Technique: The successful injection must be placed just underneath the transverse carpal ligament. Injection of anesthesia into the fibrous tissue above the ligament requires moderate pressure. As the needle is advanced through the ligament, a pop or a giving-way sensation is often felt. As soon as the carpal tunnel is entered, the medications should flow with a minimum of pressure. The patient may experience a temporary median nerve irritation when the needle enters the tunnel. Note: If the patient continues to feel nerve irritation with injection, either reposition the needle or withdraw ⅛".

INJECTION AFTERCARE

1) *Rest* for 3 days, avoiding all wrist movement, finger motion, and exposure to vibration.

2) *Ice* (15 minutes every 4 to 6 hours) and *Tylenol ES* (1000 mg twice a day) for soreness.

3) *Protect* the wrist for 3 to 4 weeks with a Velcro wrist immobilizer with a metal stay and by limiting grasping, pinching, gripping, and exposure to vibration.

4) Reemphasize the need to make ergonomic adjustments at the work station.

5) Begin passive *stretching exercises* of the fingers in extension at 3 to 4 weeks.

6) Repeat the *injection* at 6 weeks if symptoms have not improved by 50%.

7) Obtain a *consultation* with a surgical orthopedist if two injections fail to provide at least 4 to 6 months of symptomatic relief or if loss of motor function intervenes.

SURGICAL PROCEDURE.   Release of the transverse carpal ligament is the treatment of choice for both persistent symptoms and motor involvement (recurrent median nerve involvement).

PROGNOSIS.   Medical therapy provides long-term control of symptoms in fewer than half of patients. A local injection is highly effective in the short term (months), but only 25 to 30% have long-term benefit over years. Symptoms often persist because of secondary factors, especially repetitive wrist and hand use, uncontrollable factors on the job, and unavoidable exposure to vibration.

Surgery is indicated for persistent or slowly progressive nerve dysfunction or motor loss such as loss of grip and specific loss of thumb opposition. Surgical release of the transverse carpal ligament is successful in 90% of cases; 10% of cases fail to improve because of nerve damage, postoperative neuritis, or recurrent compression due to scar tissue formation.

Radiocarpal Joint Arthrocentesis

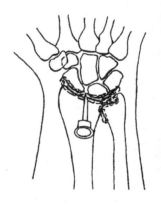

Enter the joint between the distal radius and the navicular, just on the radial side of the extensor tendon of the index finger.

Needle: ⅝", 25 gauge for anesthesia and injection (21 gauge for aspiration)

Depth: ½" to ensure an intra-articular injection.

Volume: 1 ml of anesthetic and ½ ml of K40

Note: If bone is encountered at ¼", then withdraw through the radionavicular ligaments, use skin traction to redirect the needle, and reenter the joint.

Figure 4–5.   Arthrocentesis of the wrist joint

DESCRIPTION.   Arthritis affecting the radiocarpal joint is not common. Osteoarthritis of the wrist is uncommon and nearly always results from injury (multiple wrist sprains, fracture of the navicular or distal radius, or dislocation of the carpal bones). Aspiration of the wrist and synovial fluid analysis are indicated to differentiate posttraumatic monoarticular arthritis, crystal-induced arthropathy, rheumatoid arthritis, and the uncommon septic arthritis. Persistent swelling at the radiocarpal joint can lead to secondary carpal tunnel symptoms.

SYMPTOMS.   The patient complains of pain, swelling, and loss of range of motion at the wrist. The patient often rubs over the dorsum of the wrist when describing the condition.

"I can't bend my wrist."
"My wrist is swollen."
"I cannot perform my usual assembly job. The constant turning of my wrist has become too painful."

"I've sprained my wrist so many times that I've lost count. Over the last few years of basketball coaching my wrist has slowly begun to stiffen."

EXAM. Each patient is examined for dorsal wrist swelling, for tenderness over the proximal navicular bone, and for pain and loss of range of motion in dorsiflexion and volar flexion.

EXAM SUMMARY

1. Tenderness at the intersection of the navicular, radius, and extensor tendon
2. Loss of range of motion and endpoint stiffness or pain with forced flexion or extension
3. Swelling over the dorsum
4. Associated bony enlargement, ganglion, or prominent carpal bones over the dorsum

(1) Joint line tenderness is located at the intersection of the distal radius and to the radial side of the extensor tendon of the first finger. Firm pressure is applied over the navicular with or without passive flexion of the finger. Local tenderness may be palpable in the proximal snuffbox, as well. (2) Loss of range of motion and endpoint stiffness will be present with passive flexion and extension of the wrist. The normal range of motion is 90 and 80 degrees for flexion and extension, respectively. Severe wrist involvement shows only 45 degrees of flexion and extension. (3) Swelling of the wrist is best appreciated over the dorsum of the wrist. Subtle swelling will fill in the depression over the navicular. Moderate to severe swelling of the joint will cause a visible bulging or convexity over the navicular. (4) Advanced osteoarthritis of the wrist may cause bony enlargement dorsally.

X-RAYS. X-rays of the wrist (including PA, lateral, and oblique) are always recommended. The normal thickness of the articular cartilage between the radius and navicular is 2 to 3 mm. Rheumatoid arthritis causes a symmetric loss of cartilage and the characteristic thinning of the bones (juxta-articular osteoporosis). Osteoarthritis of the wrist causes an asymmetric loss of cartilage, sclerosis of the radius and navicular bones, and gradual resorption of the navicular bone (shrinkage).

SPECIAL TESTING. Synovial fluid analysis is indicated when septic arthritis and crystal-induced arthritis must be excluded.

DIAGNOSIS. The diagnosis of rheumatoid arthritis or osteoarthritis is strongly suggested by the physical exam findings of loss of range of motion and local tenderness. The diagnosis can be confirmed by intra-articular injection of local anesthesia. If septic arthritis or gout/pseudogout is suspected, synovial fluid analysis must be performed.

TREATMENT. The goals of treatment are to reduce the inflammation and restore the range of motion of the joint. Aspiration of fluid for lab analysis is often unsuccessful. Ice and a Velcro wrist immobilizer are the treatments of choice for mild wrist involvement. Local corticosteroid injection is the treatment of choice for moderate to severe involvement of the nonseptic effusion. Septic arthritis is rare.

Step 1: Measure the range of motion in flexion and extension (volar flexion and dorsiflexion, respectively) and order plain x-rays of the wrist (including PA, lateral, and oblique views).

Aspirate, flush the joint with saline, and send the fluid for diagnostic studies if septic arthritis is suspected: Gram stain and culture, uric acid crystal analysis, and cell count and differential.

Apply ice over the dorsum of the wrist for 15 minutes several times a day.

Avoid repetitious movement.

Prescribe a Velcro wrist immobilizer with a metal stay (p. 288).

Prescribe an NSAID (e.g., ibuprofen [Advil, Motrin]) for 3 to 4 weeks.

Step 2 (1 to 3 days after lab analysis): If septic arthritis is not a consideration and the patient has already tried an oral anti-inflammatory medication, perform an intra-articular injection of K40 for the rheumatoid or osteoarthritic effusion.

Continue the Velcro wrist immobilizer with metal stay.

Begin range-of-motion exercises to restore full flexion and extension.

Step 3 (3 to 4 weeks for persistent cases): Repeat the local injection of K40 if there is persistent swelling and pain.

Continue range-of-motion exercises to restore full flexion and extension.

Step 4 (3 months for chronic cases): If symptoms persist and at least half of the normal range of motion has been lost, consider an orthopedic consultation for joint fusion.

PHYSICAL THERAPY.   Physical therapy plays a minor role in the active treatment of radiocarpal arthritis and a significant role in the prevention of future arthritic flares. *Ice* applications and phonophoresis with a hydrocortisone gel are effective for the temporary control of pain and swelling. As soon as the acute symptoms have been controlled, gentle *range-of-motion exercises* are performed passively.

Isometric toning exercises of gripping and wrist flexion and extension are performed after all symptoms have resolved. Increasing the resting tone of the extensor muscles—restoring the balance between the strength of the flexor muscles and the extensor muscles—should provide the best protection against future arthritic flares.

PHYSICAL THERAPY SUMMARY   ● ● ● ● ● ● ● ● ● ● ● ● ● ● ●

1. Ice over the dorsum of the wrist
2. Phonophoresis with a hydrocortisone gel
3. Toning exercises of gripping, isometrically performed
4. Toning exercises of wrist extension, isometrically performed

INJECTION.   Local corticosteroid injection is commonly used when ice, restricted use, immobilization, and an oral NSAID fail to control symptoms.

Positioning: The hand and wrist are to be placed in the prone position. The wrist is flexed to 30 degrees and held in place with a rolled-up towel.

Surface Anatomy and Point of Entry: The extensor tendon of the index finger is identified and marked as it crosses the radius. The very edge of the distal radius is palpated and marked. The point of entry is on the radial side of the tendon and the distal edge of the radius.

Angle of Entry and Depth: The needle is inserted perpendicular to the skin. The depth is ½″. If the firm resistance of bone or ligament is encountered at a superficial depth (¼ to ⅜″), the needle must be withdrawn back through the ligament and repositioned with the aid of skin traction!

Anesthesia: Ethyl chloride is sprayed on the skin. Local anesthetic is placed in the subcutaneous fat (½ ml), in the firm resistance of the radiocarpal ligament (½ ml), and in the joint (½ ml).

Technique: The *dorsal approach* is preferred. The successful injection will carefully enter the ¼″ space between the radius, navicular, and lunate at a depth of ½″. The 25-gauge needle is advanced perpendicularly through the radionavicular ligament and into the wrist. The needle must be redirected if bone is encountered at ¼″. If fluid is not obtained with the 25-gauge needle, a 22-gauge needle can be used to aspirate. If aspiration is still negative, the joint can be irrigated with 1 to 2 ml of sterile saline and sent for Gram stain and culture. For the aseptic effusion, the needle is left in place and the joint is injected with ½ ml of K40.

INJECTION AFTERCARE

1) *Rest* for 3 days, avoiding repetitious motion and tension across the wrist.

2) *Ice* (15 minutes every 4 to 6 hours) and *Tylenol ES* (1000 mg twice a day) for soreness.

3) *Protect* the wrist for 3 to 4 weeks with a Velcro wrist brace worn continuously for the first week.

4) Begin *isometric toning exercises* of wrist flexion and extension at 3 weeks.

5) Repeat *injection* at 6 weeks if swelling persists or chronic synovial thickening develops.

6) Advise on the long-term protection of the joint.

7) Obtain a *consultation* with a surgical orthopedist if symptoms persist, if 50% of normal range of motion has been lost, and if the patient is willing to undergo surgical fusion.

SURGICAL PROCEDURE. Patient with severe restrictions of motion (over 50% loss) and persistent symptoms can be considered for fusion of the wrist (arthrodesis). The patient has to be willing to accept the loss of wrist motion in exchange for pain control. Although this surgery is very effective in controlling symptoms, few patients will want to sacrifice the last remaining motion of the joint.

PROGNOSIS. Intra-articular injection is very effective in the palliation of symptoms arising at the radiocarpal joint from rheumatoid arthritis or osteoarthritis. Patients often experience months of relief from pain and swelling and improvement in function from the combination of a properly placed injection of corticosteroid and isometric toning exercises.

DESCRIPTION. A dorsal ganglion is an abnormal accumulation of synovial or tenosynovial fluid. Subtle abnormalities in the wrist or the extensor tendon sheath cause an overproduction of fluid that leaks into the subcutaneous tissue. The fluid, rich in protein content, irritates the tissues and leads to cyst formation. Other names for this common condition include Bible cyst, wrist cyst, or dorsal tendon cyst. Volar synovial cysts occur but are distinctly less common, occurring in a ratio of 1 to 20 or less.

SYMPTOMS. Most patients complain of a painless lump at the wrist. However, some patients have symptomatic cysts when pressure is exerted on an adjacent structure (pressure on the carpal bones, neuritic complaints when pressure occurs on the superficial branch of the radial nerve, and so forth).

Dorsal Ganglion

Enter at the base of the palpable cyst, paralleling the skin and avoiding the adjacent veins and tendons.

Needle: ⅝", 25 gauge for anesthesia; 1½", 18 gauge for aspiration

Depth: variable but rarely below ⅜"

Volume: ½ ml of anesthetic in the subcutaneous tissue adjacent to the cyst wall plus ½ ml of K40 into the cyst

Note: A 10-ml syringe is necessary to obtain enough vacuum pressure to aspirate the highly viscous fluid.

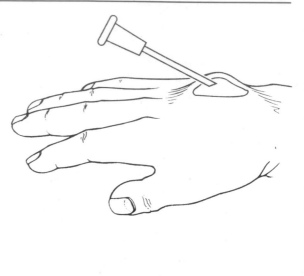

Figure 4–6.   Ganglion aspiration and injection

"I noticed this swelling over my wrist. My brothers have all died of cancer, and I was very worried about it."
"I developed this really ugly swelling over the back of my hand. I want it taken off."
"I type all day long. Over the last several months I have noticed this lump on the back of my hand."
"I've had this bump on the back of my wrist for years, but it recently has grown bigger."

EXAM.   The characteristics (such as size, mobility, and compressibility) of the cyst are evaluated and an assessment is made of the wrist joint and of the function of the dorsal tendons that cross the wrist.

EXAM SUMMARY

1. A highly mobile, fluctuant cyst overlying the wrist
2. Minimal tenderness
3. Normal wrist motion in most cases
4. A characteristic highly viscous aspirate

(1) A 1- to 2-cm, highly mobile, fluctuant to tense cyst is palpable in the subcutaneous tissue. It should not be grossly adherent to the underlying tissue. (2) Tenderness is minimal unless the cyst is pressing against one of the cutaneous nerves (a superficial branch of the radial nerve; causes numbness or paresthesias over the back of the hand and fingers). (3) Wrist motion is painless and full unless underlying carpal or radiocarpal arthritis is present. (4) The diagnosis is confirmed by aspirating the thick, highly

viscous, nearly colorless fluid from the cyst (the consistency of Karo syrup or 90-weight lubricating oil).

X-RAYS. X-rays of the wrist are not necessary for the diagnosis. Most x-rays are normal unless there is underlying carpal or radiocarpal arthritis.

SPECIAL TESTING. None.

DIAGNOSIS. The diagnosis is confirmed by demonstrating the typical thick, non-bloody aspirate.

TREATMENT. The goals of treatment are to reassure the patient that this is not a serious problem, to decompress the cyst, and to prevent recurrent cyst formation. The treatment of choice is simple aspiration.

Step 1: Observe the cyst, which may diminish with time.

Educate the patient: "This may resolve spontaneously."

Do a simple aspiration.

Limit wrist motions, especially repetitious use.

Use a Velcro wrist brace (p. 288).

Step 2 (8 to 10 weeks for persistent cases): Repeat aspiration and inject with K40.

Continue the wrist brace.

Step 3 (12 weeks or longer for chronic cases): Consider a repeat injection with K40 (if the first treatment was partially successful).

Perform gripping and wrist-toning exercises (p. 262).

Consider an orthopedic consultation for removal.

Educate the patient: "Some cases may recur even after surgical removal, depending on whether you continue to produce too much lubricating fluid."

PHYSICAL THERAPY. The role of physical therapy is limited in the treatment and prevention of ganglia. Wrist-strengthening exercises are indicated if there is clinical evidence of underlying radiocarpal arthritis. Generally, isometric toning exercises are performed to strengthen wrist extension and flexion in patients who work intensively with their hands.

INJECTION. Aspiration is the treatment of choice for ganglia that fail to resolve with time. At least half of them will respond to simple aspiration. Corticosteroid injection is the treatment of choice for ganglia that cause pressure on a superficial branch of the radial nerve (dysesthetic pain on the dorsum of the hand and fingers) and for recurrent cysts that are larger than 1" in diameter.

Positioning: The hand and wrist are to be placed in the prone position. The wrist is flexed to 30 to 45 degrees and held in place with a rolled-up towel.

Surface Anatomy and Point of Entry: Most dorsal ganglia are located directly over the navicular and are more prominent when the wrist is flexed. The point of entry is at the proximal base of the cyst, away from any local vein or tendon.

Angle of Entry and Depth: The 18-gauge needle is advanced into the center of the cyst, paralleling the skin. The depth is rarely more than ¼ to ⅜" from the surface.

Anesthesia: Ethyl chloride is sprayed on the skin. Local anesthetic is placed in the subcutaneous fat adjacent to the cyst (the cyst wall has few if any nerve endings).

Technique: Success of injection depends on complete cyst aspiration and subsequent injection through the same needle. Optimal aspiration is at the *base* of the ganglion. An 18-gauge needle attached to a 10-ml syringe is advanced into the center of the cyst. The bevel of the needle is rotated 180 degrees and the highly viscous fluid is removed. Manual pressure applied from either side may assist in the removal of the fluid. With the needle left in place, the cyst is injected with ½ ml of K40.

INJECTION AFTERCARE

1) *Rest* for 3 days, avoiding repetitious motion and tension across the wrist.

2) *Ice* (15 minutes every 4 to 6 hours) and *Tylenol ES* (1000 mg twice a day) for soreness.

3) *Protect* the wrist for 3 to 4 weeks by avoiding repetitive lifting, gripping, grasping, and vibration.

4) Suggest that a Velcro wrist brace be worn if advanced wrist arthritis is present.

5) Begin *isometric toning exercises* of wrist flexion and extension at 3 weeks.

6) Repeat *injection* at 6 weeks with corticosteroid if fluid reaccumulates.

7) Consider an intra-articular injection of the radiocarpal joint to reduce the overproduction of joint fluid (especially with significant radiocarpal joint disease).

8) Obtain a *consultation* with a surgical orthopedist if the patient has pressure symptoms, radial nerve paresthesias, or swelling that interferes with normal wrist motion.

SURGICAL PROCEDURE.   Excision of the cyst and sinus tract.

PROGNOSIS.   The results of aspiration and injection are variable. Simple aspiration is effective in 50% of cases. Aspiration must be combined with corticosteroid injection to resolve an additional 30% of cases. Approximately 20% of patients fail to respond to aspiration with corticosteroid injection because of constant overproduction of fluid (chronic arthritis, chronic tenosynovitis, tendon scarring, and so forth). Surgical removal of the cyst and the sinus tract can be offered to these patients.

chapter 5

Hand

Trigger Finger

Enter just distal to the metacarpal head, directly over the center of the tendon.

Needle: ⅝″, 25 gauge

Depth: ¼ to ⅜″ flush against the tendon

Volume: ½ ml of anesthetic plus ¼ ml of D80

Note: Never inject with hard pressure (within the body of the tendon).

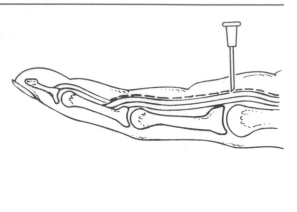

Figure 5–1.   Trigger finger injection

DESCRIPTION.   Trigger finger is an inflammation of the flexor tendons of the finger as they cross the metacarpophalangeal (MCP) head in the palm. Repetitive gripping and grasping or pressure over the palm causes swelling and inflammation of the tendon and the tendon sheath (tenosynovitis). As the swelling increases, the two flexor tendons lose their smooth motion under the A-1 pulley, the specialized ligament that anchors the tendon to the bone. If the tendon continues to swell, the finger begins to catch or lock (triggering).

SYMPTOMS.   The patient complains of a painful finger or of loss of smooth motion of the finger when gripping or pinching. The patient rubs over the tendon in the palm or actually demonstrates the locking phenomenon when describing the condition.

"My finger keeps catching."
"I wake up in the morning and my finger is locked."
"My finger has started to tie up again."
"The dumb thing locks down."
"I had to stop knitting because my finger hurts all the time."
"If I use scissors or fingernail clippers, I get this sharp pain in my finger (pointing to the base of the finger in the palm)."
"I just thought that this was arthritis! I ignored the pain for the longest time. I didn't know that it could be treated."

EXAM.   Each patient is examined for active tenosynovitis of the flexor tendons of the finger along with the degree of mechanical locking.

EXAM SUMMARY   ● ● ● ● ● ● ● ● ● ● ● ● ● ● ●

1.   Local tenderness at the MCP head
2.   Pain aggravated by stretching the finger in extension, passively performed
3.   Pain aggravated by resisting finger flexion, isometrically performed
4.   Mechanical locking of the proximal interphalangeal (PIP) joint (fingers) and the interphalangeal (IP) joint (thumb)

(1) Local tenderness is present at the base of the finger, directly over the tendon as it courses over the metacarpal head. There is also subtle, palpable swelling in 10% of cases. (2) Pain is aggravated by stretching the tendon in extension or (3) by resisting the action of flexion isometrically. (4) Clicking or locking with active flexion may or may not be present, depending on the time of day or how long the patient has been symptomatic.

X-RAYS. Plain x-rays of the hand are not necessary. Calcification of the tendon rarely occurs.

SPECIAL TESTING. None.

DIAGNOSIS. The diagnosis is based on a history of locking and on an exam showing three of the four principal signs—locking, local tenderness at the MCP head, painful stretching in extension, or isometrically resisted flexion. A regional anesthetic block is rarely necessary to make the diagnosis, except in the case of tenosynovitis complicating an early presentation of Dupuytren contracture.

TREATMENT. The goals of treatment are to reduce the swelling and inflammation in the flexor tendon sheath, to allow smoother movement of the tendon under the A-1 pulley, and to perform stretching exercises in extension to prevent recurrent tenosynovitis. Immobilization using buddy-taping is the treatment of choice in the first 4 to 6 weeks. Corticosteroid injection is the treatment of choice for patients with symptoms that have been present beyond 6 weeks.

Step 1: Assess the degree of mechanical locking and the degree of active tenosynovitis.

> Restrict gripping and pinching.

> Demonstrate for the patient the technique of buddy-taping to the adjacent finger (p. 293).

> Suggest ice applications over the metacarpal head.

> Recommend a metal finger splint if buddy-taping is poorly tolerated or unsuccessful (p. 294).

> Recommend antivibration padded gloves (Sorbothane).

Step 2 (4 to 6 weeks for persistent cases): Perform a local injection of D80.

> Repeat the injection at 6 weeks if symptoms have not improved by at least 50%.

Step 3 (10 to 12 weeks for chronic cases): Recommend padded or oversized tools.

> Advise reducing the tension when gripping or pinching.

> Begin gentle stretching exercises in extension of the fingers (p. 262).

> Consider surgical release if symptoms are not relieved by two injections.

PHYSICAL THERAPY. Physical therapy plays a minor role in the overall management of trigger finger. Stretching exercises in extension are used to prevent recurrent tenosynovitis and to rehabilitate the tendons in the postoperative recovery period. Sets of 20 gentle stretches are performed daily to maintain flexor tendon mobility and to reduce the contracture over the MCP head. Physical therapy is not appropriate for active tenosynovitis.

INJECTION. Local injection is the anti-inflammatory treatment of choice. Indications for injection include failure of simple immobilization, severe locking on presentation, and treatment of symptoms that have been present for over 6 to 8 weeks.

Positioning: The hand is placed flat on the exam table with the palm up and the fingers outstretched.

Surface Anatomy and Point of Entry: The proximal volar crease of the finger or the distal volar crease over the MP joint of the thumb is identified. The point of entry for the finger is just proximal to the first volar crease in the midline. The point of entry for the thumb is at the distal volar crease in the midline.

Angle of Entry and Depth: The needle is inserted perpendicular to the skin. The depth of injection is ¼ to ⅜″ for trigger finger and ⅛ to ¼″ for trigger thumb.

Anesthesia: Ethyl chloride is sprayed on the skin. Local anesthetic is placed in the subcutaneous tissue.

Technique: A *volar approach* directly over the center of the tendon is preferred. The needle is advanced down to the firm resistance of the flexor tendon, a rubbery sensation. The needle is held flush against the tendon, utilizing just the weight of the syringe. Without advancing the needle, the corticosteroid is injected just atop the tendon and, hence, underneath the tenosynovial sheath.

INJECTION AFTERCARE

1) *Rest* for 3 days, avoiding all gripping and grasping.

2) Buddy-tape the adjacent two fingers for the first few days.

3) *Ice* (15 minutes every 4 to 6 hours) and *Tylenol ES* (1000 mg twice a day) for soreness.

4) *Protect* the fingers for 3 to 4 weeks by avoiding repetitive gripping, grasping, pressure over the MCP heads, and vibration.

5) Begin passive *stretching exercises* of the fingers in extension at 3 weeks.

6) Repeat *injection* at 6 weeks with corticosteroid if tenosynovitis or locking persists.

7) Suggest padded gloves or padded tools for long-term prevention in recurrent cases.

8) Obtain a *consultation* with surgical orthopedist if two consecutive injections fail to provide at least 6 months of relief.

SURGICAL PROCEDURE.   Surgery is indicated when locking and tenosynovitis persist despite two consecutive local corticosteroid injections. Percutaneous release and open surgical release of the A-1 pulley ligament are equally effective.

PROGNOSIS.   A local injection with D80 is highly effective. Two thirds of cases require only one injection for long-term benefit. One quarter of cases require reinjection within 1 year. Only 10% will fail medical therapy and require surgical release. This outpatient surgery is safe and effective. The fascial tissue over the tendon at the MCP head is sharply dissected. Recovery may take 3 to 4 weeks.

RESULTS.   These results were published in the Archives of Internal Medicine 151:153–156, 1991 (Table 5–1).

TABLE 5-1. CLINICAL OUTCOMES OF 74 CASES OF TRIGGER FINGER TREATED WITH DEPO-MEDROL 80*

Resolved with 1 injection	45 (61%)
Recurrence requiring 1 to 3 additional injections	20 (27%)
Failed to respond completely (surgical release, 5; chronic tenosynovitis, 4)	9 (12%)
Total	74

*Follow-up: 4.2 years

Tendon Cyst

Enter directly over the palpable nodule.

Needle: ⅝″, 25 gauge or 1″, 21 gauge

Depth: ¼ to ⅜″ into the cyst

Volume: ½ ml of anesthetic for the initial treatment; ¼ ml of D80 for the second puncture, if necessary

Note: After treatment, apply manual pressure from either side to decompress the cyst.

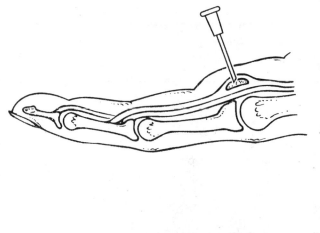

Figure 5–2.   Tendon cyst puncture and decompression

DESCRIPTION.   A tendon cyst is an abnormal collection of tenosynovial fluid, either within the tendon or adjacent to it. Direct, nonpenetrating trauma causes damage to the tendon or tendon sheath which, in turn, leads to an overproduction of fluid and the formation of the cyst. Despite its size (5 to 8 mm in diameter), the nodule rarely interferes with the function of the tendons (normal flexion) or the mobility of the MCP joint.

SYMPTOMS.   The patient complains of a lump in the palm of the hand, which is mildly tender to compression. The patient points to the area when describing the problem.

"I have this small knot right here (pointing to the base of the finger in the palm)."
"Feel this thing, kind of like a little marble or B.B."
"When I use my little scissors and place pressure over my finger, I get a sharp pain."
"My doctor told me that I have a cyst in my tendon, but I'm not so sure that I believe her. I'm worried about it."
"Ever since I hit the countertop with my hand, I've felt this lump in my palm (pointing to the base of the finger)."
"I'm a professional percussionist. My favorite instrument is the tambourine. About four weeks ago, I noticed a pain along my fourth finger every time I tried to hold my tambourine. There's a small lump there now."

EXAM.   The location and size of the nodule relative to the position of the tendon and metacarpal head are assessed in each patient.

EXAM SUMMARY

1. A smooth, firm nodule 5 to 8 mm in diameter that is palpable in the palm
2. Very mild tenderness to firm compression
3. Absence of mechanical locking, triggering, or palmar fascial thickening
4. Decompression with simple cyst puncture

(1) A firm nodule is palpable in the palm, usually adjacent to the distal metacarpal head. If the nodule is inside the tendon, passive motion of the finger in flexion and extension will cause it to move. If the nodule is adjacent to the tendon, the nodule is less likely to move directly with passive motion. (2) Mild tenderness may be present over the nodule. Firm pressure exerted toward the underlying bone will cause pain; it is most pronounced in the first few months. With time, this tenderness becomes less prominent. (3) The flexor tendons are free of mechanical catching or locking (that is, the MCP and PIP joints should have full, smooth flexion and extension).

X-RAYS.   Plain x-rays of the hand are not necessary. Calcification of the cyst is rare. Significant underlying bony changes do not occur.

SPECIAL TESTING.   None.

DIAGNOSIS.   A presumptive diagnosis is based on the size and location of the nodule in the palm. A simple puncture with decompression confirms the diagnosis and differentiates this kind of cyst from the solid cyst, "giant cell tumor." Those cysts that fail to decompress with simple puncture may need to have their diagnoses confirmed surgically.

TREATMENT.   The goal of treatment is to decompress the abnormal accumulation of fluid. Simple puncture with manual decompression is the treatment of choice for cysts that are symptomatic and that have not resolved spontaneously.

Step 1: Observe the condition over weeks to months for spontaneous resolution.

> Educate the patient: "This is simply a cyst of the tendon. Many times this kind of cyst will resolve without any specific treatment."

Step 2 (4 to 8 weeks for persistent cases): Perform simple puncture and decompression.

> Repeat the procedure if the cyst recurs.

> Reduce gripping and grasping tension; use padded tools or antivibration gloves (Sorbothane).

Step 3 (months for chronic cases): Consider surgical decompression for tendon cysts that continue to interfere with gripping or grasping.

PHYSICAL THERAPY.   Physical therapy does not have a significant role in the treatment of tendon cysts.

INJECTION.   Simple puncture with manual decompression is the injection procedure of choice.

Positioning: The hand is placed flat on the exam table with the palm up and the fingers outstretched.

Surface Anatomy and Point of Entry: The proximal volar crease of the finger or the distal volar crease over the MP joint of the thumb is identified. The point of entry is centered directly over the cyst.

Angle of Entry and Depth: The needle is inserted perpendicular to the skin. The depth of injection is ¼ to ⅜".

Anesthesia: Ethyl chloride is sprayed on the skin. Local anesthetic is placed in the subcutaneous tissue.

Technique: The cyst is identified by placing a fingertip above it and a fingertip below it. While holding the cyst firmly in place, the needle is centered over the nodule and passed down into the cyst at least twice. The bevel of the needle is kept parallel to the tendon fibers (separating the tendon fibers rather than cutting them!). To ensure the accurate placement inside the cyst, the tendon can be passively flexed and extended; the needle should move with the cyst. Aspiration of the small amount of highly viscous fluid is usually unsuccessful. Manual pressure using the barrel of a syringe in a rolling fashion or with digital pressure will decompress most cysts. Fewer than 10% will not decompress with simple puncture (those that have very little fluid within the cyst cavity). Repeat the procedure with a 21-gauge needle if the nodule is not reduced in size.

INJECTION AFTERCARE

1) *Rest* for 3 days, avoiding all gripping, grasping, and direct pressure.

2) Buddy-tape the adjacent two fingers for the first few days.

3) *Ice* (15 minutes every 4 to 6 hours) and *Tylenol ES* (1000 mg twice a day) for soreness.

4) *Protect* the fingers for 3 to 4 weeks by avoiding repetitive gripping, grasping, pressure over the MCP heads, and vibration.

5) Repeat *injection* at 6 weeks with corticosteroid if the cyst fluid reaccumulates.

6) Suggest padded gloves or padded tools for long-term prevention in recurrent cases.

7) Observe it; commonly, the cyst will slowly diminish in size over several months.

8) Obtain a *consultation* with a surgical orthopedist if two consecutive procedures and time fail to resolve the condition; advise the patient of the possibility of postoperative scarring over the MCP joint that could adversely affect the range of motion of the finger!

SURGICAL PROCEDURE.   For problem cysts that remain symptomatic (pressure pain, interference with gripping and grasping, persistent anxiety), excision of the cyst can be considered. (Note that surgery performed on the hand can cause significant scarring over the tendon or adjacent joint, limiting the movement of the finger in extension.)

PROGNOSIS.   Simple puncture is highly effective. Surgical excision is indicated if the nodule persists and hand function is interfered with. Surgery for cosmetic results is to be discouraged. Postoperative scarring may develop; at times it is larger than the original size of the cyst and limits the mobility of the finger.

DESCRIPTION.   Dupuytren contracture is a progressive fibrosis of the palmar fascia. Tissue thickening envelops the flexor tendons—typically, the fourth and fifth tendons—and leads to the gradual contracture of the fingers into the palm. The condition develops insidiously over decades. The initial tendon-thickening, often going unnoticed and undiagnosed, causes joint stiffness and a loss of full extension. Over the years, the stiffness is followed by continued scarring and finger contracture. The majority of cases are idiopathic, although the occurrence is statistically higher in patients of northern European descent.

SYMPTOMS.   The patient complains of finger stiffness, thickening in the palm, loss of motion of the affected finger or fingers, or all three. The patient often rubs the palm and fingers in an attempt to straighten them out as the condition is described.

"I've got these knots in my palm."
"I can't straighten my ring and little fingers."
"My fingers have slowly drawn down into my hand."
"I can't hold my hammer and small tools anymore. I can't open my hand enough."

Dupuytren Contracture

Enter adjacent to the nodular thickening in the midline over the flexor tendon: hold the needle vertically. Injection is indicated only when tenosynovitis accompanies the fibrosis process.

Needle: ⅝″, 25 gauge

Depth: ¼ to ⅜″

Volume: ½ ml of anesthetic plus ¼ ml of K40 (for the accompanying flexor tenosynovitis only).

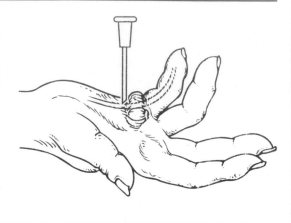

Figure 5–3. Dupuytren contracture injection

EXAM. Each patient is examined for the extent and location of the palmar fibrosis, for the impairment of flexion and extension in the affected fingers (that is, the degree of flexion contracture of the fingers), and for any concurrent tenosynovitis.

(1) Discrete nodules are visible and palpable along the course of the flexor tendons. Passive extension of the affected fingers will demonstrate the puckering of the tendon as it courses over the MCP head. The tendons of the fourth and fifth fingers are most commonly involved. (2) The flexibility of the MCP and PIP joints is reduced, leading to fixed flexion contractures (loss of full extension). (3) Signs of active inflammation are notably absent in most cases. Specifically, local tenderness, swelling, and pain with passive flexion and extension are absent unless a concurrent tenosynovitis is present (uncommon except in the earliest cases).

EXAM SUMMARY ● ● ● ● ● ● ● ● ● ● ● ● ● ●

1. Puckering of the skin over flexor tendon in the palm with forced extension of the finger
2. Painless palmar nodules
3. Fixed flexion contracture of the affected fingers (usually the fourth and fifth fingers)
4. Signs of active tenosynovitis are uncommon (tenderness, pain, or locking).

X-RAYS. Plain films of the hand are not necessary. Calcification of the tendons does not occur.

DIAGNOSIS. The diagnosis is based on the history of painless stiffness of the fingers and on the characteristic physical findings of peritendinous thickening and flexor tendon deformity. Note that on rare occasions, Dupuytren contracture can be painful. In the early stages, tenosynovitis can be present.

TREATMENT. The goals of treatment are to educate the patient regarding the slowly progressive nature of the condition, to improve the flexibility of the flexor tendons, and to evaluate the need for surgery. Passive stretching of the flexor tendons after lanolin massage is the treatment of choice for early disease. Surgery is the treatment of choice for advanced tendon contracture.

Step 1: Educate the patient: "The process slowly worsens over many years, even over decades."

> Heat the hand, massage the tendons with a heavy lanolin–based cream, and gently stretch the tendons in extension. "If the scarring process is inevitable, at least attempt to keep the scarring process from contracting the finger."

Step 2 (months to years for persistent or progressive cases): If the pain of tenosynovitis occurs, a local injection of K40 can be performed.

Step 3 (years for cases with flexion contractures): Consider surgical release if the contracture process progresses and causes poor function of the affected fingers.

> Educate the patient: "Surgery will not cure the problem, only improve function temporarily."

PHYSICAL THERAPY. Physical therapy stretching exercises remain the treatment of choice for the early stages of this condition. Passive stretching exercises in extension are used to prevent flexion contractures and to rehabilitate the postoperative patient.

INJECTION. Fewer than 5% of cases have concomitant tenosynovitis. Local injection with corticosteroid is performed infrequently (see "Trigger Finger," p. 86).

SURGICAL PROCEDURE. Partial fasciectomy is the procedure of choice to débride and release the fibrotic tissue enveloping the tendon or tendons.

PROGNOSIS. Dupuytren contracture is a slow, progressive scarring of the flexor tendons of the hand. All treatments are palliative. No therapy has been shown to stop the scarring process. However, it is important to advise the patient on the proper stretching exercises to retard the development of flexion contracture.

When function has been impaired significantly, surgical removal of the fascial thickening is the treatment of choice. Fasciotomy and fasciectomy are usually successful in the near term. Unfortunately, despite careful technique and meticulous dissection, in many cases, the condition progresses. It is not uncommon to recommend long-term stretching exercises or even a second operation in the case of recurrent fibrosis and progressive contracture.

DESCRIPTION. Isolated arthritic involvement of the metacarpophalangeal (MCP) joints is uncommon. The second and third MCP joints are affected most commonly. Swelling and inflammation of the joint are usually the result of remote and often unrecognized trauma—"posttraumatic monoarticular arthritis." Involvement of multiple MCP joints is more likely to be caused by rheumatoid arthritis. Septic arthritis of the MCP joint is rare; it is usually caused by a penetrating injury. Aspiration of the joint is difficult and produces a low yield.

SYMPTOMS. The patient complains of pain and swelling of the affected joint or of the inability to make a closed fist. The patient often attempts to make a fist when describing the condition.

"My knuckle is swollen."
"I can't close my hand."
"I can't hold on to my hammer because my knuckle hurts too much."
"When I close my hand, it feels like the tendons are slipping."

Metacarpophalangeal Joint Arthrocentesis

Enter over the joint line just distal to the metacarpal head, staying on the dorsal half of the joint.

Needle: ⅝", 25 gauge

Depth: ¼ to ⅜" flush against the bone

Volume: ½ ml of local anesthetic plus ¼ ml of K40

Note: The joint will not accept more than ¼ ml; place the anesthetic in the subcutaneous tissue and the steroid just under the synovial membrane.

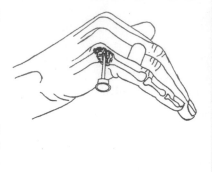

Figure 5—4.   Arthrocentesis and injection of the MCP joint

EXAM.   Each patient is examined for tenderness and swelling of the individual MCP joints and for a loss of full flexion and extension.

EXAM SUMMARY

● ● ● ● ● ● ● ● ● ● ● ● ● ●

1.   Swelling and tenderness of the affected MCP (loss of the normal hills and valleys of the knuckles)
2.   A positive MCP squeeze sign
3.   Inability to make a closed fist

(1) Swelling and tenderness are located over the dorsum of the affected MCP joint or joints. With the MCP joints flexed to 90 degrees, the normal contours formed by the knuckles are obliterated. (2) Pain is aggravated by squeezing the MCP joints together. Pressure is applied across the MCP joints while simultaneously holding the joints in line with the opposite hand. (3) Severe swelling prevents full flexion. A full fist cannot be made. (4) Multiple MCP joint swelling in a symmetric pattern is highly suggestive of inflammatory arthritis or other rheumatologic conditions that cause a symmetric small-joint polyarthritis.

X-RAYS.   X-rays of the hand (including PA and lateral views) are not necessary in the case of monoarticular arthritis of a single MCP joint. However, patients with multiple MCP joint involvement have a greater likelihood of having inflammatory arthritis and thus should be evaluated with bilateral hand x-rays (see "Rheumatoid Arthritis," p. 99).

DIAGNOSIS.   The diagnosis can be made based on the characteristic swelling and loss of range of motion of the MCP joint. Occasionally, local anesthetic block is required to confirm the diagnosis and distinguish this localized joint problem from flexor tenosynovitis or injury to the supporting ligaments.

TREATMENT.   Reducing joint swelling and increasing the range of motion are the goals of treatment. When joint swelling is moderate to severe, local corticosteroid injection is the treatment of choice for nonseptic effusion.

Step 1: Document the number of fingers that are involved and the degree of loss of range of motion, and estimate the strength of gripping.

Restrict gripping and grasping.

Recommend the use of oversized tools and grips and the incorporation of other occupation-oriented adjustments.

Prescribe 3 weeks of immobilization using a radial gutter splint (p. 289) for the first or second MCP joint or an ulnar splint (p. 289) for involvement of the third or fourth MCP joint.

A 4-week course of an NSAID (e.g., ibuprofen [Advil, Motrin]) can be tried, but it has limited efficacy in this small joint.

Step 2 (3 to 4 weeks for persistent cases): Perform a local injection of D80.

Repeat the injection after 4 to 6 weeks if symptoms have not decreased by 50%.

Perform range-of-motion exercises in flexion and extension.

Step 3 (2 to 3 months for chronic cases): Consider a consultation with a hand surgeon for implant arthroplasty.

PHYSICAL THERAPY. Physical therapy plays a minor role in the treatment of monoarticular involvement of the MCP joint. Ice and *phonophoresis with a hydrocortisone gel* can provide temporary relief of pain and swelling. In the recovery phase, passively performed stretching exercises in flexion and extension are used to restore full range of motion.

INJECTION. Corticosteroid injection is the preferred anti-inflammatory treatment for the nonseptic effusion. Note that the response to local corticosteroid injection depends on the extent of injury to the joint. If synovitis is accompanied by damage to the articular cartilage (pitted, fissured, or eroded articular cartilage) then injection will provide temporary benefit only.

Positioning: The hand is placed flat on the exam table with the palm down and the fingers outstretched.

Surface Anatomy and Point of Entry: The distal metacarpal head and the MCP joint line are identified by subluxing the proximal phalangeal bone dorsally (¼" beyond the prominence of the MCP knuckle). A 25-gauge needle is inserted into the skin over the distal metacarpal head adjacent to the joint line. For the second and fifth digits, the point of entry will be just above the midplane, but not in the neurovascular bundle. For the third and fourth digits, the point of entry will be halfway between the MCP heads.

Angle of Entry and Depth: The needle is inserted perpendicular to the skin for the second and fifth digits and at a 45-degree angle for the third and fourth digits. The depth of injection is ¼ to ⅜".

Anesthesia: Ethyl chloride is sprayed on the skin. Local anesthetic is placed in the subcutaneous tissue (½ ml).

Technique: A *dorsal approach* is preferable. The needle is advanced until the firm resistance of the supporting ligament and joint capsule is encountered. Anesthesia is injected just outside this layer (⅛"). Then the needle is advanced to the hard resistance of the bone (¼") and ¼ ml of K40 is injected under the synovial membrane. Note that the small joints of the hand can accommodate only a small volume of medication. If the pressure of injection increases, withdraw ¹⁄₁₆".

INJECTION AFTERCARE

1) *Rest* for 3 days avoiding all gripping, grasping, extremes of motion, vibration, and cold.

2) *Ice* (15 minutes every 4 to 6 hours) and *Tylenol ES* (1000 mg twice a day) for soreness.

3) *Protect* the fingers for 3 to 4 weeks by avoiding repetitive gripping, grasping, pressure over the MCP heads, and vibration, or use a Velcro wrist immobilizer with a metal stay for advanced disease.

4) Begin passively performed range-of-motion *stretching exercises* in flexion and extension at 2 to 3 weeks.

5) Begin isometrically performed *gripping exercises* at 4 to 5 weeks.

6) Repeat *injection* at 6 weeks with corticosteroid if swelling persists or if range of motion is still affected.

7) Suggest padded gloves or padded tools for long-term prevention in recurrent cases.

8) Obtain a *consultation* with a surgical orthopedist if two consecutive injections fail to resolve the condition.

SURGICAL PROCEDURE. Metacarpophalangeal joint implant arthroplasty (replacement) is used in carefully selected cases. Patients with severe disease manifested by a loss of 50% of range of motion and near total loss of the articular cartilage are the optimal candidates for replacement.

PROGNOSIS. The majority of patients respond favorably to a combination of immobilization and corticosteroid injection. However, the long-term outcome for patients with posttraumatic monoarticular involvement of the MCP is dependent on the damage suffered by the articular cartilage, the associated bony fracture with persistent deformity (poorly aligned Boxer fracture), and the physical demands placed on the joint.

Osteoarthritis of the Hand

Only the PIP joint can be injected easily; enter at the joint line, ¼" beyond the distal end of the proximal phalanges above the midplane.

Needle: ⅝", 25 gauge

Depth: ¼ to ⅜"

Volume: ¼ to ½ ml of anesthetic plus ⅛ ml of K40

Note: Use small amounts of anesthetic; the joint will accept only small volumes.

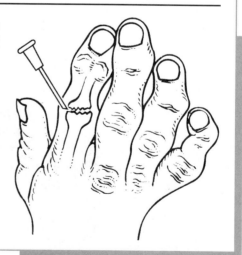

Figure 5–5.   Proximal interphalangeal (PIP) joint injection

DESCRIPTION.   Osteoarthritis of the small joints of the hand is a universal problem. It occurs as a result of age or injury or because of an imbalance in the musculoskeletal system. It is characterized by relatively painless bony enlargement and bony deformity of the small joints of the hand. Involvement of the distal interphalangeal (DIP) joints or the Heberden nodes is most common. A smaller number of patients have involvement at the proximal interphalangeal joints or Bouchard nodes. X-rays demonstrate asymmetric wear of the articular cartilage. Reactive bony osteophytes are characteristic of this wear-and-tear arthritis. A family history, heavy use, and repeated exposure to vibratory tools are all associated with an increased susceptibility.

SYMPTOMS.   Most patients complain of bony enlargement of the fingers and seek confirmation of their self-diagnosis. A small number of patients experience acute inflammatory flares that manifest as pain and swelling in a single or in multiple joints and are known as inflammatory osteoarthritis. Many patients look at their hands, describe the deformity, and rub the individual fingers as they describe the condition.

"Am I getting what my grandma called 'old-age arthritis'?"
"I hate my hands. They're so crooked and ugly."
"Look at my hands; I'm really getting older."
"I can't make a fist anymore; my fingers won't close."
"My hands are a little stiff in the morning, but they really don't hurt that much."
"I know I have arthritis, but my middle knuckle is so much bigger than the others and it won't bend."

EXAM.   Each patient is examined for bony enlargement, loss of finger flexibility, and signs of inflammation involving the DIP and PIP joints of the hand.

EXAM SUMMARY

1. Bony enlargement of the DIP and PIP joints
2. Inability to fully flex the fingers to make a fist
3. Angulation of the DIP and PIP joints
4. Relative absence of inflammatory changes (synovitis), except in the inflammatory subtype

(1) The DIP and PIP joints have bony enlargement palpable along the sides of the joints. The involvement is greater in the DIP joints in most cases. (2) As the disease progresses, the flexibility of the fingers gradually decreases, creating the typical deformities. The patient is unable to make a fist. Extension of the fingers may be impaired. The DIP joints may sublux to the ulnar side. (3) Inflammation and synovitis are notably absent, except in patients with the subtype of erosive, inflammatory osteoarthritis. This condition is typically seen in young women and presents with swelling, heat, and boggy enlargement of the DIP and PIP joints. (4) The end-stage form of the disease is characterized by large, palpable bony osteophytes, decreased range of motion of the DIP and PIP joints, ankylosis of some joints, and atrophy of the intrinsic muscles of the hand.

X-RAYS.   Routine x-rays of the hand (including the PA and lateral views) are always recommended and are diagnostic. Distribution among joints can be accurately assessed. Asymmetric narrowing of the articular cartilage and bony osteophyte formation on either side of the joint line are characteristic. Advanced cases show ever-increasing ulnar deviation, subchondral cyst formation, and ankylosis. The periarticular erosions so typical of rheumatoid arthritis are notably absent.

DIAGNOSIS.   The characteristic changes of bony enlargement with little inflammatory reaction in the typical joint distribution is highly suggestive of the diagnosis.

Confirmation of the diagnosis, especially in early presentations, is made by the typical changes seen on x-rays.

TREATMENT.   The goals of treatment are to confirm the diagnosis, to advise on proper joint protection, and to reduce acute inflammation and swelling.

Step 1: Define the joint distribution, examine for bony osteophytes, and order x-rays of the hand (PA and lateral views).

> Educate the patient: "This is wear-and-tear arthritis that results from aging."

> Advise on avoiding the extremes of position and repetitive gripping and grasping.

> Limit exposure to vibration (vacuum cleaners, lawn mowers, and tools that vibrate).

> Prescribe coated aspirin or acetaminophen as an alternative to the NSAIDs.

> Apply heat, including paraffin treatments.

> Avoid exposure to cold.

Step 2 (weeks to years for acute flares): For inflammatory flares, recommend simple immobilization with buddy-taping (p. 293) or a tube splint (p. 293).

> Perform a local injection of K40 into the fingers with prominent swelling or heat.

PHYSICAL THERAPY.   Physical therapy plays a minor role in the overall treatment of osteoarthritis, simply because most patients do not seek medical treatment or experience symptoms severe enough to justify intervention. However, application of heat to the affected joints in warm to hot water and avoidance of exposure to cold are always recommended. Gentle stretching exercises in extension and toning exercises involving gentle gripping (p. 263) are recommended to preserve function.

INJECTION.   Occasionally, an isolated small joint of the hand will present with enlargement, pain, and swelling that are disproportionate to that being experienced in the other joints of the hand (enough swelling to interfere with the full flexion of the joint). A history of trauma is often obtained. The symptoms gradually develop over weeks, as opposed to the acute presentation of a monoarticular infective arthritis that occurs over hours or days. This monoarticular traumatic arthritis is an acute flare of an underlying osteoarthritis joint and is often very responsive to intra-articular injection.

PROGNOSIS.   The course of osteoarthritis is extremely variable. The prognosis is determined by hereditary factors, exposure to vibration, and heavy repetitive use. Any treatment, including injection, is palliative. Surgery is rarely indicated and should be discouraged. Cyst removal, resection of prominent osteophytes, and other procedures on the small joints lead to significant periarticular scarring, joint stiffness, and permanent joint contracture, all of which may have a greater effect on joint function than does the arthritis itself!

DESCRIPTION.   Rheumatoid arthritis (RA) is an inflammatory arthritis that can present in a variety of ways. Classic RA presents as a symmetric, polyarticular, small-joint arthritis affecting the MCP, PIP, and MTP joints. It is characterized by fusiform swelling and by synovial thickening around these joints. Nonclassic RA may present in a single joint (monoarticular) or in several medium to large joints (pauciarticular) or as a fleeting, small-joint arthritis that affects the small joints (palindromic). All are characterized by moderately intense inflammation and swelling.

Rheumatoid Arthritis

Enter at the joint line above the mid-plane.

Needle: ⅝″, 25 gauge

Depth: ¼ to ⅜″

Volume: ⅛ to ¼ ml of K40 after minimal subcutaneous anesthesia

Note: This is an injection under the synovial membrane and not directly between the articular surfaces of the bones.

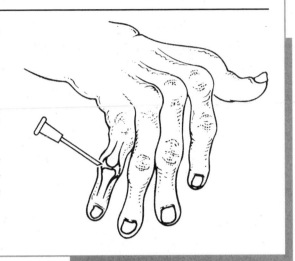

Figure 5–6.   Proximal interphalangeal joint injection

SYMPTOMS. Depending on the clinical presentation, the patient complains of fatigue and diffuse arthralgias, small-joint stiffness and swelling, or stiffness, swelling, and loss of mobility in a particular joint.

"My hands have been swelling at the knuckles."
"I have to put my hands in hot running water in the morning to get rid of the horrible stiffness."
"I'm losing my grip. I can't hold onto my tools any longer."
"My hands hurt so much that it's even hard to pull up the sheets on the bed."
"The balls of my feet are so tender, I can't wear my shoes any longer."
"Every time I go up the stairs, the balls of my feet hurt."
"My knee is swollen and feverish."
"I can't straighten my elbows all the way."

EXAM. Each patient is examined for joint inflammation, swelling, and deformity along with a careful documentation of the involvement of the small, medium, and large joints of the skeleton.

EXAM SUMMARY   • • • • • • • • • • • • • • • •

1. Early: a normal exam and subtle swelling in the MCPs, PIPs, or MTPs
2. The MCP or MTP squeeze signs create dramatic pain
3. Joint enlargement due to synovial thickening
4. Loss of joint mobility
5. Deformity: ulnar deviation, subluxation, hammer toes, and so forth

(1) The earliest findings in RA may be so subtle or so evanescent (depending on the time of day) as to escape detection by the examiner. (2) As the condition advances, swelling appears. Squeezing the MCPs or MTPs together from side to side is a useful, quick screening sign for hand and foot involvement. (3) Otherwise, individual joints

are inspected and palpated for swelling and thickening. For the PIP joints, this is best accomplished by alternating compression of the joint with four fingers. One finger is placed above the joint and one below, and a finger is placed along each side of the joint. Pressure is alternated back and forth to feel for synovial thickening. (4) As the condition progresses, finger flexibility becomes impaired, the hand becomes doughy and loose due to ligamentous laxity, and the intrinsic muscles of the hand begin to waste. (5) Ulnar deviation of the MCPs eventually develops. The hand generally loses its strength.

Early involvement of the wrist is associated with subtle swelling dorsally and dramatic degrees of pain when passively moving the joint to the extremes of full dorsiflexion and volarflexion. Involvement of the elbow is associated with a loss of full extension and lateral joint line swelling (the "bulge sign" appears halfway between the olecranon process and the lateral epicondyle). Early involvement of the ankle is associated with general swelling anteriorly, loss of the contours around the medial and lateral malleoli, and pain at the extremes of full plantarflexion and dorsiflexion. Knee involvement is almost always associated with a moderate suprapatellar effusion, warmth anteriorly, and loss of full flexion.

X-RAYS.   X-rays of the hand (including PA and lateral views) are always indicated. Early plain x-rays are often normal or show only subtle juxta-articular osteoporosis. As the condition progresses, osteoporosis becomes more obvious, symmetric loss of articular cartilage develops, and joint erosions form close to the lateral margins of the joints, usually the MCP and PIP joints.

DIAGNOSIS.   The diagnosis of RA may be elusive early in the course of the disease. It is based on the clinical findings of a symmetric, small-joint pattern of stiffness, pain, and swelling (classic RA) or on the demonstration of an inflammatory effusion (pauciarticular or monoarticular RA). In some cases, reexamination and reevaluation may be necessary at 1- to 2-month intervals until the case "blossoms." Plain films of the hand can be helpful in determining the extent and severity of the disease but cannot replace the clinical clues from the history and on examination.

Note that the RA factor should *not* be relied on as a screening test for patients presenting with arthralgia or arthritis. It may take 6 to 9 months for this serologic marker to become positive, and at least 15% of patients with a clinical diagnosis of RA are seronegative.

TREATMENT.   The goals of treatment are to confirm the diagnosis, to stage the extent of the disease, and to begin step-by-step care to reduce pain and inflammation. Systemic treatment with oral medication is the treatment of choice.

Step 1: Define the distribution among joints, examine for acute synovitis, and order x-rays of the hand (PA and lateral views).

Reduce repetitive, fine finger motions and heavy gripping and grasping.

Modify the work schedule, adding rest periods in between periods of repetitive handwork.

Encourage the patient to remain active, balancing periods of rest with activity.

Recommend gentle, passive stretching exercises (p. 263).

Avoid exposure to vibration (vacuum cleaners, lawn mowers, and tools that vibrate).

Offer salicylates, extra-strength Tylenol, or an NSAID for moderate disease.

Recommend heat to reduce stiffness (warm water, shower, paraffin treatments, and so forth).

Minimize the use of narcotics.

Step 2 (months to years for persistent or progressive disease): Alternate between chemical classes of the NSAIDs to maintain efficacy.

Perform a local injection for flares in isolated joints (always performing synovial fluid analysis to exclude infection if one joint is disproportionately inflamed).

Consider a consultation with a rheumatologist in the case of progressive disease.

Perform an intramuscular injection of 2 ml of K40 to reduce the mild to moderate flare.

Prescribe gold salts, hydroxychloroquine (Plaquenil), penicillamine, or metho-trexate for the progressive or advanced case.

Use a moderate dose of oral prednisone for 1 to 2 months, with a slow taper to reduce the intensity of a moderate to severe flare (30 to 40 mg per day, tapering by 5 mg until 10 to 15 mg is reached and then by 1 to 2 mg increments until the course is completed; when tapering, never reduce the dose by more than 10 to 15%).

Limit narcotics to severe flares and to a specified number per week or month.

Avoid chronic use of oral corticosteroids.

Step 3 (years for chronic arthritis): Request an orthopedic consultation for joint replace-ment when severe deformity accompanies dramatic functional impairment.

PHYSICAL THERAPY: Physical and occupational therapy play a very important role in the overall management of RA, especially in the late stages.

PHYSICAL THERAPY SUMMARY • • • • • • • • • • • • • • • •

1. Ice for any acutely inflamed joint
2. Phonophoresis with a hydrocortisone gel applied to the small joints of the hands
3. Heating to reduce morning stiffness
4. Gentle, passively performed stretching exercises to preserve range of motion
5. Isometrically performed toning exercises, especially for the large and medium-sized joints
6. Occupational therapy (specialized splints, occupational aids)
7. Low-impact aerobic exercises as tolerated

Acute Period.   *Ice* and *phonophoresis* using a hydrocortisone gel provide temporary relief of pain and swelling. Immobilization (wrist splinting, buddy-tape, and so forth) enhance the effectiveness of these treatments.

Recovery/Rehabilitation.   *Heating,* often discovered and used regularly by the pa-tient, is used to reduce the gel phenomenon and morning stiffness. *Range-of-motion* exercises are mandatory to preserve joint flexibility and to guard against tendon contracture. Medium and large joints must be supported by well-toned muscles. If the patient has lost significant motor function due to chronic arthritis or deformity, *isometric toning exercises* must be used as a substitute for regular activities. *Occupational therapy* consultation should be considered if chronic arthritis or deformity interferes with the activities of daily living. Low-impact *aerobic exercising* is recommended for general conditioning.

INJECTION: Many patients with early presentations of rheumatoid arthritis, especially the monoarticular and pauciarticular forms, can be successfully managed with local corticosteroid injection.

Positioning: The hand is placed flat, with the palm down and the fingers extended.

Surface Anatomy and Point of Entry: The distal portion of the proximal phalanges is located and marked. The point of entry is above the midplane of the finger, ¼" distal to the proximal phalanges at the joint line.

Angle of Entry and Depth: The needle is inserted perpendicular to the skin. The depth of injection is ¼ to ⅜".

Anesthesia: Ethyl chloride is sprayed on the skin. Because the depth of the synovial membrane is so superficial, injection of local anesthetic in the subcutaneous tissue (¼ ml) is optional.

Technique: These small joints can accommodate only a small volume, so anesthesia should be kept to a minimum. The 25-gauge needle is advanced through the synovial membrane and down to the adjacent bone. Note that the joint is *not* entered directly. Passing a needle into the center of the joint is difficult, painful, and potentially dangerous (cartilage damage)! With the needle held flush against the bone, the medication is injected under the synovial membrane. Moderate pressure may be needed. If excess pressure or pain is experienced with injection, the needle is withdrawn 1/16".

INJECTION AFTERCARE:

1) *Rest* for 3 days, avoiding all gripping, grasping, and pinching.

2) Use buddy-taping to the adjacent PIP joint for the first few days.

3) *Ice* (15 minutes every 4 to 6 hours) and *Tylenol ES* (1000 mg twice a day) for soreness.

4) Suggest padded gloves or padded tools for long-term prevention in recurrent cases.

5) *Protect* for 3 to 4 weeks by limiting repetitive gripping, grasping, and pinching.

6) Begin passive range-of-motion *stretching exercises* in flexion and extension at 2 to 3 weeks.

7) Begin isometrically performed *gripping exercises* at 4 to 5 weeks.

8) Repeat *injection* at 6 weeks if swelling persists or if range of motion is still affected.

SURGICAL PROCEDURE: Patients with refractory inflammatory change, severe loss of articular cartilage, or dramatic functional impairment should be offered surgical consultation. Synovectomy for the large joints, arthroscopic débridement for medium and large joints, arthroplasty for the shoulder, hip, and knee, and implant arthroplasty (replacement) for the small joints are the procedures most often recommended.

PROGNOSIS: Most patients with early presentations of rheumatoid arthritis, especially the monoarticular and pauciarticular forms, can be successfully managed with local corticosteroid injection. However, as the disease progresses to multiple joint involvement, systemic treatment with oral medication should be initiated. The decision to start hydroxychloroquine (Plaquenil), gold, penicillamine, or methotrexate should not be delayed. These "remitting" drugs may take months to have an appreciable clinical effect.

Patients with progressive deformity and severe functional impairment should be evaluated by an orthopedic surgeon for synovectomy (large joints), arthroscopic débridement (medium and large joints), arthroplasty (shoulder, hip, and knee), or implant arthroplasty (small joints).

chapter 6

Chest

Sternochondritis/Costochondritis

Enter atop the center of the rib; angle the syringe perpendicular to the skin.

Needle: ⅝″, 25 gauge

Depth: ½ to 1″, depending on the site

Volume: 1 to 2 ml of local anesthetic and ½ ml of either D80 or K40

Note: The injections should be placed flush against the costochondral junction, using mild pressure.

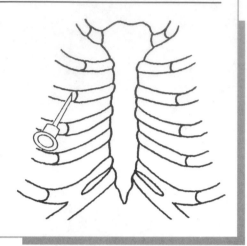

Figure 6–1.   Costochondritis injection

DESCRIPTION.   Costochondritis is the term most clinicians use when referring to the inflammation of the cartilage of the chest wall. Specifically, costochondritis is the inflammation that occurs at the junction of the rib and the costal cartilage. In contrast, sternochondritis is the term applied to the inflammation that occurs at the junction of the sternum and the costal cartilage. Most cases are of unproven cause (idiopathic), although a rare case follows open-heart surgery. Tietze syndrome, often used synonymously with costochondritis, is a distinct form of it. This rare disorder is characterized by dramatic bulbous swelling in addition to the local inflammatory changes. The majority of cases resolve spontaneously over several weeks.

SYMPTOMS.   Most patients complain of anterior chest pain or anterior chest pain overshadowed by the classic symptoms of anxiety (unfortunately, patients are likely to confuse this pain with coronary pain, especially if they have a positive family history of heart disease). Patients often rub the anterior chest wall when describing the condition.

"I think I'm having a heart attack!"
"It hurts right here (pointing to the parasternal area with one or two fingers) whenever I cough or take a deep breath."
"I can't sleep on my left side at night . . . whenever I roll over onto my side, I get this sharp pain in my chest."
"Ever since my bypass, I've had this sharp pain along the side of my incision."
"Coughing just kills me."
"It's like there is sandpaper between the ends of my ribs. It feels like the flesh has pulled away from the bone."

EXAM.   Each patient is examined for localized tenderness and swelling at the costochondral or the sternochondral junctions and for pain aggravated by chest wall compression.

1. Localized tenderness either 1″ from the midline of the sternum or at the costochondral junctions
2. Pain reproduced by chest wall compression (the rib compression test)
3. Pain relief with regional anesthetic block just over the cartilage

(1) Localized tenderness is palpable at the junction of the sternum and the costal cartilage or at the junction between the rib and the costal cartilage. The intercostal spaces should be nontender. The sternochondral junctions are ¾ to 1″ lateral to the midline. The costochondral junctions vary from 3 to 4″ from the midline. (2) Compression of the rib cage usually reproduces the patient's local chest wall pain. Pressure applied in the anteroposterior direction or from either side reproduces the discomfort. Similarly, a deep cough should recreate the pain. (3) The diagnosis is confirmed by a regional anesthetic block just atop the junction of the cartilage and bone.

X-RAYS.   The patient's expectations for x-rays or special studies are always high with this condition. Routine chest x-rays and plain films of the ribs are often ordered, but they are normal in the majority of cases. No specific changes are seen. Similarly, special testing is often ordered (bone scan, MRI, and so forth) to exclude bony pathology or disease inside the chest. Once again, no specific abnormalities are seen that would assist in the diagnosis of costochondritis.

SPECIAL TESTING.   Local anesthetic block is diagnostic!

DIAGNOSIS.   The diagnosis is suggested by a history of localized chest pain and by an exam showing local tenderness aggravated by chest compression. The diagnosis can be confirmed by regional anesthetic block. The rapid control of chest pain with this simple, superficially placed injection is particularly useful in the anxious patient.

TREATMENT.   The goals of treatment are to reassure the patient that this is not a life-threatening heart problem and to reduce the local inflammation. Observation and restriction of chest expansion and direct pressure are the treatments of choice for the patient with mild symptoms that have been present only 4 to 6 weeks. Corticosteroid injection is the treatment of choice for the patient with persistent or dramatic symptoms.

Step 1: Perform a careful exam of the chest wall, heart, and lungs, identify the chondral junctions that are most involved, and order a chest x-ray and ECG for the anxious patient.

Educate the patient: "This is not a heart pain!" "Most cases resolve on their own."

Reassure the patient that the condition is benign.

Perform a regional anesthetic block to confirm the diagnosis or to reassure the severely anxious patient.

Observe for 2 to 3 weeks.

Prescribe a cough suppressant when indicated.

Prescribe a rib binder or a neoprene waist wrap (p. 295) or a snug-fitting bra (do not use for the debilitated patient or for a patient older than 65 years of age).

Restrict lying on the sides, lifting, and strenuous activity.

Step 2 (3 to 4 weeks for persistent cases): Perform a local anesthetic block and inject ½ ml of D80.

Continue the restrictions.

Step 3 (3 to 4 weeks for persistent cases): Repeat the injection in 6 weeks if pain continues.

Combine the injection with a rib binder.

Continue the restrictions.

PHYSICAL THERAPY.   Physical therapy does not play a significant role in the treatment of costochondritis. Phonophoresis with a hydrocortisone gel has questionable value.

INJECTION.   Local anesthetic injection is used to differentiate the pain arising from the chest wall from coronary artery chest pain, pleuritic chest pain, or other causes of anterior chest pain. Corticosteroid injection is used to treat symptoms that persist beyond 6 to 8 weeks.

Positioning: The patient is to be in the supine position.

Surface Anatomy and the Point of Entry: The point of maximum tenderness atop the cartilage is carefully palpated. The center point of the cartilage is identified by placing one finger above and one finger below the cartilage in the intercostal spaces. The point of entry for sternochondritis is 1″ from the midline of the sternum, directly over the center of the cartilage. The point of entry for costochondritis is over the point of maximum tenderness along the rib, directly over the center of the cartilage.

Angle of Entry and Depth: The needle is inserted perpendicular to the skin. The depth of injection is ½″ for sternochondritis and ½ to 1″ for costochondritis.

Anesthesia: Ethyl chloride is sprayed on the skin. Local anesthetic is placed in the subcutaneous tissue (½ ml) and just above the firm resistance of the cartilage or the hard resistance of the bone.

Technique: Successful treatment depends on the identification of the most involved costal cartilage and the accurate localization of the junction of the cartilage and the bone. The most seriously affected costal cartilage is identified either by careful palpation of the most painful junction or by local anesthetic block. The needle is centered over the rib and is gently advanced down to the firm resistance of the cartilage or the hard resistance of the bone. With the needle left in place, ½ ml of K40 or D80 is injected flush against the cartilage.

INJECTION AFTERCARE

1) *Rest* for 3 days, avoiding lying on the sides, lifting, and strenuous activities.

2) Combine the injection with a rib binder (or wide bra) for the first few days (especially for persistent or recurrent cases).

3) *Ice* (15 minutes every 4 to 6 hours) and *Tylenol ES* (1000 mg twice a day) for soreness.

4) *Protect* the chest wall for 3 to 4 weeks by limiting lying on the sides, lifting, and strenuous activities and by aggressively treating coughing and sneezing.

5) Repeat *injection* at 6 weeks if local irritation continues.

SURGICAL PROCEDURE.   None.

PROGNOSIS.   Since most cases resolve spontaneously within 4 to 6 weeks, specific treatments may not be necessary. In the small number of cases that persist beyond 4 to 6 weeks, local injection can provide excellent palliation of symptoms.

Sternoclavicular Joint

Enter atop the center of the proximal clavicle, with the needle perpendicular to the skin.

Needle: ⅝", 25 gauge

Depth: ⅜ to ½"

Volume: 1 ml of local anesthetic and ½ ml of K40

Note: The injection should be placed flush against the periosteum of the bone under the synovial membrane of the joint.

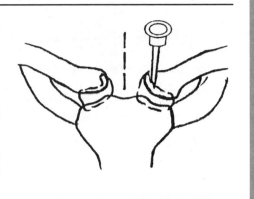

Figure 6–2. Sternoclavicular joint injection

DESCRIPTION. Anterior swelling and inflammation of the sternoclavicular (SC) joint are uncommon. Septic arthritis with severe swelling, redness, and pain is an unusual complication of intravenous drug abuse. Moderate inflammatory change can occur in Reiter disease. Mild to moderate swelling of the joint and pseudoenlargement of the proximal end of the clavicle can occur as a long-term consequence of trauma.

SYMPTOMS. The patient complains of pain, swelling, or enlargment of the joint. The patient rubs over the swollen joint when describing the condition.

"My bone is growing."
"I can't sleep on my right side. The pain over my breast bone wakes me up."
"My breast bone is sore and swollen."
"I hate those stupid shoulder belts. I had a mild head-on collision and ever since the accident, my collar bone has been swollen."

EXAM. The patient is examined for swelling, tenderness, and subluxation of the sternoclavicular joint.

EXAM SUMMARY ● ● ● ● ● ● ● ● ● ● ● ● ● ● ●

1. Tenderness and swelling over the joint
2. Pseudoenlargement of the proximal end of the clavicle
3. Pain aggravated by adducting the arm across the chest, passively performed
4. Local anesthetic block to confirm the diagnosis

(1) The SC joint is tender and swollen ¾ to 1" lateral to the midline, directly across from the sternal notch. (2) The proximal end of the clavicle often appears enlarged; this is the pseudoenlargement of the joint. Swelling of the joint gives the appearance of bony enlargement but also contributes to anterior subluxation of the clavicle. (3) Pain arising from the SC joint is predictably aggravated by passive adduction of the arm across the chest. This forces the clavicle against the sternum,

compressing the joint. (4) Finally, local anesthesia placed at the joint will confirm the diagnosis.

X-RAYS.   Apical lordotic x-rays of the upper chest will adequately assess the clavicle and sternum bones. Careful comparison of the contours of the sternum and the size and relative shape of the proximal ends of the clavicles should not disclose any asymmetry.

SPECIAL TESTING.   Because of the obvious enlargement of the joint and the appearance of enlargement of the proximal end of the clavicle, many patients are evaluated with bone scanning, CT scanning, or even MRI. None of these tests is diagnostic of sternoclavicular arthritis.

DIAGNOSIS.   The diagnosis is suggested by the typical findings of exam (local tenderness and swelling at the joint) and is confirmed by local anesthetic block placed just atop the joint. X-rays and special testing are used to rule out infection and tumor.

TREATMENT.   The goal of treatment is to reduce the local swelling that has led to the pseudoenlargement of the joint. For the patient with mild symptoms that have been present only 4 to 6 weeks, direct application of ice is combined with restrictions on shoulder adduction and sleeping on the affected side. For the patient with persistent or dramatic symptoms, local anesthetic block combined with corticosteroid injection is the treatment of choice.

Step 1: Order apical lordotic x-rays of the chest, confirm the diagnosis with local anesthesia, and reassure the patient that this is simply an enlargement of the joint due to swelling and subluxation.

Recommend ice over the joint to temporarily reduce pain and swelling.

Advise avoiding to-and-fro motions of the upper arm.

Avoid sleeping on the affected shoulder.

Prescribe an antitussive if an acute cough develops.

Step 2 (4 to 6 weeks for persistent cases): Perform a local injection of K40.

Reemphasize the restrictions.

Step 3 (8 to10 weeks for persistent cases): Repeat the local injection of K40 if the first injection does not reduce swelling and pain by 50%.

Combine the injection with a shoulder immobilizer for 2 to 3 weeks.

PHYSICAL THERAPY.   Physical therapy does not play a significant role in the treatment or rehabilitation of this condition. Ice can be applied directly over the top of the joint for temporary control of symptoms. *General shoulder conditioning* is recommended after the acute symptoms have resolved. In order to avoid aggravating the joint, military press, bench press, and pectoralis exercises should be limited.

INJECTION.   Local anesthetic injection is used to identify the SC joint as the source of anterior chest wall swelling and pain. This is especially necessary when the patient complains that the "bone is growing"—the pseudoenlargement of the proximal clavicle. Corticosteroid injection is used to treat symptoms that have persisted beyond 6 to 8 weeks.

Positioning: The patient is to be in the supine position.

Surface Anatomy and the Point of Entry: The midline, the sternal notch, and the center of the proximal clavicle are identified and marked. The point of entry is ¾ to 1" from the midline, directly over the center of the proximal clavicle.

Angle of Entry and Depth: The needle is inserted perpendicular to the skin. The depth of injection is ⅜ to ½".

Anesthesia: Ethyl chloride is sprayed on the skin. Local anesthetic is placed in the subcutaneous tissue (¼ ml) and just above the firm to hard resistance of the periosteum of the bone (¼ ml).

Technique: The success of treatment depends on the accurate localization of the point of entry. After confirming the diagnosis with local anesthesia, the syringe containing the anesthetic is replaced with the second syringe containing ½ ml of K40. The needle is advanced down to the hard resistance of the bone. With just the weight of the syringe against the periosteum, the corticosteroid is injected flush against the bone.

INJECTION AFTERCARE

1) *Rest* for 3 days, avoiding sleeping on the affected side, reaching, lifting, and all strenuous activities.

2) *Ice* (15 minutes every 4 to 6 hours) and *Tylenol ES* (1000 mg twice a day) for soreness.

3) *Protect* for 3 to 4 weeks by limiting sleeping on the affected side, reaching, lifting, and all strenuous activities.

4) Combine the injection with a shoulder immobilizer for 3 to 7 days for persistent or recurrent cases.

5) Repeat the *injection* at 6 weeks if swelling persists or if range of motion is still affected.

SURGICAL PROCEDURE.   None.

PROGNOSIS.   Most patients that present with swelling in the SC joint are concerned that the bone is growing. Apical lordotic views will confirm the normal size of the proximal clavicles. CT scanning and MRI of the chest are not necessary. Local anesthetic block is an integral part of the diagnosis and is very helpful in allaying the patient's anxiety (*"The bone appears larger because of the deep swelling that forces the bone outward!"*).

chapter 7

Back

Lumbosacral Strain

Occasionally a patient presents with very localized tenderness in the erector spinae muscle; dramatic relief with local anesthesia is the best indication for corticosteroid injection.

Needle: 1½", 22 gauge

Depth: 1¼ to 1½"

Volume: 2 to 3 ml of anesthesia plus 1 ml of D80

Note: Place the anesthesia at the first tissue plane—the erector spinae fascia—and then enter the muscle three times to cover an area of approximately 1".

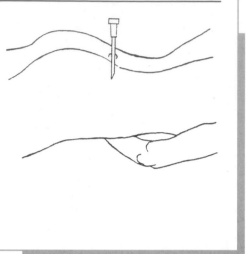

Figure 7–1.   Acute lumbosacral back muscle injection

DESCRIPTION.   Lumbosacral (LS) strain is a spasm and irritation of the supporting muscles of the lumbar spine and is the end result of many different conditions. Repetitive use of improperly stretched and toned muscles is the most common cause of this reactive muscle spasm. Other causes include poor posture, scoliosis, spondylolisthesis, advanced osteoarthritis (spinal stenosis), compression fracture, radiculopathy from any cause, and so forth. It is the body's natural reaction to the threat of injury to the spinal nerve, root, or cord. Severe and persistent muscle spasm can lead to secondary problems, including acquired scoliosis (reversible), a loss of the normal lumbosacral kyphotic curve, "sensory" sciatica (common and reversible), and trochanteric or gluteus medius bursitis (the principal cause of these conditions).

SYMPTOMS.   The patient complains of a well-localized lower back pain and muscle stiffness. The patient often rubs the lower back and flank when describing the condition.

"Oh, my aching back."
"My back is so stiff in the morning I can hardly straighten up . . . I have to take a long hot shower to loosen up."
"I used to be able to touch my toes."
"I get these terrible back spasms right here (using the hand to rub the side of the lower back)."
"I can't find a comfortable chair to sit in anymore . . . I've tried everything from hardbacks to recliners."
"I can't bend forward without my back killing me."
"I can't find a comfortable position in bed, let alone a comfortable mattress."
"I don't want to end up like my father, all hunched over and unable to bend over."

EXAM.   Each patient is examined for the degree of paraspinal muscle spasm and tenderness, and an assessment is made of the loss of range of motion of the back.

EXAM SUMMARY ● ● ● ● ● ● ● ● ● ● ● ● ● ● ●

1. Paraspinal muscle tenderness and spasm
2. Straightening of the LS curve
3. Decreased LS flexion (abnormal Schober measurement) and lateral bending
4. A normal neurologic exam, unless there is concomitant radiculopathy

(1) The maximum paraspinal muscle tightening is 1 1/2" off the midline, adjacent to L3–L4. A second common trigger point is at the origin of the erector spinae, just above the sacroiliac joint. (2) The normal LS lordotic curve is straightened in the case of severe muscle spasm. If the strain is unilateral, the back may tilt to the affected side (an "acquired," or reversible, scoliosis). (3) Measurements of LS flexion and lateral bending are impaired. The Schober test, measuring LS flexion, is abnormal in most cases. With the patient standing as erect as possible, 2 lines, 10 cm apart, are marked in the midline just above a line drawn between the iliac crests. The patient is asked to flex forward at the waist. At full LS flexion, the marks are remeasured. A 50% increase to 15 cm is normal. The patient is asked to report any symptoms when flexing forward. In addition, measurements of lateral bending add to the objective measurement of back mobility. Two lines, 20 cm apart, are marked along the flank above the most lateral point of the iliac crest and should increase to 26 cm (a 33% increase) when bending to the side. (4) The neurologic exam of the lower extremity should be normal, unless concomitant radiculopathy is present.

X-RAYS.   LS spine x-rays with oblique views can be very helpful in defining the degree of spondylolisthesis, the severity of the scoliosis, the degree of degenerative disk disease, or the presence of advanced osteoarthritis or in estimating the degree of osteoporosis. Uncomplicated cases of lumbar strain—those unassociated with scoliosis, old compression fractures, and so forth—should have normal x-rays.

SPECIAL TESTING.   Special testing with CT scanning or MRI is indicated when the local back symptoms are accompanied by moderate to severe radicular symptoms, particularly when neurologic symptoms and signs are prominent and the motor system is involved (see "Lumbar Radiculopathy," p. 116).

DIAGNOSIS.   The diagnosis of an uncomplicated lumbosacral strain is based on the presence of pain, tenderness, and spasm localized to the lower back and on the absence of any other significant underlying back processes, such as acute compression fracture, radiculopathy, or epidural processes. If the lumbar strain presentation is atypical (severity of symptoms, intermittent but severe radicular symptoms and signs, unusual injury, and so forth), a work-up for an underlying process should not be delayed.

TREATMENT.   The goals of therapy are to reduce the acute erector spinae muscle spasm, to reduce the tendency of recurrent muscle spasm by stretching and toning exercises, and to treat any underlying structural back condition. Bedrest combined with physical therapy exercises and a muscle relaxant are the treatments of choice.

Step 1: Thoroughly examine the back and perform a complete lower extremity neurologic exam; perform the Schober measurements, order plain x-rays of the LS spine with oblique views, and order a CT scan or an MRI if radicular symptoms are prominent and involve the motor system (refer to "Lumbar Radiculopathy," p. 116).

Avoid twisting and extremes of bending and tilting.

Advise on proper lifting: hold the object close to the body, bend at the knee and not with the back, never lift in a twisted position, carry heavier objects as close as possible to the body.

Reinforce the importance of correct posture; suggest a lumbar support for the office chair and vehicle.

Begin gentle stretching exercises to maintain flexibility (p. 266).

Prescribe a muscle relaxant to be taken at night.

Prescribe an NSAID, but note that the drug may have limited benefit as inflammation is not a significant part of the process.

Use an appropriate amount of narcotics for the first week, but limit their use thereafter.

Apply ice, alternating with heat, to the low back.

Order therapeutic ultrasound from a physical therapist for deep heating.

Recommend 3 to 4 days of bedrest for the acute, severe case.

Use crutches if pain and spasm are severe.

Step 2 (2 to 4 weeks for persistent cases): Reevaluate the neurologic exam and back motion.

Begin strengthening exercises (p. 268).

Begin water aerobics, low-impact walking, or swimming to reestablish general conditioning without stressing the recovering back muscles.

Reduce the use of medication.

Resume normal activities gradually, but with continued attention to proper care of the back.

Step 3 (6 to 8 weeks for chronic cases): If symptoms are chronic, use an LS corset for external support (p. 295).

Order a TENS unit.

Consider the use of a tricyclic antidepressant.

Refer to a pain clinic.

PHYSICAL THERAPY.   Physical therapy is a fundamental part of the treatment of acute and chronic low back strain and is the main treatment for rehabilitation and prevention.

PHYSICAL THERAPY SUMMARY   ● ● ● ● ● ● ● ● ● ● ● ● ● ● ●

1. Ice alternating with heat
2. Aerobic exercises, low impact
3. Stretching exercises for erector spinae, the sacroiliac joint, and the gluteus muscles, passively performed
4. Toning exercises of the back and abdominal muscles, performed with minimal movement of the back
5. Lumbar traction

Acute Period. Cold, heat, and gentle stretching exercises are used in the early treatment of lumbar strain to reduce acute muscular spasm and to increase lumbar flexibility.

Cold, heat, and cold alternating with heat are effective in reducing pain and muscular spasm. Recommendations are based on individual clinical responses. *Stretching exercises* are fundamental for maintaining flexibility, especially in patients with structural back disease. Side-bends, knee-chest pulls, and pelvic rocks—the Williams flexion exercises—are designed to stretch the paraspinal muscles, the gluteus muscles, and the sacroiliac joints (p. 266). These exercises should be started after the hyperacute symptoms have resolved. Stretching is performed after heating the body. Initially, these exercises should be performed while the patient is lying down. As pain and muscular spasm ease, stretching can be performed while the patient is standing. Each exercise is performed in sets of 20. Stretching should never exceed the patient's level of mild discomfort.

Recovery/Rehabilitation. To continue the recovery process and to reduce the possibility of a recurrence, toning exercises are added at 3 to 4 weeks. *Toning exercises* are performed after the acute muscular spasms have subsided. Modified sit-ups, weighted side-bends, and gentle extension exercises (p. 268) are performed after heating and stretching. Aerobic exercise is one of the best ways to prevent recurrence. Swimming, cross-country ski machine workouts, low-impact water aerobics, fast walking, and light jogging are excellent fitness exercises that will be unlikely to aggravate the back.

Traction is used infrequently for acute LS strain. Patients with acute facet syndrome or persistent acute lumbar strain (despite home bedrest, medication, and physical therapy) may respond dramatically to 25 to 35 lb of lumbar traction in bed. In addition, traction can be used at home in combination with traditional stretching exercises (p. 267). *Vertical traction* can be achieved by suspending the legs between two bar stools or leaning against a countertop, or by using inversion equipment. The weight of the body is used to pull the lumbar segments apart. It is used primarily for prevention. It is not appropriate for hyperacute strain.

Chronic back strain unresponsive to traditional physical therapy may require a TENS unit for control of chronic pain.

INJECTION. Local injection of the paraspinal muscles or the lumbar facet joints is infrequently performed and is of questionable overall value. Occasionally a patient will present with very localized tenderness in the erector spinae and respond to local anesthesia. Dramatic relief with anesthesia is the best indication for corticosteroid injection.

Positioning: The patient is to be in the prone position, completely flat.

Surface Anatomy and the Point of Entry: The spinous processes of the LS spine are marked. The point of entry is 1 1/2" from the midline, directly at the point of maximum muscle tenderness at the convexity of the paraspinous muscle.

Angle of Entry and Depth: The needle is inserted perpendicular to the skin. The depth of injection is 1 1/4 to 1 1/2".

Anesthesia: Ethyl chloride is sprayed on the skin. Local anesthetic is placed in the subcutaneous tissue (1/2 ml), just above the moderate resistance of the outer fascia of the muscle (1 ml), and in the muscle belly itself (1 to 2 ml).

Technique: The success of treatment depends on the accurate *intramuscular* injection. A 22-gauge 1 1/2" needle is passed vertically down to the firm, rubbery resistance of the outer fascia of the muscle, approximately 1 to 1 1/4" deep. The muscle is entered three times in an area the size of a quarter. A total of 2 or 3 ml of local anesthetic is injected. The needle is withdrawn and the local tenderness is reevaluated. Local anesthetic injection is sufficient in most cases.

It can be combined with D80 in patients with dramatic improvement after local anesthesia.

INJECTION AFTERCARE

1) *Rest* for 3 days, avoiding all walking, standing, bending, and twisting.

2) Advise bedrest for 3 days and crutches with touch-down weightbearing for severe cases.

3) *Ice* (15 minutes every 4 to 6 hours) and *Tylenol ES* (1000 mg twice a day) for soreness.

4) *Protect* the back for 3 to 4 weeks by limiting prolonged standing, unnecessary walking, repetitive bending, lifting, and twisting.

5) Prescribe a lumbosacral corset for the first 2 to 3 weeks for severe cases.

6) Begin passive *stretching exercises* in flexion (the Williams exercises) when the acute pain has begun to resolve (knee-chest pulls, pelvic rocks, and side-bends).

7) Repeat *injection* at 6 weeks with corticosteroid if pain and muscle spasm persist.

8) Begin active *toning exercises* of the abdominal and lower back muscles once flexibility has been restored.

9) Obtain *plain x-rays, CT scans, or an MRI* to identify the subtle disk, progressive spondylolisthesis, or other correctable conditions in the patient with chronic symptoms.

SURGICAL PROCEDURE.   Surgery is not indicated for the patient with an uncomplicated LS strain. If a correctable, underlying cause is identified (subtle disk, spondylolisthesis, scoliosis, and so forth) and the chance of substantial overall improvement is likely, surgery should be considered.

PROGNOSIS.   The course of low back strain is dependent on the underlying cause and on the patient's willingness to do regular exercises. A patient with persistent symptoms requires evaluation for an underlying cause (often an L4-L5 disk or spinal stenosis). Surgery is indicated when a correctable underlying condition is uncovered.

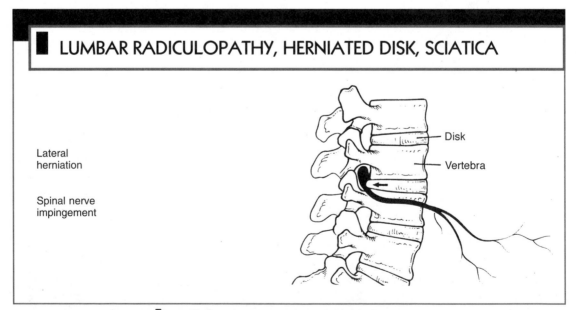

■ LUMBAR RADICULOPATHY, HERNIATED DISK, SCIATICA

Lateral
herniation

Spinal nerve
impingement

Disk

Vertebra

Figure 7–2.   Herniated disk of the lumbar spine

DESCRIPTION.   Sciatica is the term commonly used to describe the pain associated with the abnormal function of the LS nerve roots or of one of the nerves of the LS plexus. Pressure on the nerve from a herniated disk, from bony osteophytes (narrowed lateral recess or spinal stenosis), a compression fracture, or any other extrinsic pressure (for example, epidural process, pelvic mass, or "wallet sciatica") causes progressive sensory, sensorimotor, or sensorimotor visceral loss.

SYMPTOMS. The sciatica pain pattern varies considerably depending on the degree of nerve compression. The patient may complain of pain in the buttock area, pain radiating a variable distance down the lateral or posterior leg, or pain in an isolated part of the lower leg. In addition, the patient may also describe a loss of feeling or an abnormal sensation in the feet (sensory sciatica), weakness or clumsiness of the lower leg (sensorimotor sciatica), or loss of control of bowel or bladder function (visceral involvement).

"I have this shooting pain down my leg. It starts in my hip and goes all the way to my toes."
"My feet feel like they're coming out of Novocain, they're tingling."
"I'm dragging my leg."
"My leg feels weak."
"If I cough, I get this electric shock down my leg."
"If I sit too long, my toes go numb."
"It feels as if I have this burning steel rod in the center of my calf."

EXAM. Each patient is examined for the degree of lower extremity neurologic impairment (sensory, sensorimotor, or sensorimotor visceral) and an evaluation of its underlying cause is made.

EXAM SUMMARY

1. Abnormal straight-leg raising
2. Percussion tenderness over the spinous processes
3. Abnormal neurologic exam: sensory loss, loss of deep tendon reflex, motor weakness, loss of bowel or bladder control
4. Signs of LS strain
5. Signs reflecting the underlying cause

(1) The hallmark sign of sciatica is pain with the straight-leg–raising maneuver. The maneuver should be reproducible in a given position and angle and should reproduce the patient's radicular symptoms in the lower extremity. Forced dorsiflexion of the ankle may be necessary to bring out a subtle case. (2) Percussion tenderness over the spinous processes may be present in cases of acute herniated disks, epidural processes, and other acute vertebal bony processes; however, it is an unreliable sign in spinal stenosis or any process that is outside the vertebral column. (3) Neurologically, loss of sensation in a radicular pattern is the most subtle and earliest sign of nerve dysfunction. Light touch, pinprick, and two-point discrimination are lost early. Advanced conditions may also show loss of deep tendon reflexes, loss of strength of involved muscle groups (foot dorsiflexion and plantarflexion, most commonly), or loss of bowel and urinary control (cauda equina syndrome). (4) Signs of LS muscular strain may accompany sciatica (p. 112). Local paraspinous muscle tenderness and spasm and loss of normal LS flexibility may be present. (5) Finally, signs reflecting the underlying process must be sought if the primary process is not readily evident at the spinal level.

X-RAYS. LS spine x-rays with oblique views can be very helpful in determining the integrity of the vertebral bones, the degree of spondylolisthesis, the presence of compression fractures, and an estimation of the degree of osteoarthritis (exuberant osteophytes or extreme degrees of facet joint sclerotic bone can provide a strong clue to the presence of spinal stenosis. However, plain x-rays of the spine are not effective in determining the specific cause of sciatica.

SPECIAL TESTING.   Defining the exact cause of lumbar radiculopathy requires a CT scan or an MRI. These imaging techniques are mandatory when considering the diagnosis of epidural metastasis or abscess. They provide accurate anatomic measurements of the diameter of the spinal canal (spinal stenosis), the width of the lateral recess exit foramina, the degree of disk herniation along with the presence of nerve compression or spinal cord indentation, the presence of scar tissue from previous laminectomy, the integrity of the vertebral bodies, and the presence of fibrotic tissue associated with spondylolisthesis.

Patients who present with intermediate symptoms and signs and inconclusive imaging may require an electromyogram for evaluation of specific nerve root dysfunction.

DIAGNOSIS.   The diagnosis of sciatica is often based solely on the description of a radicular pain provided by the patient. One of the best neurologic correlates is the patient's description of the location of the pain: down the posterior leg (L5–S1) or down the lateral leg (L4–L5). The neurologic examination is used to stage the severity of the problem (that is sensory, sensorimotor, or sensorimotor visceral). However, definitive diagnosis requires specialized testing!

TREATMENT.   The goals of treatment are to confirm the diagnosis, to reduce the pressure over the nerve, to improve neurologic function, to reduce any accompanying low back strain, and to evaluate for the need for surgery. The treatments of choice vary according to the neurologic findings. Three days of bedrest combined with physical therapy exercises and a muscle relaxant are the treatments of choice for patients with sensory radiculopathy and those with mild motor involvement. Patients with dramatic motor signs can be managed similarly but should undergo early imaging and neurosurgical consultation. Patients with sensorimotor visceral involvement should be hospitalized, seen by the neurosurgeon, and imaged the day of admission.

Step 1: Thoroughly examine the back, perform a Schober measurement, and assess the neurologic function of the lower extremities.

Perform LS spine x-rays or order a CT scan or an MRI, depending on the severity of the signs and symptoms.

Order bedrest for 3 to 5 days for acute symptoms.

Limit walking and standing to 30 to 45 minutes each day.

Advocate the use of crutches to avoid pressure on the back (from bed to the bathroom and back).

Prescribe a muscle relaxant—strong enough to cause mild to moderate sedation—and an appropriate dose of a potent narcotic.

Apply ice to the lower back muscles.

Hospitalize and consult with a neurosurgeon if the patient has bilateral symptoms, extreme motor weakness, incontinence of stool or urine, or urinary retention.

Step 2 (7 to 14 days acute follow-up): Reevaluate the patient's neurologic and back exams.

Begin gentle stretching exercises while the patient is still at bedrest (p. 265).

Use hand-held weights in bed to keep the upper body toned.

Liberalize the amount of time spent out of bed, still relying on crutches.

Use a simple LS corset while out of bed (p. 295).

Consider an injection of the erector spinae muscle with local anesthetic, corticosteroid, or both for muscle spasms that are interfering with the recovery process.

Step 3 (2 to 3 weeks for persistent cases): Reevaluate the patient's neurologic and back exam.

Consider a moderate dose of oral corticosteroid for persistent sensory sciatica (prednisone at 30 to 40 mg for several days, followed by a rapid taper).

Reduce the use of medications.

Begin muscle toning exercises of the lower back (p. 268).

Advise swimming to tone muscles and recondition the cardiovascular system.

Use crutches to assist in ambulation until the patient has recovered sufficient muscle tone of the back.

Emphasize proper care of the back.

Step 4 (3 to 6 weeks for persistent cases or worsening symptoms): Order a neurosurgical consultation if motor symptoms intervene, persist, or progress.

Refer the patient to an anesthesiologist for an epidural steroid injection in the case of persistent sensory sciatica.

Resume normal activities gradually, but with continued attention to proper care of the back.

If symptoms are chronic, use an LS corset for external support (p. 295), order a TENS unit, consider the use of a tricyclic antidepressant, or refer to a pain clinic.

PHYSICAL THERAPY. Physical therapy plays an integral part in the active treatment and prevention of recurrent sciatica (see "Low Back Strain," p. 112). Greater emphasis is placed on bedrest for the hyperacute symptoms, on crutches to assist in ambulation, and on general muscular toning when at bedrest.

INJECTION. Local injection of the paraspinal muscles or of the lumbar facet joints is infrequently performed and of questionable overall value. Occasionally, a patient will present with very localized tenderness in the erector spinae and respond dramatically to local anesthesia, corticosteroid injection, or both (see "Lumbosacral Strain," p. 112).

SURGICAL PROCEDURE. Large disk herniations, fragmented disk herniations, or osteoarthritic changes causing persistent pressure on the spinal nerve, root, or cord should be considered for diskectomy, decompression laminectomy (spinal stenosis), surgical fusion (unstable vertebral body), and so forth. Surgery is not indicated for intermittent sciatic pain, minor disk bulges, radicular symptoms that do not correlate directly with scan results, and so forth.

PROGNOSIS. Patients with sensory complaints only or with very minimal motor findings do very well with medical treatment. The vast majority (75 to 80%) respond to nonsurgical conservative therapy. Surgical consultation is always indicated for progressive neurologic deficits, large disk herniations associated with dramatic motor loss or incontinence, and fragmented disks with fragments lodged in the neuroforamina and for patients with persistent sensorimotor symptoms that correspond with the anatomic abnormalities on scan.

DESCRIPTION. Sacroiliac strain is an irritation and inflammation of the articulation between the sacrum and the ilium. Symptoms can result from mechanical irritation caused by improper lifting, twisting injuries, direct trauma, or the inflammation

Sacroiliac Strain

Enter 1″ caudal to the posterior superior iliac spine and 1″ lateral to the midline; advance at a 70 degree angle to the firm resistance of the posterior supporting ligaments. Note: the injection should be placed flush against the periosteum at the junction of the sacrum and the ileum and at the maximum depth.

Needle: 1½″, 22 gauge or 3½″, 22 gauge

Depth: 1½ to 2½″

Volume: 1 to 2 ml of local anesthetic and 1 ml of K40

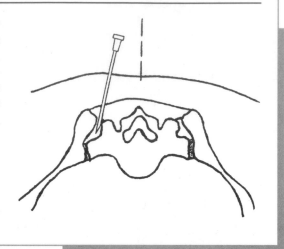

Figure 7–3.   Sacroiliac joint injection

associated with the spondyloarthropathies (Reiter disease, ankylosing spondylitis, or ulcerative-colitis–associated arthritis). This unique cause of low back pain is generally very well localized to the lower lumbosacral spine but can refer pain into the gluteal area or even down the leg, mimicking sciatica.

SYMPTOMS.   The patient complains of a very well-localized pain and stiffness in the bottom of the lumbosacral spine or of pain referred to the gluteal area or down the leg. The patient often rubs the iliac crest and gluteal area when describing the symptoms.

"I have this sharp pain in my buttock every time I twist."
"I'm losing the flexibility in my lower back."
"Sitting has become very painful down here on my left side (pointing to the left lower buttock)."
"It feels like an ice pick is being shoved into my lower back."
"I can't climb into bed very easily, let alone find a comfortable position for any length of time."

EXAM.   Each patient is examined for local irritation of the sacroiliac joint, for flexibility of the lumbosacral spine, and for secondary inflammation of the trochanteric or gluteus medius bursae.

EXAM SUMMARY   • • • • • • • • • • • • • • • •

1. Local tenderness directly over the sacroiliac joint
2. Tenderness aggravated by compression or by pelvic torque (fabere maneuver)
3. Stiffness to the lumbosacral spine (abnormal Schober measurement)
4. Secondary trochanteric or gluteus medius bursa tenderness
5. Dramatic relief with local anesthetic block

(1) Sacroiliac joint tenderness is best identified with the patient lying prone. A quarter-sized area of tenderness is located 1″ medial and 1″ inferior to the posterior superior iliac spine (PSIS). This is in contrast to the local tenderness of the erector spinae muscle located superior to the PSIS and extending well up into the lumbosacral curve. (2) Sacroiliac pain should be aggravated by compression or by the application of torque across the joint. Compression can be accomplished by pushing down on the pelvis when the patient is lying in the lateral decubitus position. Torque can be applied to the joint by placing the hip in a figure-of-four position (p. 270) and simultaneously pushing on the contralateral anterior superior iliac spine (ASIS) and the ipsilateral knee—the Patrick, or fabere (*f*lexion, *ab*duction, *e*xternal *r*otation of the hip), test. (3) As with lumbosacral strain, the patient with sacroiliac irritation may have an abnormal Schober test (p. 113). (4) Trochanteric and gluteus medius bursal irritation can accompany chronic sacroiliac strain. (5) The diagnosis is complete when dramatic relief is achieved with local anesthetic block.

X-RAYS.   A standing AP pelvis x-ray is an excellent screening test for sacroiliitis as well as for leg length discrepancy, osteoarthritis of the hip joint, bony abnormalities of the pelvis and femur, and conditions of the lower lumbosacral spine. If sacroiliitis or sacroiliac strain is likely, oblique views of the pelvis should be obtained for greater anatomic detail. A lumbosacral spine series is indicated if concurrent scoliosis, spondylolisthesis, or other cause of structural back disease is suspected.

SPECIAL TESTING.   Nuclear medicine joint scans or an MRI will provide more detailed information of synovitis or bony erosive disease.

DIAGNOSIS.   The diagnosis of sacroiliac joint disease requires a history of localized lower back pain and an exam demonstrating sacroiliac joint tenderness. The specific diagnosis of sacroiliac strain requires confirmation by local anesthetic block. The specific diagnosis of sacroiliitis requires an elevated sedimentation rate combined with typical changes on plain x-rays (erosive disease) or an abnormal nuclear medicine joint scan. A ratio of radionuclide uptake of the sacroiliac joint to the surrounding iliac bone greater than 1.3 is highly suggestive of sacroiliitis.

TREATMENT.   The goals of treatment are to reduce local inflammation in the sacroiliac joint and to increase the flexibility of the lumbosacral spine and sacroiliac areas. Rest and physical therapy exercises are the treatments of choice for unilateral localized sacroiliac strain. Oral anti-inflammatory medication is the treatment of choice for patients with inflammatory sacroiliitis. Corticosteroid injection is the treatment of choice for patients with persistent or dramatic symptoms of sacroiliac strain.

Step 1: Thoroughly examine the sacroiliac joint, the lumbosacral spine, and the two large bursae at the hip, perform a Schober measurement of lumbosacral flexibility, and order a standing AP pelvis x-ray.

Avoid twisting and extremes of bending and tilting.

Advise on proper lifting involving the knees: hold the object close to the body, bend at the knee and not with the back, never lift in a twisted position, carry heavier objects particularly close to the body.

Reinforce the need to maintain correct posture; suggest a lumbar support for the office chair and vehicle.

Suggest a sacroiliac belt to be worn during the day (p. 295).

Begin William flexion exercises to maintain muscle flexibility (p. 266).

Recommend a muscle relaxant at night if concurrent lumbosacral muscle spasm is present.

Prescribe an NSAID if sacroiliitis is suspected.

Recommend 3 to 4 days of bedrest for the acute, severe case.

Use crutches if pain and spasm are severe.

Step 2 (2 to 4 weeks for persistent cases): Perform a local anesthetic block and inject 1 ml of K40.

Recommend 3 to 4 days of bedrest following the injection.

Continue the restrictions.

Step 3 (6 to 8 weeks for persistent cases): Repeat the corticosteroid injection if symptoms have not improved by at least 50%.

Begin strengthening exercises (p. 268).

Begin general conditioning of the back and gradually increase water aerobics, low-impact walking, or swimming.

Resume normal activities gradually, but with continued attention to proper care of the back.

Step 4 (10 to 12 weeks for chronic cases): Use an LS corset for external support (p. 295).

Order a TENS unit.

Consider the use of a tricyclic antidepressant.

Refer to a pain clinic.

PHYSICAL THERAPY.   Physical therapy plays a fundamental part in the treatment of conditions affecting the sacroiliac joint and is essential for rehabilitation and prevention.

PHYSICAL THERAPY SUMMARY   ● ● ● ● ● ● ● ● ● ● ● ● ● ●

1.   Ice over the sacroiliac joint
2.   Williams flexion exercises (knee-chest, side-bends, and pelvic rocks), performed passively
3.   Toning exercises of erector spinae and the abdominal muscles, performed with minimal motion of the lower spine

Acute Period.   Cold, heat, and gentle stretching exercises are used in the early treatment of sacroiliac strain to reduce the acute muscular spasm that accompanies this localized lower back irritation.

Cold, heat, and cold alternating with heat are effective in reducing pain and muscular spasm. Recommendations are based on individual clinical responses. *Stretching exercises* are fundamental to maintaining sacroiliac and lower back flexibility. Side-bends, knee-chest pulls, and pelvic rocks—the Williams flexion exercises—are designed to stretch the paraspinal muscles, the gluteus muscles, and the sacroiliac joints (p. 266). These exercises should be started after the hyperacute symptoms have resolved. Stretching is performed after the body is heated. Initially, these exercises should be performed while the patient is lying down. As pain and muscular spasm ease, stretching can be performed while the patient is standing. Each exercise is performed in sets of 20. Stretching should never exceed the patient's level of mild discomfort.

Recovery/Rehabilitation.   To continue the recovery process and to reduce the possibility of a recurrence, toning exercises are added at 3 to 4 weeks. *Toning exercises* are performed after the acute muscular spasms have subsided. Modified sit-ups, weighted side-bends, and gentle extension exercises (p. 267) are performed after heating and stretching. Aerobic exercise is one of the best ways to prevent recurrence. Swimming, cross-country ski machine workouts, low-impact water aerobics, fast walking, and light jogging are excellent fitness exercises that will be unlikely to aggravate the back.

Chronic pain arising from the sacroiliac joint unresponsive to traditional physical therapy may require a TENS unit for control of chronic pain.

INJECTION.   Local injection with anesthesia can be used to differentiate conditions affecting the sacroiliac joint from the local irritation and spasm of the paraspinal muscles (the origin of erector spinae), pain arising from the LS spine, or pain arising from the lower LS roots. Corticosteroid injection is used to treat the persistent inflammation of the SI joint that fails to respond to rest, physical therapy exercises, and bracing.

Positioning: The patient is to be in the prone position, perfectly flat.

Surface Anatomy and the Point of Entry: The PSIS is identified and marked. A line is drawn in the midline. The point of entry is 1" caudal to the PSIS and 1" lateral to the midline.

Angle of Entry and Depth: The angle of entry is 70 degrees, with the needle directed outward. The depth of injection is 1 1/2" to 2 1/2" depending on the weight of the patient.

Anesthesia: Ethyl chloride is sprayed on the skin. Ideally, 1 ml of local anesthesia is placed at the joint, the greatest possible depth. However, depending on the sensitivity of the patient, 1/2-ml–volume increments may be injected at the periosteum of the ileum or sacrum as the needle is advanced and redirected to the joint.

Technique: The successful injection of the sacroiliac joint requires a careful passage of the needle to the maximum depth allowable between the iliac and sacral bones (they form an inverted cone, the sacrum and ileum representing the sides and the SI joint representing the apex). The needle is advanced downward until the firm resistance of the periosteum is encountered. If bone is encountered at 1 1/2" the needle is withdrawn 1", redirected approximately 5 degrees, and advanced until the maximum depth is achieved. If the injection is placed accurately, the local anesthetic effect should permit improved flexibility and decreased pain.

INJECTION AFTERCARE

1) *Rest* for 3 days, avoiding all walking, standing, bending, and twisting.

2) Advise bedrest for 3 days and crutches with touch-down–weightbearing.

3) *Ice* (15 minutes every 4 to 6 hours) and *Tylenol ES* (1000 mg twice a day) for soreness.

4) *Protect* the joint for 3 to 4 weeks by limiting prolonged standing, unnecessary walking, and repetitive bending, lifting, and twisting.

5) Prescribe a lumbosacral corset or sacral belt for the first 2 to 3 weeks for severe cases.

6) Begin passive *stretching exercises* in flexion (the Williams exercises) when the acute pain has begun to resolve (knee-chest pulls, pelvic rocks, and side-bends).

7) Repeat *injection* at 6 weeks with corticosteroid if pain and muscle spasm persist.

8) Begin active *toning exercises* of the abdominal and lower back muscles at 4 to 6 weeks.

9) Obtain *plain x-rays* of standing PA pelvis for leg length discrepancy and nuclear medicine bone scan, CT scan, or MRI to identify the sacroiliitis, short leg, and so forth.

SURGICAL PROCEDURE.   None.

PROGNOSIS.   Sacroiliac strain and sacroiliitis uniformly respond to the combination of anti-inflammatory medication and physical therapy exercises. Recurrent irritation often depends on the presence of concomitant lumbosacral conditions.

Patients with scoliosis, spondylolisthesis, compression fracture, and so forth need to perform maintenance stretching and toning exercises to reduce the possibility of recurrence.

chapter 8

Hip

Trochanteric Bursitis

Enter over the midtrochanter in the lateral decubitus position; lightly advance the needle to the firm resistance of the gluteus medius tendon and then ½" farther to the femur.

Needle: 1½", 22 gauge, or a 22-gauge spinal needle

Depth: 1½ to 3", down to the periosteum

Volume: 2 ml of anesthetic and 1 ml of K40

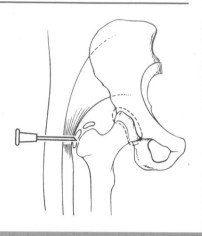

Figure 8–1.   Trochanteric bursa injection

DESCRIPTION.   Trochanteric bursitis is an inflammation of the lubricating sac located between the midportion of the trochanteric process of the femur and the gluteus medius tendon/iliotibial tract. Repetitive flexing of the hip and direct pressure aggravate this condition. A disturbance in gait causes 95% of the cases of trochanteric bursitis. Abnormal patterns of walking and standing lead to increased friction and uneven contraction of the gluteus medius tendon resulting in irritation of the bursa. Common causes of altered gait include underlying lumbosacral back disease (75%), leg length discrepancy (10%), sacroiliac joint disorders (5%), or a lower leg gait disturbance (10%). Osteoarthritis of the hip with its decreased hip motion is a rare cause of bursitis.

SYMPTOMS.   The patient complains of hip pain over the outer thigh or difficulty with walking. The patient often rubs the outer thigh when describing the condition.

"Whenever I roll over onto my right side, this sharp pain in my hip wakes me up."
"I get this achy pain in my hip (pointing to the upper outer thigh) when I walk too much in the mall."
"I can't stand for very long."
"I have this sharp pain in my hip (rubbing the outer thigh) that I feel clear down the outside of my leg to my knee."
"Climbing up the stairs has become impossible."
"My back has hurt me for years. Lately, I've had a sharper pain right here (pointing to the upper outer thigh) whenever I lie on a hard surface."

EXAM.   Each patient is examined for the degree of local tenderness at the greater trochanter, and an assessment is made of the gait, the flexibility of the lower back, and the degree of involvement of the sacroiliac joint.

(1) Local tenderness is present at the midportion of the greater trochanter. This is best identified in the lateral decubitus position with the knees flexed to 90 degrees (identification of the midportion and the superior portion of the trochanteric process is easier in this position). The maximum tenderness is 1 1/2″ below the superior portion of the trochanter, directly over the maximum lateral prominence. (2) Stiffness or mild discomfort may be experienced at the extremes of internal or external rotation of the hip. This is present in approximately 50% of cases but is not as specific as the site of local tenderness. (3) Isometrically resisted hip abduction may aggravate the pain in 25% of cases. (4) The range of motion of the hip in an uncomplicated case should be normal. (5) Signs of an underlying back condition, an underlying leg length discrepancy, or a sacroiliac condition should be sought.

X-RAYS. X-rays of the hip are strongly recommended. A standing AP pelvis x-ray and specific views of the hip and back are used to evaluate for leg length discrepancy, disease affecting the sacroiliac joint, and structural back disease. Plain films show calcification in 5% of cases.

SPECIAL TESTING. Bone scanning, CT scans, or MRIs are used to evaluate for underlying conditions at the lumbosacral spine, the sacroiliac joint, the femur, or the pelvic bones.

DIAGNOSIS. The diagnosis of an uncomplicated case of trochanteric bursitis is based on the clinical findings of outer thigh pain, local tenderness at the midtrochanter, and pain relief with regional anesthetic block. Regional anesthetic block may be very helpful in differentiating the pain of trochanteric bursitis from referred pain from the gluteus medius bursa (p. 130) or the lumbosacral spine and from the dysesthetic pain of meralgia paresthetica (p. 136). Complicated cases with a suspected underlying cause require specialized testing for a definitive diagnosis.

TREATMENT. The goals of treatment are to reduce the inflammation in the bursa, to correct any underlying disturbance of gait, and to prevent recurrent bursitis by proper hip and back stretching exercises. The cross-leg stretching exercise of the gluteus medius combined with specific treatment of the primary gait disturbance are the treatments of choice.

Step 1: Define the site of local tenderness, order a standing AP pelvis x-ray, and evaluate and correct any underlying gait disturbance (e.g., a shoe lift, low back stretching exercises, a knee brace, high-top shoes for ankle support, custom-made foot orthotics for ankle pronation, etc.).

Reduce weightbearing (e.g., a lean bar, sitting vs. standing, crutches temporarily, weight loss for the chronic case, etc.).

Restrict repetitious bending (e.g., climbing stairs, getting out of a chair).

Advise on avoiding direct pressure.

Recommend daily stretching exercises for the gluteus medius tendon (p. 273).

Suggest sitting with the leg moderately abducted and externally rotated to lessen the pressure over the bursa.

Prescribe an NSAID (e.g., ibuprofen [Advil, Motrin]) for 4 weeks at full dose.

Step 2 (6 to 8 weeks for persistent cases): Reevaluate for an underlying cause (e.g., CT scan of the back, bone scan).

Obtain a standing AP pelvis x-ray to evaluate for leg length discrepancy.

Inject the bursa with K40.

Repeat the injection in 4 to 6 weeks if symptoms have not decreased by 50%.

With improvement, emphasize the stretching exercises of the hip and back.

Avoid direct pressure.

Step 3 (10 to 12 weeks for chronic cases): Perform a more thorough search for or treatment of the underlying gait disturbances.

Use deep ultrasound for persistent cases.

Recommend a TENS unit for chronic pain.

PHYSICAL THERAPY.   Physical therapy plays an important role in the active treatment of trochanteric bursitis and a major role in preventing recurrent bursitis.

PHYSICAL THERAPY SUMMARY

1. Heat
2. Stretching exercises for the gluteus medius tendon and muscle, passively performed
3. Stretching exercises for the lumbosacral spine and sacroiliac joint, passively performed
4. Ultrasound for deep heating
5. A TENS unit for chronic pain

Acute Period.   Heat treatments and passive stretching exercises are used in the first few weeks to reduce the pressure over the bursal sac.

Heat is applied to the outer thigh for 15 to 20 minutes to prepare the area for stretching. *Stretching exercises of the gluteus medius tendon* are recommended to reduce the pressure over the bursa. While in the sitting position, cross-leg pulls are performed in sets of 20 (p. 273). The maximum amount of stretch is obtained when the buttocks—both ischial tuberosities—are kept flat on a hard surface. These are followed by *low back and sacroiliac stretches* (p. 266). Stretching all three areas increases flexibility through the lower spine, the sacroiliac joints, and the hips. *Therapeutic ultrasound* treatments provide deep heating to the area and can be combined with stretching. A *TENS unit* may be necessary for patients with chronic bursitis secondary to structural back disease or chronic neurologic impairment.

Recovery/Rehabilitation.   Several weeks after the local symptoms have resolved, daily stretching exercises are cut back to three times a week. Maintaining low back, sacroiliac, and hip flexibility will reduce the chance of recurrent bursitis.

INJECTION.   For an uncomplicated case of bursitis—one that is not associated with a correctable underlying gait disturbance—local injection is the preferred anti-inflammatory treatment.

Positioning: The patient is to be in the lateral decubitus position with the affected side up and the knees flexed to 90 degrees (the trochanter is most prominent in this position).

Surface Anatomy and the Point of Entry: The superior, posterior, and anterior edges of the trochanteric process are palpated and marked. The point of entry is directly over the center point of the trochanter, 1 1/2″ below the superior trochanter. Alternatively, the point of entry is at the crown of the trochanter, viewed tangentially.

Angle of Entry and Depth: The needle is inserted perpendicular to the skin. The depth is 1 to 2 1/2″ to the gluteus medius and 1 1/2 to 3″ to the femur (the gluteus medius tendon/iliotibial band is 3/8 to 1/2″ thick).

Anesthesia: Ethyl chloride is sprayed on the skin. Local anesthetic is placed at the gluteus medius tissue plane (1 ml) and at the periosteum of the femur (1/2 to 1 ml).

Technique: The success of treatment depends on an accurate injection of the bursa at the level of the femur. The needle is held very lightly and advanced through the low resistance of the subcutaneous fat to the firm, rubbery resistance of the gluteus medius tissue plane. Following anesthesia at this level, the needle is advanced (firm pressure) 1/2 to 5/8″ farther to the periosteum of the femur. *Caution:* the patient will usually experience sharp pain as soon as the needle touches the periosteum! Injection at this deeper level requires firm pressure. If excessive pressure is encountered, the needle should be rotated 180 degrees or withdrawn ever so slightly. If the trochanter tenderness is significantly relieved, then 1 ml of K40 is injected through the same needle.

INJECTION AFTERCARE

1) *Rest* for 3 days, avoiding direct pressure and repetitive bending.

2) Advise 3 days of bedrest and crutches (touch-down–weightbearing) for severe cases.

3) *Ice* (15 minutes every 4 to 6 hours) and *Tylenol ES* (1000 mg twice a day) for soreness.

4) *Protect* the hip for 3 to 4 weeks by limiting direct pressure, repetitive bending, prolonged standing, and unnecessary walking.

5) Begin cross-leg *stretching exercises* for the gluteus medius on day 4.

6) For those with accompanying structural back disease, begin flexion *stretching exercises* of the lower back (the Williams exercises) after the acute pain has begun to resolve.

7) Repeat *injection* at 6 weeks with corticosteroid if pain persists.

8) Obtain *plain x-rays* of standing AP pelvis for leg length discrepancy and a *CT scan* or an *MRI* to identify a short leg, a subtle disk, spondylolisthesis, or other condition.

9) Advise long-term restrictions for the patient with chronic bursitis (5%).

SURGICAL PROCEDURE.   Bursectomy is rarely performed. The bursa probably reforms if lateral hip friction and pressure persist.

PROGNOSIS.   Uncomplicated cases of bursitis—those unassociated with a chronic or fixed gait disturbance—usually respond dramatically to one or two corticosteroid injections 6 weeks apart. A poor response to local injection suggests either a chronic bursal thickening or an undiscovered underlying cause. The prognosis for recovery depends greatly on the underlying cause, the patient's steadfastness in performing the stretching exercises, and the degree of obesity. Intractable symptoms are seen in patients with extreme obesity, severe structural back disease, or chronic neurologic impairment.

Gluteus Medius Bursitis/Piriformis Syndrome

Enter 1″ above the superior edge of the trochanter process in the lateral decubitus position; advance the needle down to the gluteus tendon and then to the periosteum of the femur.

Needle: 1½″ or 3½″ spinal needle, 22 gauge

Depth: 1½ to 3″ (down to periosteum)

Volume: 2 ml of anesthetic and 1 ml of K40

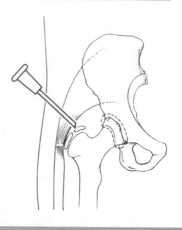

Figure 8–2.   Gluteus medius bursitis injection

DESCRIPTION.   Gluteus medius bursitis (also referred to as deep trochanteric bursitis) is an inflammation of the bursal sac that is located between the top of the superior trochanteric process and the gluteus medius tendon. It serves to lubricate the gluteus medius tendon, the piriformis muscle insertion, and the lateral aspect of the femur. Repetitive flexing of the hip and direct pressure aggravate this condition. It is identical to trochanteric bursitis in symptoms, presentation, and treatment (see p. 126). Osteoarthritis of the hip and bursitis rarely coexist.

SYMPTOMS.   The patient complains of hip pain or difficulties in walking identical to those that occur in trochanteric bursitis.

"Whenever I roll over onto my right side, this sharp pain in my hip wakes me up."
"I get this achy pain in my hip (pointing to the upper outer thigh) when I walk too much in the mall."
"I can't stand very long."
"I have this sharp pain in my hip (rubbing the outer thigh) that I feel clear down the outside of my leg to my knee."
"Climbing up the stairs has become impossible."
"My back has hurt me for years. Lately, I've had a sharper pain right here (pointing to the upper outer thigh) whenever I lie on a hard surface."

EXAM.   Each patient is examined for local tenderness at the superior portion of the greater trochanter; the range of motion of the hip and lumbosacral spine is measured, gait is assessed, and the sacroiliac joints are evaluated.

EXAM SUMMARY   • • • • • • • • • • • • • •

1. Local tenderness directly over the superior portion of the trochanteric process
2. Pain aggravation at the extremes of hip rotation
3. Pain aggravated by resisted hip abduction (75% of cases), isometrically performed
4. Normal range of motion of the hip
5. Associated gait disturbance, leg length discrepancy, back or sacroiliac disease

(1) Maximum tenderness is located just superior to the trochanteric process of the femur, directly in the midline. This is best identified in the lateral decubitus position with the knees flexed to 90 degrees (the superior portion of the trochanteric process is more prominent in this position). (2) Stiffness or mild discomfort may be experienced at the extremes of internal or external rotation of the hip. This is present in approximately 50% of cases but is not as specific as the local point of tenderness. (3) Isometrically resisted hip abduction may aggravate the pain in 75% of cases. (4) The range of motion of the hip in an uncomplicated case should be normal. (5) Signs of an underlying lumbosacral back condition, leg length discrepancy, lower extremity gait disturbance, or sacroiliac condition are present in the majority of cases!

X-RAYS.   X-rays of the hip are strongly recommended. A standing AP pelvis x-ray and specific views of the hip and back are used to evaluate for the underlying cause—leg length discrepancy, disease affecting the sacroiliac disease, or structural back disease. Plain films may show calcification in fewer than 5% of cases.

SPECIAL TESTING.   Bone scanning, CT scanning, and MRI are used to evaluate for underlying conditions at the lumbosacral spine, sacroiliac joint, femur, and pelvic bones.

DIAGNOSIS.   The diagnosis of an uncomplicated case of gluteus medius bursitis is based on the clinical findings of outer thigh pain, local tenderness at the superior portion of the greater trochanter, and pain relief with regional anesthetic block. Regional anesthetic block may be very helpful in differentiating the pain of gluteus medius bursitis from pain referred from the trochanteric bursa (p. 126) or the lumbosacral spine and the dysesthetic pain of meralgia paresthetica (p. 136). Complicated cases with a suspected underlying cause require specialized testing for a definitive diagnosis.

TREATMENT.   The goals of treatment are to reduce the inflammation in the bursa, to correct any underlying disturbance of gait, and to prevent recurrent bursitis by teaching proper hip and back stretching exercises. The cross-leg stretching exercise of the gluteus medius combined with specific treatment of the primary gait disturbance are the initial treatments of choice for most patients. Local corticosteroid injection is the treatment of choice for patients presenting with severe symptoms and signs.

Step 1: Evaluate and correct any underlying gait disturbance (e.g., a shoe lift, low back stretching exercises, a knee brace, high-top shoes for ankle support, custom-made foot orthotics for ankle pronation, etc.).

Reduce weightbearing (e.g., a lean bar, sitting vs. standing, crutches temporarily, weight loss for the chronic case, etc.).

Restrict repetitious bending (e.g., climbing stairs, getting out of a chair).

Advise on avoiding direct pressure.

Perform daily stretching exercises for the gluteus medius tendon (p. 273).

Suggest sitting with the leg moderately abducted and externally rotated to lessen the pressure over the bursa.

Prescribe an NSAID (e.g., ibuprofen [Advil, Motrin]) for 4 weeks at full dose.

Step 2 (6 to 8 weeks for persistent symptoms): Reevaluate for an underlying cause (e.g., CT scan of the back, bone scan).

Obtain a standing AP pelvis x-ray to evaluate for leg length discrepancy.

Perform an injection of the bursa with K40.

Repeat the injection in 4 to 6 weeks if symptoms have not decreased by 50%.

With improvement, emphasize the stretching exercises for the hip and back.

Step 3 (10 to 12 weeks for chronic cases): Perform a more thorough search for, or more directed treatment of, the underlying gait disturbance.

Recommend deep ultrasound for persistent cases.

Recommend a TENS unit for chronic pain.

PHYSICAL THERAPY. Physical therapy plays an important role in the active treatment of gluteus medius bursitis and a major role in preventing recurrent bursitis.

PHYSICAL THERAPY SUMMARY ● ● ● ● ● ● ● ● ● ● ● ● ● ● ●

1. Heat
2. Stretching exercises for the gluteus medius tendon and muscle, passively performed
3. Stretching exercises for the sacroiliac joint and the lumbosacral spine, passively performed
4. Ultrasound for deep heating
5. A TENS unit for chronic bursitis

Acute Period. Heat treatments and passive stretching exercises are used in the first few weeks to reduce the pressure over the bursal sac.

Heat is applied to the outer thigh for 15 to 20 minutes to prepare the area for stretching. *Stretching exercises of the gluteus tendon* are recommended to reduce the pressure over the bursa. While in the sitting position, cross-leg pulls are performed in sets of 20 (p. 273). The maximum amount of stretching is obtained when the buttocks—both ischial tuberosities—are kept flat on a hard surface. These are followed by *low back and sacroiliac stretches* (p. 266). Stretching all three areas provides flexibility through the lower spine, the sacroiliac joints, and the hips. *Therapeutic ultrasound* treatments provide deep heating to the area and can be combined with stretching. A *TENS unit* may be necessary for patients with chronic bursitis secondary to structural back disease or chronic neurologic impairment.

Recovery/Rehabilitation. Several weeks after the local symptoms have resolved, daily stretching exercises are cut back to three times a week. Maintaining low back, sacroiliac, and hip flexibility will reduce the chance of recurrent bursitis.

INJECTION. For an uncomplicated bursitis—one not associated with a correctable underlying cause such as mechanical low back stiffness, short leg, or gait disturbance—local injection is the preferred treatment. Note: If both the gluteus and trochanteric bursa are involved, the trochanteric bursa should be treated first.

Positioning: The patient is to be in the lateral decubitus position with the affected side up and the knees flexed to 90 degrees (the trochanter is most prominent in this position).

Surface Anatomy and the Point of Entry: The superior, posterior, and anterior edges of the trochanteric process are palpated and marked. The point of entry is 3/4 to 1″ above the midpoint of the most superior portion of the trochanter.

Angle of Entry and Depth: The needle is inserted at a 45-degree angle in direct alignment with the femur. The depth is 1 to 2 1/2″ to the gluteus medius tendon and 1 1/2 to 3″ to the superior trochanter (the tendon is 1/2″ thick).

Anesthesia: Ethyl chloride is sprayed on the skin. Local anesthetic is placed at the gluteus medius tissue plane (1 ml) and at the periosteum of the femur (1/2 to 1 ml).

Technique: The success of treatment depends on an accurate injection of the bursa at the level of the femur. The needle is held very lightly and advanced through the low resistance of the subcutaneous fat to the firm, rubbery resistance of the gluteus medius tissue plane. Following anesthesia at this level, the needle is advanced (firm pressure) 1/2" farther to the periosteum of the femur. *Caution:* The patient will usually experience sharp pain as soon as the needle touches the periosteum! Injection at this deeper level requires firm pressure. If excessive pressure is encountered, the needle should be rotated 180 degrees or withdrawn ever so slightly. If the local tenderness over the trochanter is significantly relieved, then 1 ml of K40 is injected through the same needle.

INJECTION AFTERCARE

1) *Rest* for 3 days, avoiding direct pressure and repetitive bending.

2) Advise bedrest for 3 days and crutches with touch-down–weightbearing for patients with severe involvement.

3) *Ice* (15 minutes every 4 to 6 hours) and *Tylenol ES* (1000 mg twice a day) for soreness.

4) *Protect* the hip for 3 to 4 weeks by limiting direct pressure, repetitive bending, prolonged standing, and unnecessary walking.

5) Begin cross-leg *stretching exercises* for the gluteus medius on day 4.

6) For those with accompanying structural back disease, begin flexion *stretching exercises* of the lower back (the Williams exercises) after the acute pain has begun to resolve.

7) Repeat *injection* at 6 weeks with corticosteroid if pain persists.

8) Obtain plain films of standing AP pelvis for leg length discrepancy and a CT scan or an MRI to identify a short leg, a subtle disk, spondylolisthesis, or other condition in the chronic case.

9) Advise long-term restrictions for the patient with chronic bursitis (5%).

SURGICAL PROCEDURE.   Bursectomy is rarely performed.

PROGNOSIS.   Uncomplicated cases of bursitis unassociated with a chronic or fixed disturbance of gait usually respond dramatically to one or two corticosteroid injections 6 weeks apart. A poor response to an injection suggests either a chronic bursal thickening or an undiscovered underlying cause. Note that two injections of triamcinolone, with its greater effect on atrophy, have the theoretical advantage of reducing the size of chronic bursal thickening.

The prognosis for recovery depends greatly on the underlying cause, the patient's willingness to do stretching exercises, and the degree of obesity. Intractable symptoms are seen in patients with severe obesity, severe structural back disease, or chronic neurologic impairment.

DESCRIPTION.   Osteoarthritis of the hip results from wear and tear of the articular cartilage between the head of the femur and the acetabulum. Obesity, a family history of osteoarthritis, a history of systemic arthritis, or a history of severe gait disturbance are predisposing factors. It is the second most common cause of pain around the hip, second only to hip bursitis.

SYMPTOMS.   The patient complains of groin or thigh pain or both or loss of flexibility. The patient often pushes deep into the groin or grabs the upper thigh when describing the condition.

"I can't get my socks on anymore . . . and there's absolutely no way I can tie my shoe laces."
"My hip is getting stiffer and stiffer."
"My right hip is beginning to hurt just like the left hip did before I had it replaced."

■ OSTEOARTHRITIS OF THE HIP

The indications for surgical replacement of the hip are:

intractable pain,
functional loss ("I cannot put my socks on or tie my shoes"),
greater than 50% loss of internal and external rotation, and medical suitability for a 2- to 2½-hour operation; ideally, this operation should be considered after age 60.

(The average prosthesis lasts 10 to 15 years.)

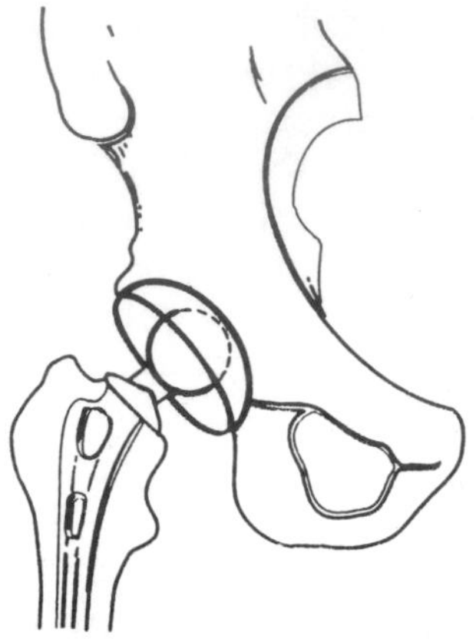

Hip prosthesis is in place.

Hip joint injection is rarely indicated.

Figure 8–3. Hip prosthesis

"I can't take my usual constitutional around the golf course any longer without having to stop two or three times (because of hip pain)."
"I've had this deep achy pain (pointing to the anterior hip area) whenever I walk a certain distance."
"I can't believe that I have arthritis in my hip. My hip has never hurt me. I feel pain in my lower thigh and knee. I thought I had arthritis in my knee."

EXAM. The patient's gait, the general function of the hip, and the range of motion of the hip are examined in each patient.

EXAM SUMMARY   • • • • • • • • • • • • • •

1. Impaired function: loss of normal gait, inability to remove socks, cross the legs, and so forth
2. Loss of internal and external rotation with endpoint stiffness and pain
3. A positive fabere maneuver (abnormal Patrick test)
4. Tenderness 1 1/2" below the inguinal ligament

(1) General hip function can be assessed by observing the patient's gait, the move from chair to exam table, the removal of shoes and socks, and the crossing of the legs. As arthritis advances, these basic functions become more and more difficult to accomplish. (2) The range of motion of the hip is restricted. Early disease shows a common pattern of loss of rotation and endpoint stiffness. Normally, a 50-year-old patient should have 45 degrees of internal and external rotation. By comparison, a young woman with supple hips may have 60 to 70 degrees of rotation in each direction. (3) The result of the fabere maneuver (also known as the Patrick test) may be positive. This test is performed by placing the hip in flexion, abduction, and external rotation (in a figure-of-four position), and pressure is applied to the anterior superior iliac spine and the knee. This stretches the anterior capsule of the hip, resulting in pain. This maneuver is associated with moderate pain in cases of acute

synovitis and with extreme pain in cases of septic arthritis. (4) Tenderness may be found 1½" below the midportion of the inguinal ligament, very close to the femoral artery.

Note that all of these findings on exam are exaggerated with inflammatory arthritis, severe with avascular necrosis of the hip, and extreme with acute septic arthritis.

X-RAYS. Specific x-rays (including standing AP, lateral, and frog-leg views) to evaluate the extent of primary disease of the hip joint are always indicated. The most useful view for screening and evaluating hip disease is the standing AP pelvis. This single x-ray exposure allows simultaneous comparison of both hips, screens for sacroiliac disease, and assesses leg length discrepancy. In addition, the standing AP pelvis is useful in determining the position of the hips. This view can be used to assess for shallow acetabulum, a form of hip dysplasia, and for an unusual complication of hip disease, protrusio acetabuli, a pathologic migration of the femoral head into the pelvis.

The early changes of osteoarthritis of the hip include a loss of joint space between the superior acetabulum and the femoral head (normally 4 to 5 mm), increased bony sclerosis of the superior acetabulum, variable degrees of osteophyte formation along the superior acetabulum, and subchondral cyst formation.

SPECIAL TESTING. An MRI is not necessary in the routine case. If subjective pain and pain with rotation of the hip on exam are extreme, an MRI may be necessary to evaluate for avascular necrosis, occult fracture, or complicating primary bone disease.

DIAGNOSIS. The diagnosis is based on the loss of hip rotation coupled with characteristic changes on plain films of the hip.

TREATMENT. The goals of treatment are to relieve pain, preserve function, and stage for surgery. A 3- to 4-week course of an NSAID and mild restrictions on weightbearing activities are the treatments of choice for mild disease. Total hip replacement surgery is the treatment of choice for advanced disease.

Step 1: Measure the patient's loss of internal and external rotation (normally 40 to 45 degrees in a 50-year-old person), obtain a standing AP pelvis x-ray and determine the patient's functional status.
Restrict jogging, Jazzersize, and other impact exercises.
Suggest padded insoles to reduce impact pressure (p. 303).
Advise on passive hip stretching exercises (p. 272) to preserve range of motion.
Prescribe an NSAID (e.g., ibuprofen [Advil, Motrin]) in full dose. Emphasize the need to take it regularly for at least 2 to 3 weeks for its anti-inflammatory effect.

Step 2 (months to years for reassessment): Assess hip rotation and evaluate functional status.
Repeat the standing AP pelvis x-ray if rotation has decreased by more than 20% or if function has changed dramatically.
Consider switching to another chemical class of NSAIDs if the current medication has lost its effectiveness.
Use narcotics cautiously!

Step 3 (months to years for progressive cases): Assess hip rotation and functional status.
Consider orthopedic consultation when (1) pain is intractable, (2) function is severely limited, (3) internal rotation has declined to 10 to 15 degrees, or (4) protrusio acetabuli has developed.
Assess the patient's surgical candidacy.

PHYSICAL THERAPY. Physical therapy plays an adjunctive role in the overall management of osteoarthritis of the hip.

PHYSICAL THERAPY SUMMARY   ● ● ● ● ● ● ● ● ● ● ● ● ● ● ● ●

1. Stretching exercises of the adductors, rotators, and gluteus muscles and tendons, passively performed
2. Toning exercises of the iliopsoas and gluteus muscles, isometrically performed
3. Occupational therapy consultation for practical aids for daily activities

Acute Period/Recovery/Rehabilitation. Stretching and toning exercises are recommended to maintain hip flexibility and to preserve the muscular tone around the hip. Figure-of-four, Indian-style sitting, and knee-chest pulls are performed daily in sets of 20 to stretch the adductors, rotators, and gluteus muscles, respectively (p. 270). Toning exercises of the iliopsoas and the gluteus muscles follow the stretching exercises. Initially, straight-leg raising is performed without weights in the supine and prone positions (p. 276). With improvement, 5- to 10-lb weights are added to the ankle to increase the tension. Advanced cases with functional impairment may benefit from an occupational therapy assessment.

INJECTION. Intra-articular injection is limited to the nonsurgical candidate with advanced disease. For optimal results, it should be performed under fluoroscopy by an orthopedic surgeon or radiologist.

SURGICAL PROCEDURE. Patients who meet the criteria for operation should be considered for total joint replacement, arthroplasty.

PROGNOSIS. Uncomplicated osteoarthritis of the hip is a slowly progressive disease. The patient should be educated about the slow progression over years, the nature of the course of arthritic flare, and the efficacy of surgery when indicated. Local injection should be restricted to the palliation of symptoms in the nonsurgical candidate.

By contrast, osteoarthritis may progress rapidly in the presence of congenital shallow acetabulum, avascular necrosis, or previous femoral neck fracture. Patients with these associated conditions should be followed closely at 2- to 4-month intervals.

DESCRIPTION. Meralgia paresthetica is a compression neuropathy of the lateral femoral cutaneous nerve as the nerve exits the pelvis and groin and enters the thigh. Obesity with an overlying panniculus, tight garments around the waist, or scar tissue near the lateral aspect of the inguinal ligament are the usual causes.

SYMPTOMS. The patient has neuritic pain in a very specific area of the anterolateral thigh. The patient often rubs the outer thigh back and forth as the condition is described.

"I have this burning pain in my thigh."
"It feels funny (pointing to the outer upper thigh) when my jeans rub over the skin."
"My skin feels numb and tingly (rubbing the skin of the outer upper thigh)."
"I think I have a pinched nerve. My leg is numb right here."
"My leg has some dead spots."

EXAM. The sensory function of the upper outer thigh is examined and a lower extremity neurologic examination is performed in each patient.

◼ MERALGIA PARESTHETICA

Hypesthetic, dysesthetic area
Injection of the lateral femoral cutaneous nerve as it enters the thigh
  next to the ASIS is uncommonly
  performed.

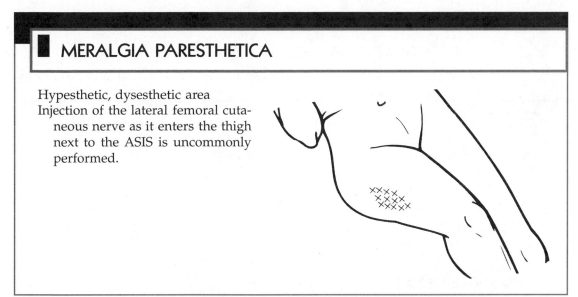

Figure 8–4.   Meralgia paresthetica

EXAM SUMMARY   ● ● ● ● ● ● ● ● ● ● ● ● ● ●

1. Hypesthetic or dysesthetic pain in the upper outer thigh
2. The lower extremity neurologic exam is normal
3. The hip, back, and sacroiliac joints are normal

1) Pinprick and light touch are abnormal in a 10 × 6″ oval-shaped area on the anterolateral thigh. Note that the distribution of the lateral femoral cutaneous nerve is not strictly lateral. It is not unusual for the nerve to provide sensation to a portion of the anterior thigh! (2) The neurologic exam of the lower extremity is otherwise normal. The straight-leg–raising sign is negative, and the deep tendon reflexes and distal motor strength are preserved. (3) There is no evidence of a hip, back, or sacroiliac joint abnormality.

X-RAYS.   Plain x-rays of the hip and pelvis are not necessary. No characteristic changes are seen on these films. When the clinical findings are equivocal, radiographic testing of the lower lumbar spine is often used to exclude spondylolisthesis, spinal stenosis, or disk disease.

SPECIAL TESTING.   None.

DIAGNOSIS.   The diagnosis is based on the unique description of the pain, its characteristic location, the sensory abnormalities on exam, and the conspicuous absence of neurologic abnormalities in the lower leg.

TREATMENT.   The goals of treatment are to reassure the patient that this is not a serious condition and to recommend ways to reduce pressure over the nerve in the groin. Education of the patient (reassure that "This isn't a pinched nerve!") combined with measures to reduce the pressure in the groin are the treatments of choice. Local corticosteroid injection is used infrequently in patients with refractory symptoms and signs.

Step 1: Educate the patient: "This is not a serious back problem; it is not a pinched nerve!"

Avoid tight garments.
Discuss the need for weight loss.
Suggest abdominal toning exercises to tighten the groin.

Step 2 (months for persistent symptoms): Reexamine the dysesthetic area to confirm the local nature of the problem.
Consider carbamazepine (Tegretol) or phenytoin (Dilantin) to reduce the dysesthetic pain (advise that "This relatively minor problem should not be treated with harsh and potentially harmful medications!").
Consider a consultation with an anesthesiologist for a local nerve block.

Step 3 (months to years for chronic symptoms): Consider a neurosurgical consultation for intractable dysesthetic cases.

PHYSICAL THERAPY.   Physical therapy does not play a significant role in the treatment of meralgia paresthetica. Abdominal muscle toning exercises may reduce the pressure over the lateral femoral cutaneous nerve but is of unproven value.

SURGICAL PROCEDURE.   Rarely, neurolysis.

PROGNOSIS.   Meralgia paresthetica is a self-limited, benign disease in most patients. Neurologic symptoms are restricted to sensory changes only (the nerve does not contain motor fibers). The most troublesome cases involve dysesthetic pain. If oral medication does not control symptoms, then local anesthetic block can be considered. A rare case of severe and disabling dysesthetic pain can be considered for neurolysis.

chapter 9

Knee

■ PATELLOFEMORAL DISEASES

The patellofemoral family of conditions includes
    patellofemoral syndrome,
    patellofemoral subluxation,
    patellofemoral arthritis,
    patellar dislocation, and patella alta.
These are all characterized by abnormal tracking
    of the patella in the femoral groove.
Intra-articular corticosteroid injection is indicated
    in patients with refractory symptoms and in
    those with joint effusion.
Note: Injection must be combined with physical
    therapy.

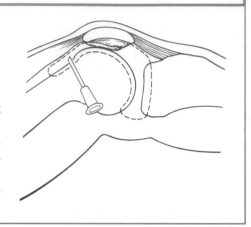

Figure 9–1.   Injection for patellofemoral osteoarthritis

DESCRIPTION.   Patellofemoral syndrome represents the family of conditions that cause symptoms at the patellofemoral joint, including chondromalacia patella (the term describing the pathology), patellar subluxation (the mechanical term that describes the abnormal patellofemoral tracking), patella alta (excessive length of the patellar tendon), and patellofemoral arthritis (the end result of years of symptoms). Although some cases are caused by direct trauma, most cases result from the repetitive irritation of abnormal tracking of the patella in the femoral groove. Arthroscopically, the undersurface of the patella shows defects in the articular cartilage (pits and cracks). Over many years, diffuse irregularities of the articular cartilage occur (e.g., osteoarthritis). Poor muscle tone, overdeveloped vastus lateralis, an abnormal Q angle, repetitive squatting and kneeling, and direct trauma predispose to the condition.

SYMPTOMS.   The patient complains of knee pain (in front of the knee), a "noisy" knee, and, occasionally, swelling. The patient often rubs the entire area around the patella or attempts to demonstrate the noise when describing the condition.

"My knee caps ache after I run."
"I can't squat or kneel anymore."
"I have this grinding sound when I bend my knee."
"My knees have always had this grinding noise, but now they're swelling."
"I can't sit Indian-style anymore."
"Whenever I use the stairstepper or do Jazzersize, both my knees will ache that evening."
"Two years ago, I rammed my knees into the dashboard. Ever since then, my knees ache after skiing."

EXAM.   The patellofemoral articulation is examined for local irritation, alignment, and abnormal tracking, and the knee is examined for signs of effusion.

EXAM SUMMARY   ● ● ● ● ● ● ● ● ● ● ● ● ● ●

1.   Painful retropatellar crepitation (squatting, patellar compression, Insall maneuver)
2.   Full range of motion but with abnormal patellofemoral tracking (clicking with passive flexion and extension)
3.   Negative apprehension sign for patellar dislocation
4.   Knee effusion (uncommon)

(1) Painful retropatellar crepitation is best detected by passively moving the patella back and forth across the femoral groove. The leg is placed in the extended position, and the patient is asked to relax the quadriceps muscle. With the examiner's fingers on all four poles and with firm downward pressure, the patella is forced onto the lateral and medial femoral condyles and down into the inferior patellofemoral groove. Note that crepitation may be palpable only in the inferior portion of the groove, where the disease most often first develops. (2) Patellofemoral alignment and tracking are assessed by inspection, by measurement of the Q angle, and by passive flexion and extension of the knee. The patella may be visibly subluxed (laterally displaced in the femoral groove) when the knee is in the extended position. The Q angle (the angle formed by the anterior superior iliac spine, the midpatella, and the midtibial tubercle) should be less than 20 degrees. (3) With the palm placed over the center of the patella, a patellar click may be palpable as the knee is passively flexed and extended. (4) The apprehension sign (pressure applied medially to laterally to reproduce patellar dislocation) should be absent. (5) Knee effusion is not common. Moderate to large effusion suggests severe exacerbation or advanced disease (p. 143). In the absence of a knee effusion, uncomplicated patellofemoral syndrome should have full range of motion.

X-RAYS. Four views of the knee, including the sunrise (also referred to as the merchant view), standing PA, lateral, and tunnel views are always recommended. Typical changes include lateral subluxation, a narrowing of the lateral patellofemoral articular cartilage, sclerosis of the lateral aspect of the patella (the reaction to the constant lateral pressure) and, in the advanced case, osteoarthritic changes, including osteophytes, severe sclerosis, and the subchondral cyst formation of osteoarthritis. Note that early disease may show only subluxation.

DIAGNOSIS. The diagnosis of patellofemoral syndrome is based on clinical findings. Anterior knee pain associated with painful patellar crepitation and subluxation on x-rays is highly suggestive. Regional anesthetic block may be necessary to differentiate the articular pain arising from the patella from a complicating periarticular process such as anserine bursitis. Arthroscopy to exclude osteochondritis dissecans, loose body, or meniscal tear is indicated when patellofemoral syndrome presents with a greater degree of mechanical symptoms or with a large knee effusion (1 to 2%).

TREATMENT. The goals of treatment are to improve patellofemoral tracking and alignment, reduce pain and swelling, and retard the development of patellofemoral arthritis. Restriction of repetitive flexion combined with isometrically performed straight-leg raising with the leg externally rotated (toning of the vastus medialis) is the treatment of choice.

Step 1: Evaluate the baseline quadriceps tone, perform a heel-to-buttock measurement to assess knee flexibility, and order x-rays of the knee.

Apply ice and elevate the knee, especially with effusion.

Emphasize the absolute need to avoid squatting and kneeling.

Recommend swimming, NordicTrack, and fast walking in place of jogging, bicycling, and the stop-and-go sports that involve too much bending and impact.

Begin isometrically performed straight-leg raises with the leg externally rotated to increase the tone of the vastus medialis and thereby improve patellofemoral tracking.

Step 2 (4 to 8 weeks for persistent cases): Reinforce restrictions and exercises.

Prescribe an NSAID (e.g., ibuprofen [Advil, Motrin]) at full dose for 3 weeks and with a taper at week 4.

Recommend a patellar strap (p. 297) or a Velcro patellar restraining brace (p. 297), especially for patients active in sports.

Step 3 (3 to 4 months for persistent cases): Perform a local corticosteroid injection with K40, especially for the patient with knee effusion.

Repeat the injection at 4 to 6 weeks if symptoms have not been reduced by 50%.

Step 4 (4 to 6 weeks for chronic cases): Reemphasize the need to continue daily or thrice weekly straight-leg–raising exercises.

Make the restrictions of use and motion a long-term recommendation.

Consider orthopedic referral for persistent pain and dysfunction or in cases associated with patella alta, or Q angles greater than 20 degrees.

PHYSICAL THERAPY. Physical therapy exercises are the cornerstone of treatment for patellofemoral disorders.

PHYSICAL THERAPY SUMMARY

1. Ice
2. Straight-leg–raising exercises with the leg externally rotated to increase the quadriceps tone of the vastus medialis, isometrically performed
3. Active exercises and apparatus that minimize impact and repetitive bending

Acute Period. Ice and elevation are used when symptoms are acute. *Ice* is an effective analgesic and may help to reduce swelling.

Recovery/Rehabilitation. Exercises are combined with activity restrictions to reduce patellofemoral irritation. *Muscle toning exercises* help to stabilize the knee joint, reduce subluxation and dislocation, and improve patellofemoral tracking. Daily straight-leg–raising exercises in the supine and prone positions are performed in sets of 20 (p. 276). These exercises are performed initially without weights. With improvement, 5- to 10-lb weights are added at the ankle. *Active exercises,* especially on equipment, must be performed with caution. Stationary bicycle exercise, rowing machines, and universal gym requiring full-knee flexion must be avoided initially. Fast walking, swimming, and NordicTrack cross-country ski machines are preferable because of their low impact and the minimal bending required.

INJECTION. The indications for local corticosteroid injection are limited. Injection can be considered for intractable pain, large knee effusion, or the patient who fails to respond to exercise or NSAIDs (see "Knee Effusion" for injection technique, p. 143).

SURGICAL PROCEDURE. Lateral retinacular release, tibial tubercle transposition, or arthroscopic débridement are used in selected cases. All of these procedures attempt to reduce patellar irritation either directly (débridement) or indirectly by attempting to correct abnormal patellofemoral tracking (lateral retinacular release and tibial tubercle transposition). Surgery, like injection therapy, is not a substitute for regular quadriceps toning.

PROGNOSIS.   Symptomatic flares of pain or swelling can last for months. Preventive exercises cannot be overemphasized. Improvement in quadriceps and hamstring tone should retard the progression of the disease.

Knee Effusion

Enter laterally between the lines formed by the underside of the patella and the middle of the iliotibial track; gently advance the needle to the mild resistance of the lateral retinaculum, angling toward the superior pole of the patella.

Needle: 1½", 18 gauge or 3½" spinal needle

Depth: ½ to 3"

Volume: 1 to 2 ml of anesthesic plus 1 ml of K40

Note: Continuously aspirate with mild pressure as the needle is advanced.

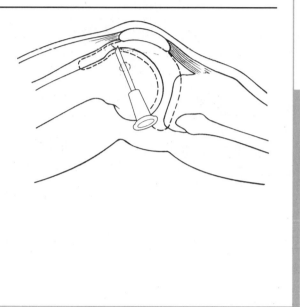

Figure 9–2.   Aspiration of the knee from the lateral approach

DESCRIPTION.   A knee effusion is an abnormal accumulation of synovial fluid. It is classified as noninflammatory or inflammatory, depending on the cellular content (see Appendix, p. 311). Osteoarthritis, inflammatory arthritis, patellofemoral syndrome, and infection such as gonococcal, staphylococcal, and so forth are the most common causes. Increasing amounts of fluid interfere with the normal motion of the knee, restricting flexion first and eventually extension. The hydraulic pressure of repetitive bending forces the synovial fluid into the popliteal space, limiting flexion, and over time it leads to the formation of a Baker cyst in approximately 10 to 15% of cases.

SYMPTOMS.   The patient complains of knee swelling, tightness in the knee, or restricted range of motion. The patient often rubs over the front of the knee with both hands when describing the condition.

"My knee is swollen."
"I feel an egg behind my knee whenever I bend it back."
"My right knee seems to be so much bigger than the left."
"My whole knee feels achy and tight."
"At the end of the day the swelling is so great that I limp. It feels like it's going to burst."
"My knee is giving out. It feels like it won't hold my weight."
"I have a fever inside my knee."
"My knee has become so swollen that I can't bend it back or fully straighten it."

EXAM.   Maneuvers to detect knee swelling are combined with an objective measurement of the range of motion of the knee.

(1) With the knees in the extended position and the quadriceps muscle relaxed, the size and shape of both knees are compared and the medial and lateral peripatellar dimples are inspected. Small effusions (5 to 10 ml) will fill in these normal anatomic landmarks and create a general fullness to the knee. (2) For small effusions with high viscosity, the synovial milking sign may be positive. Pressure is held over the medial dimple (over the medial patellar retinaculum) to force the synovial fluid into the lateral compartment. When pressure is released and a milking motion is applied to the lateral dimple (over the lateral patellar retinaculum), the fluid reappears medially. Note that this test is practical only in asthenic patients with high-viscosity fluid. (3) The ballottement sign is positive with 10 to 15 ml of fluid. With the examiner using both hands, the synovial fluid is milked into the center of the knee from all four quadrants. With the index finger, the patella is forcibly snapped down against the femur. A moderate effusion is associated with a clicking or tapping sensation. (4) Large effusions (20 to 30 ml) fill the suprapatellar space. This area just above the superior pole of the patella is usually flat or slightly concave. Large effusions cause a convexity above the patella and a bulging under the distal vastus lateralis muscle and fascia. (5) Joint aspiration is the definitive test for knee effusion. This is especially true for the obese patient or for the patient with unusually large peripatellar fat pads. (6) A joint effusion should always be suspected if the affected knee is enlarged and lacks full flexion. Flexion can be compared between one side and the other or measured in degrees (0 degrees at full extension, 90 degrees with the knee bent at a right angle). A simple observation that provides an objective measurement of flexion is the heel-to-buttock distance. The knee is gently forced into full flexion, and the distance between the heel and the point on the buttock the heel would ordinarily come into contact with is measured. This measurement correlates very well with the acute effusion. It also is abnormal with previous surgical treatment of the knee (total knee replacement, anterior cruciate ligament repair, and so forth) and with neuromuscular disorders that have affected the lower extremities. The measurement may not be abnormal in chronic effusion, as chronic effusions gradually dilate all the supporting structures.

X-RAYS.   X-rays of the knee (including weightbearing PA, lateral, sunrise, and tunnel views) are always recommended. The weightbearing view is used to determine the widths of the cartilage of the medial and lateral compartments as well as of the valgus carrying angle of the knee. The sunrise, or merchant, view is used to determine the degree of patellofemoral disease. The tunnel view is used to evaluate for osteochondritis dissecans and intra-articular loose bodies. The lateral view, with good soft-tissue technique, can provide clues to the presence of a large joint effusion, the location of bony lesions, and soft-tissue calcifications.

SPECIAL TESTING.   Synovial fluid analysis is an integral part of the evaluation of knee effusion.

DIAGNOSIS.   A presumptive diagnosis of a knee effusion can be made on the basis of physical signs; however, a definitive diagnosis requires synovial fluid analysis obtained by aspiration. Joint aspiration is mandatory whenever infection is in the differential diagnosis (see Appendix, p. 311).

TREATMENT. The goals of treatment are to diagnose the underlying cause of the effusion, to reduce swelling and inflammation, and to restore the stability of the joint. Joint aspiration is the treatment of choice for tense hemarthrosis and tense effusions causing instability of the knee. Joint aspiration combined with injection is the treatment of choice for large nonseptic effusions. Hospitalization and intravenous antibiotics are the treatments of choice for the septic effusion.

Step 1: Perform a heel-to-buttock measurement, aspirate the effusion for diagnostic studies (e.g., cell count and differential, crystals, glucose, Gram stain, and culture), and order standing PA, lateral, and sunrise views of the knees.

Hospitalize and begin intravenous antibiotics empirically (covering for staphylococcal organisms) if infection is suspected.

Apply ice and elevate the knee.

Suggest crutches with touch-down–weightbearing for severe cases.

Minimize squatting and kneeling.

Prescribe a patellar restraining brace if the knee is grossly unstable (giving out excessively).

Begin straight-leg–raising exercises without weights as soon as the acute symptoms resolve.

Step 2 (days to 4 weeks acute follow up): Reaspirate tense effusions.

Reemphasize the importance of straight-leg–raising exercises in restoring quadriceps support to the knee (with weights as tolerated).

Prescribe an NSAID (e.g., ibuprofen [Advil, Motrin]) for 4 weeks at full dose with a taper beginning at 3 weeks.

Step 3 (3 to 6 weeks for persistent cases): Reaspirate and inject the knee with K40.

Repeat the injection at 4 to 6 weeks if symptoms are not reduced by 50%.

Reemphasize the importance of weighted straight-leg raises.

Step 4 (2 to 4 months for chronic cases): Repeat plain x-rays or perform an MRI for cases that have failed to respond to treatment and especially for cases associated with symptoms of mechanical locking or severe giving out.

Consider orthopedic consultation, depending on the underlying cause (e.g., meniscal tear, loose body, advanced osteoarthritis).

PHYSICAL THERAPY. Physical therapy plays an essential role in the active treatment and prevention of knee effusion.

PHYSICAL THERAPY SUMMARY

1. Application of ice and elevation of the knee
2. Crutches with touch-down–weightbearing
3. Straight-leg–raising exercises to restore support and stability, isometrically performed
4. Gradual resumption of active exercises, with caution

Acute Period. For the first few days apply ice, elevate the knee, and restrict weight-bearing. *Ice* and elevation are always recommended for acute knee effusions. An ice bag, a bag of frozen corn, or an iced towel from the freezer applied for 10 to 15 minutes is effective for swelling and analgesia. *Crutches*, a *walker*, or a *cane* may be necessary during the first few days.

Recovery/Rehabilitation. After the acute symptoms have subsided, toning exercises are begun and are combined with restricted use. *Straight-leg–raising* exercises are always recommended to restore muscular support to the knee (p. 274). Initially they are performed without weights in sets of 20, with each held 5 seconds. With improvement in strength, a 5- to 10-lb weight is added to the ankle. These exercises are performed in the prone and supine positions to tone the quadriceps femoris and hamstring muscles. *Active exercises,* especially on apparatus, must be included with caution. Exercise on a stationary bicycle, a rowing machine, or a universal gym may be irritating to an inflamed and recently distended joint. Fast walking, swimming, a NordicTrack-like glide machine, and other limited-impact exercise apparatus or exercises requiring much less flexion are preferred.

INJECTION. Aspiration of synovial fluid is performed to relieve the pressure of tense effusions and to allow a fluid analysis to be made for diagnosis. Injection of local anesthetic can be used to differentiate articular from periarticular conditions affecting the knee. Corticosteroid injection is used to treat the nonseptic effusion such as osteoarthritis, rheumatoid arthritis, pseudogout, and so forth.

Positioning: The patient is to be in the prone position with the leg extended.

Surface Anatomy and the Point of Entry: The midline of the iliotibial band, the lateral edge of the patella, and the superior pole of the patella are palpated and marked. Gently push the patella laterally to palpate its edge. The point of entry is along a line drawn halfway between the iliotibial band (the center of the femur) and the lateral edge of the patella and 1/2" below the superior pole of the patella (see Figure 9–2). This provides the safest and easiest access to the superolateral portion of the suprapatellar pouch.

Angle of Entry and Depth: The needle is angled up toward the superior pole of the patella. The lateral retinaculum (the first tissue plane) is as much as 2 1/2" deep. The superior pouch of the synovial cavity is always 1/2" beyond the lateral retinaculum.

Anesthesia: Ethyl chloride is sprayed on the skin. Local anesthetic is placed at the retinaculum (1 ml) and intra-articularly.

Technique: A *lateral approach* is easiest and safest. The needle is advanced at a 70-degree angle toward the suprapatellar pouch (just above the superior pole of the patella) until the resistance of the rubber-like tissue of the lateral retinaculum—the first tissue plane—is felt. One ml of anesthesia is placed just outside the synovial lining. The needle is withdrawn.

Next, an 18-gauge, 1 1/2" needle attached to a 20-ml syringe is advanced down to the retinaculum and then into the joint (a giving-way sensation or pop is often felt and the patient feels discomfort). Gentle pressure against the medial retinaculum and joint line may shift the synovial fluid laterally. If the fluid is relatively clear (the examiner should be able to read newsprint through a low–cell-count fluid), 1 ml of K40 is injected through the same needle.

If the first pass into the joint does not yield synovial fluid, the needle is slowly withdrawn with constant low suction. If fluid is not obtained with the slow withdrawal of the needle, the needle is redirected to the level of the superior pole of the patella. Aspiration is attempted at this site. If the second attempt is unsuccessful, a dry tap knee injection is recommended (see p. 148).

INJECTION AFTERCARE

1) *Rest* for 3 days, avoiding all squatting, kneeling, and bending beyond 90 degrees.

2) Advise crutches with touch-down–weightbearing for 3 to 7 days for severe cases.

3) *Ice* (15 minutes every 4 to 6 hours) and *Tylenol ES* (1000 mg twice a day) for soreness.

4) *Protect* the knee for 3 to 4 weeks by limiting repetitive bending, prolonged standing, and unnecessary walking; continue to restrict squatting and kneeling.

5) Begin *straight-leg–raising exercises* for the quadriceps muscle on day 4.

6) Combine with a patellar restraining brace if quadriceps tone is poor and the patient has experienced repeated episodes in which the knee has given out.

7) Repeat *injection* at 6 weeks with corticosteroid if swelling persists.

8) In the chronic case, obtain *plain x-rays* (standing PA of knees, bilateral, and sunrise views) or *MRI* to identify advanced degenerative arthritis, high-degree subluxation of the patellofemoral joint, degenerative or traumatic meniscal tear, and so forth.

9) Advise long-term restrictions on bending of the knee (30 to 45 degrees) for the patient with advanced arthritis.

10) Request a *consultation* with a surgical orthopedist for a second opinion if two consecutive injections fail to provide 4 to 6 months of improved function and decreased swelling.

SURGICAL PROCEDURE.   Surgical procedures vary according to the underlying pathology. Arthroscopic débridement can be considered for severe, protracted osteoarthritis flare. Meniscectomy is performed for the degenerative or traumatic meniscal tear (see p. 166). Synovectomy is used for rheumatoid arthritis that has failed to respond to systemic therapy and intra-articular corticosteroids.

PROGNOSIS.   The response to aspiration and injection depends on the underlying cause. Mild to moderate inflammatory effusions (cell counts from 1000 to 20,000) respond most dramatically, with 6 to 18 months of relief. Noninflammatory effusions (cell counts in the 100s) respond less predictably. Poor response to intra-articular steroids (4 to 6 weeks or fewer suggests either a noninflammatory process or a mechanical process such as a loose body or meniscal tear. Any patient who fails to respond to two consecutive intra-articular injections should be evaluated further with repeat plain x-rays, MRI, or arthroscopy.

DESCRIPTION.   The lateral approach to the suprapatellar pouch did not yield synovial fluid. This is an alternative injection technique to ensure an intra-articular placement of corticosteroid. The symptoms, examination, plain x-rays, treatment protocol, and physical therapy are identical to information for knee effusion (see p. 143).

INJECTION.   In order to assure an intra-articular injection, an injection will have to be placed immediately adjacent to articular cartilage. A *lateral approach* to the patella is preferred. It is less likely to damage articular cartilage than either a medial or a lateral joint line injection. The neurovascular structures are smaller over the lateral knee. The lateral patella is closer to the skin. And the lateral approach avoids the obstacle of the contralateral leg.

Positioning: The patient is to be in the prone position with the leg extended.

Surface Anatomy and the Point of Entry: The midline of the iliotibial band, the lateral edge of the patella, and the superior pole of the patella are palpated and marked. The patella should be gently subluxated laterally to palpate its lateral edge. The point of entry in the horizontal plane is halfway between the iliotibial band and the lateral edge of the patella and 1/2" caudal to the superior pole of the patella in the craniocaudal axis.

Dry Tap Injection of the Knee

The point of entry for the aspiration of a knee effusion (p. 143) is used for this injection; direct the needle toward the undersurface of the patella.

Needle: 1½" to 3½" spinal 22 gauge or 18 gauge for viscous fluid

Depth: until the soft resistance of the patellar cartilage is felt—1 to 3¼"

Volume: 1 to 2 ml of local anesthesia plus 1 ml of K40

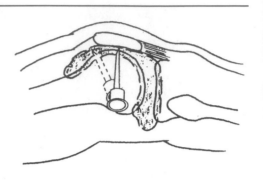

Figure 9–3.   Dry tap injection of the knee

Angle of Entry and Depth: The needle is angled up toward the undersurface of the patella. The lateral retinaculum (first tissue plane) ranges from 1/2 to 2 1/2" deep. The articular cartilage of the patella is 1/2 to 3/4" beyond the firm tissue resistance of the retinaculum.

Anesthesia: Ethyl chloride is sprayed on the skin. Local anesthetic is placed at the retinaculum (1 ml) and intra-articularly.

Technique: A *lateral approach* is easiest and safest. The same point of entry used for knee aspiration (see p. 143) is used to perform the dry tap injection. The needle is directed and advanced to the undersurface of the patella. Mild subluxation of the patella will facilitate this injection. Firm pressure is necessary to "pop" into the joint. The bevel of the needle should be turned up so that the angle of the patella matches the bevel (less likely to damage the articular cartilage!). Then the needle is advanced cautiously to the undersurface of the patella. The depth of injection is assessed by gently rocking the patella back and forth (pressure is applied from the medial edge of the patella). The medially applied pressure should be felt by the tip of the needle. At this exact point, 1 to 2 ml of anesthetic can be injected (diagnostic local anesthetic block for an intra-articular process) along with 1 ml of K40.

INJECTION AFTERCARE

1) *Rest* for 3 days, avoiding all squatting, kneeling, and bending beyond 90 degrees.

2) Advise crutches with touch-down–weightbearing for 3 to 7 days for severe cases.

3) *Ice* (15 minutes every 4 to 6 hours) and *Tylenol ES* (1000 mg twice a day) for soreness.

4) *Protect* the knee for 3 to 4 weeks by limiting repetitive bending, prolonged standing, and unnecessary walking; continue to restrict squatting and kneeling.

5) Begin *straight-leg–raising exercises* for the quadriceps muscle on day 4.

6) Combine with a patellar restraining brace if quadriceps tone is poor and the patient has experienced repeated episodes in which the knee has given out.

7) Repeat *injection* at 6 weeks with corticosteroid if swelling persists.

8) For the persistent or chronic case, obtain the following *plain x-rays*: standing PA of knees and bilateral sunrise views or CT scans or MRI to identify advanced

degenerative arthritis, high-degree subluxation of the patellofemoral joint, degenerative or traumatic meniscal tear, and so forth.

9) Advise *long-term restrictions* on bending for the patient with advanced arthritis.

10) Request a *consultation* for a second opinion with a surgical orthopedist if two consecutive injections fail to provide 4 to 6 months of improved function and decreased swelling.

PROGNOSIS. The response and long-term outcome depend on the degree of inflammation, the stage of osteoarthritis (whether early or advanced), and the association of mechanical dysfunction (poor quadriceps tone, ligamentous instability, degenerative meniscal tear, and so forth). Injection should provide 6 to 18 months of relief, on average.

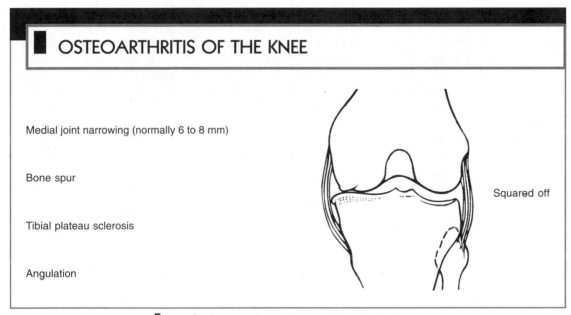

OSTEOARTHRITIS OF THE KNEE

Medial joint narrowing (normally 6 to 8 mm)

Bone spur

Tibial plateau sclerosis

Angulation

Squared off

Figure 9–4.   Wear-and-tear arthritis of the knee

DESCRIPTION.   Osteoarthritis of the knee is a wear-and-tear, noninflammatory arthritis that affects the three compartments of the joint—the medial, lateral, and patellofemoral compartments. A family history, obesity, genu valgum and genu varum, previous meniscectomy, and previous fractures of the distal femur and proximal tibia predispose to this condition. Pathologically, there is asymmetric wear of the articular cartilage, bony osteophyte formation, and sclerosis of the subchondral bone and subchondral cyst formation.

SYMPTOMS.   The patient complains of knee pain, swelling, or deformity. The patient often rubs the inner aspect of the joint (medial compartment involvement is most common) when describing the condition.

"My knee gets stiff and painful at the end of the day."
"I can't do my 'folks walks' anymore . . . my knees ache so bad."
"I'm too embarrassed to wear dresses anymore . . . my knees look so bony."
"My knees make this awful sound every time I kneel down to pray in church."
"My knees have ached for a long time . . . now they swell really badly and they give out all the time . . . I'm afraid to even go to the store."
"I can't bend my knees anymore."
"When I was 22, I had the cartilage removed from my right knee. It swelled and popped a lot then. Now the whole thing just aches."

EXAM. Each patient is examined for local joint-line tenderness, loss of smooth mechanical function (crepitation), loss of range of motion, and joint effusion.

EXAM SUMMARY

● ● ● ● ● ● ● ● ● ● ● ● ● ● ● ●

1. Joint-line tenderness (medial, lateral, or at the patella)
2. Loss of smooth mechanical motion (crepitation with passive or active motion)
3. Palpable bony osteophytes
4. Loss of full flexion or extension
5. Knee effusion

---

(1) Tenderness is present at the joint line, more commonly on the medial side. The joint lines are identified at the level of the lower third of the patella when the knee is in the extended position and the quadriceps muscle is relaxed. (2) The hallmark of osteoarthritis is crepitation of the knee, palpable at the joint line when the knee is passively flexed and extended. This is in contrast to the crepitation felt anteriorly that is seen with patellofemoral syndrome and the single popping sensation felt at the joint line that occurs with a meniscal tear. (3) Advanced cases have palpable bony osteophytes at the joint line. The enlargement is greatest at the medial tibial plateau. (4) As the condition progresses, the bony osteophytes and the damage to the articular cartilage interfere with full range of motion. (5) Knee effusion commonly complicates osteoarthritis. Effusions that develop acutely and knee effusion over 20 to 25 ml interfere with full flexion. (6) Occasionally, an acute change in the mechanical function of the knee occurs. Popping, locking, or other mechanical symptoms may suggest a degenerative meniscal tear.

X-RAYS. X-rays of the knee (including standing PA, lateral, sunrise, and tunnel views) are always recommended. Standing weightbearing PA views are used to determine the widths of the cartilage of the medial and lateral compartments as well as the valgus carrying angle of the knee. The distance between the medial tibial plateau and the medial femoral condyle is normally 6 to 8 mm. As the condition progresses, this space gradually narrows. Serial measurements can be used to predict when surgical consultation is necessary. Note that the radiographic diagnosis of arthritis does *not* have to be accompanied by osteophytes, subchondral sclerosis, or subchondral cyst formation!

The sunrise, or merchant, view is used to determine the degree of patellofemoral arthritic involvement. The tunnel view is used to evaluate for osteochondritis dissecans and intra-articular loose bodies. The lateral view with good soft-tissue technique can provide clues to the presence of a large joint effusion, the location of bony lesions, and soft tissue calcifications.

SPECIAL TESTING. If mechanical symptoms dominate the clinical findings, an MRI is obtained to evaluate for a degenerative meniscus tear or intra-articular loose body.

DIAGNOSIS. A presumptive clinical diagnosis based on joint-line tenderness, crepitation, bony enlargement, and joint effusion should be confirmed by standing weightbearing x-rays. Occasionally, a regional anesthetic block is used to differentiate the pain arising from the joint from the pain arising from the periarticular structures.

TREATMENT. The goals of treatment are to relieve pain, treat the accompanying effusion, preserve function, and evaluate the appropriateness of surgical referral. Restrictions of bending and impact combined with isometrically performed straight-leg–raising exercises are the treatments of choice for mild disease. Corticosteroid injection is the treatment of choice for osteoarthritis accompanied by a large effusion. Total knee replacement is the treatment of choice for advanced arthritis.

Step 1: Perform a heel-to-buttock measurement, aspirate the effusion for diagnostic studies (e.g., cell count and differential, crystals, glucose, Gram stain, and culture), and order standing PA, lateral, sunrise, and tunnel views of the knees. Suggest ice applications and elevation of the knee.

Recommend crutches with touch-down–weightbearing for severe cases.

Minimize squatting and kneeling.

Advise on the importance of weight loss.

Recommend heat in the morning and ice for swelling after activities.

Prescribe a patellar restraining brace if the knee is grossly unstable (giving out frequently).

Begin straight-leg–raising exercises without weights as soon as the acute symptoms resolve and advance to weighted exercises as tolerated.

Prescribe an NSAID (e.g., ibuprofen [Advil, Motrin]) for 4 weeks at full dose with a taper beginning at 3 weeks.

Step 2 (3 to 6 weeks for persistent cases): If symptoms are persistent, prescribe a 3- to 4-week course of a second NSAID (from a different chemical class) or give a local corticosteroid injection for persistent effusion.

Repeat the injection at 4 to 6 weeks if symptoms are not reduced by 50%.

Reemphasize the importance of weighted straight-leg–raising exercises.

Step 3 (2 to 4 months for chronic cases): Repeat plain films or perform an MRI for cases that have failed to respond to treatment and especially for cases associated with mechanical locking or severe giving-out.

Consider orthopedic consultation for patients who do not have any medical contraindications for surgery and if (1) pain is intractable, (2) function is severely compromised, (3) 80 to 90% of the articular cartilage has worn away, or (4) progressive angulation of the lower extremity has occurred.

Order a Velcro patellar restraining brace, a walker, or a wheelchair for the patient with advanced osteoarthritis who cannot undergo surgical replacement.

PHYSICAL THERAPY.   Physical therapy plays an essential role in the active treatment and prevention of osteoarthritis of the knee.

PHYSICAL THERAPY SUMMARY

1. Ice and elevation of the knee
2. Crutches with touch-down weightbearing
3. Straight-leg–raising exercises to restore support and stability, performed isometrically
4. Gradual resumption of active exercises, with caution

Acute Period.   For the first few days apply ice, elevate the knee, and restrict weightbearing. *Ice* and elevation are always recommended for acute arthritic flares. An ice bag, a bag of frozen corn, or an iced towel from the freezer applied for 10 to 15 minutes is effective for swelling and analgesia. *Crutches,* a *walker,* or a *cane* may be necessary in the first few days.

Recovery/Rehabilitation.   After the acute symptoms subside, toning exercises are combined with restricted use. *Straight-leg–raising* exercises are always recommended to restore muscular support to the knee (p. 276). Initially, these are performed without weights in sets of 20, with each held 5 seconds. With improvement in strength, a 5- to 10-lb weight is added to the ankle. These exercises are performed in the prone and supine positions to tone the quadriceps femoris and hamstring muscles. *Active exercises*, especially on apparatus, must be used with caution. Exercise on a stationary bicycle, a rowing machine, or a universal gym may be irritating to an inflamed and recently distended joint. Fast walking, swimming, a NordicTrack-like glide machine, and other limited-impact exercise apparatus or exercises requiring much less flexion are preferred.

INJECTION. Local corticosteroid injection can provide dramatic short-term relief and is indicated when (1) the NSAIDs are contraindicated, (2) the NSAIDs are poorly tolerated, (3) inflammation and effusion fail to improve, (4) symptom palliation is necessary for a patient who has advanced disease and cannot undergo surgery, or (5) the patient prefers it (see "Knee Effusion", p. 143). Note that a lateral approach for aspiration and injection (p. 143) may not be suitable for all patients, especially those with severe hypertrophic patellofemoral disease. In these cases, a medial approach can be performed that is analogous to the lateral approach. The point of entry is halfway between the medial edge of the patella and the midplane of the leg, centered over the femur.

SURGICAL PROCEDURE. Surgery is indicated for advanced disease. Arthroscopic débridement is indicated for degenerative meniscal tears and loose bodies. High tibial osteotomy is the procedure of choice for patients under age 62 to correct the loss of the normal 8- to 9-degree valgus angle and to shift the weightbearing pressure to the preserved lateral-compartment articular cartilage. Total knee replacement (TKR) is the procedure of choice for patients over the age of 62.

PROGNOSIS. Osteoarthritis of the knee is a relentlessly progressive problem that is characterized by periodic flares of pain and swelling. Medication by mouth or by injection should be reserved for these exacerbations. Dramatic changes in clinical findings or rapid progression of wear and tear may reflect a degenerative meniscal tear, the poorly tolerated effects of increased angulation of the knee, developing underlying rheumatic disease, or the dramatic complication of septic arthritis. In these cases, x-rays should be repeated to remeasure the valgus carrying angle, fluid should be obtained for synovial analysis to exclude a complicating hemarthrosis or infection, or an MRI should be ordered to rule out a degenerative tear.

DESCRIPTION. Prepatellar bursitis is an inflammation of the bursal sac located between the patella and the overlying skin. The most common cause is trauma as a result of a fall or the direct pressure and friction of repetitive kneeling (90% "housemaid's knee"). It is one of two bursae in the body that can become infected (5% due to *Staphylococcus aureus*) or inflamed by urate crystals (5% due to acute gout). Normally the bursa is paper-thin, simply a potential space. With chronic bursal irritation and inflammation, the bursal walls dilate, thicken, and become fibrotic—the pathologic condition of chronic bursitis.

SYMPTOMS. The patient complains of knee swelling and knee pain just over the front of the knee. The patient often rubs over the bursa or points at the swelling when describing the condition.

"My knee is swollen."
"I'm a housekeeper. I have to work on my knees a lot. Even though I am careful and wear knee pads, my right knee has begun to swell. Is this arthritis, doctor?"
"My knee is inflamed."
"I have a bump over my knee cap."
"I bumped my knee against the kitchen cabinet and within hours it had swollen up."
"It feels like a bunch of little marbles just under the skin."

Prepatellar Bursitis

The bursa is entered at the base, paralleling the patella; the needle is passed into the center of the sac. Alternatively, the needle can be advanced to the lower third of the periosteum of the patella for injection of the small or chronically thickened bursa.

Needle: 1½", 18 gauge

Depth: ¼ to ⅜"

Volume: 1 ml of anesthetic plus 1 ml of K40

Note: If the needle touches the periosteum of the anterior patella, the injection is intrabursal!

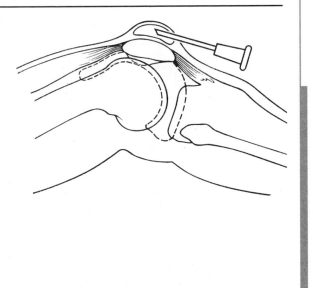

Figure 9–5. Prepatellar bursa aspiration

EXAM. The degree of swelling and inflammation, the amount of bursal fluid, and the range of motion of the knee are examined in each patient.

(1) A cystic collection of fluid is palpable directly over the patella. Inflammatory signs are variable, depending on the cause and the length of time symptoms have been present. (2) Tenderness is present over the entire sac in acute cases. Tenderness may be minimal in the chronically effused or thickened case (10%).

EXAM SUMMARY ● ● ● ● ● ● ● ● ● ● ● ● ● ● ●

1. Swelling and inflammation directly over the inferior portion of the patella
2. Bursal sac tenderness vs. bursal sac thickening (chronic)
3. Normal range of motion of the knee (unless cellulitis accompanies)

Chronic prepatellar bursitis has a characteristic cobblestone-like roughness or palpable thickening. This is best appreciated by squeezing the bursa between two fingers and comparing the thickness to the contralateral side. (3) The range of motion of the knee should be normal in an uncomplicated case of prepatellar bursitis that is unassociated with cellulitis or an underlying articular condition. This extra-articular accumulation of fluid does not interfere with motion, as opposed to the limitation of flexion commonly seen with acute knee effusion.

X-RAYS. Plain x-rays of the knee are not necessary to make the diagnosis and they rarely affect clinical management. The lateral view of the knee demonstrates soft-tissue swelling above the patella. Calcification of the quadriceps tendon at the superior pole of the patella is not related to this condition. This calcification occurs commonly but does not indicate disease of the quadriceps mechanism.

SPECIAL TESTING.   Fluid analysis.

DIAGNOSIS.   A clinical diagnosis of prepatellar bursitis is easily made by simple inspection and palpation of the anterior structures of the knee. However, bursal fluid aspiration and analysis are necessary to determine the cause of the condition.

TREATMENT.   The goals of treatment are to identify the cause of the swelling, to reduce the swelling and inflammation, to encourage the walls of the bursa to reapproximate, and to prevent chronic bursal thickening. Aspiration and drainage combined with padding and protection are the treatments of choice for acute prepatellar bursitis.

Step 1: Aspirate the bursa for diagnostic studies: Gram stain and culture, crystals, and hematocrit.
>   Apply a compression dressing for 24 to 36 hours after aspiration.
>   Advise the patient to avoid direct pressure.
>   Recommend a neoprene pull-on knee brace (p. 297) or Velcro knee pads (p. 297).
>   Prescribe an NSAID (e.g., ibuprofen [Advil, Motrin]).

Step 2 (1 to 2 days after fluid analysis): Give an oral antibiotic for infection, do an evaluation and treatment for gout, or reaspirate and inject with K40.
>   Continue padding and protective measures.
>   Educate the patient: "Between 10 and 15% remain swollen or thickened regardless of treatment."

Step 3 (4 to 6 weeks for persistent cases): Repeat the aspiration and injection of the bursa with K40 if symptoms have not been reduced by 50%.
>   Limit squatting and kneeling.

Step 4 (months for chronic cases): Consider an orthopedic consultation for bursectomy.

PHYSICAL THERAPY.   Physical therapy does not play a significant role in the treatment of prepatellar bursitis. General care of the knee is recommended with emphasis on toning the quadriceps and hamstring muscles by doing straight-leg–raising exercises.

INJECTION.   Local corticosteroid injection is indicated for (1) recurrent nonseptic bursitis, (2) bursitis due to gout when the NSAIDs are contraindicated, (3) chronic bursal thickening (palpably thickened soft tissues above the patella—the "bursal pinch sign"), or (4) persistent postinfectious bursitis (with a negative postantibiotic culture).

Positioning: The patient is to be in the prone position with the leg fully extended.

Surface Anatomy and the Point of Entry: The superior and inferior margins of the bursa are identified and marked. The point of entry is at the base of the inferior margin.

Angle of Entry and Depth: The needle is inserted at the base of the bursa, paralleling the patella, and is advanced to the center of the bursa. Alternatively, the needle is inserted above the bursa and is advanced at a 45-degree angle down to the firm to hard resistance of the periosteum of the patella (for the chronically thickened bursa with little fluid).

Anesthesia: Ethyl chloride is sprayed on the skin. Local anesthetic is placed at the base of the bursa in the subcutaneous tissue and dermis only.

Technique: Complete aspiration combined with compression assures the best outcome. After local anesthesia, an 18-gauge needle attached to a 10-ml syringe is passed into the center of the sac. The needle is rotated 180 degrees so that the bevel faces the patella. Aspiration with gentle suction combined with manual pressure from above and on the sides will facilitate fluid removal. With the needle left in place, the syringe is replaced with the syringe containing the corticosteroid. One ml of K40 is injected. The needle is withdrawn and a gauze and Elastoplast pressure dressing is applied.

INJECTION AFTERCARE

1) *Rest* for 3 days, avoiding all direct pressure, squatting, kneeling, and bending beyond 90 degrees.

2) Wear the compression dressing for 24 to 36 hours and then replace it with a neoprene pull-on knee sleeve.

3) *Ice* (15 minutes every 4 to 6 hours) and *Tylenol ES* (1000 mg twice a day) for soreness.

4) *Protect* the knee for 3 to 4 weeks by limiting pressure, repetitive bending, squatting, and kneeling.

5) Begin *straight-leg–raising exercises* for the quadriceps muscle on day 4.

6) Repeat *injection* at 6 weeks with corticosteroid if swelling recurs or persists.

7) Request a *consultation* with a surgical orthopedist if two consecutive aspirations and injections fail to eliminate the swelling and the patient still complains of pressure pain.

SURGICAL PROCEDURE. Bursectomy is infrequently performed (in 2 to 4% of cases).

PROGNOSIS. About 50 to 60% of cases will spontaneously resolve or will respond to simple aspiration. The remaining cases will require one or two local injections of K40. Between 5 and 10% of cases fail to respond to conservative care and show persistent swelling. These can be referred for definitive bursectomy. In an additional 5% of cases, the acute swelling will resolve but demonstrate persistent bursal sac thickening (chronic bursitis). Surgical treatment of these cases is individualized. Note that this bursal sac does not interfere with the normal function of the knee. Persistent swelling or thickening of the bursal sac alone is not an indication for surgery. Patients troubled with persistent pain and irritation from repetitive kneeling (e.g., carpet layers, cement finishers, and so forth) should be considered for surgery.

Anserine Bursitis

Enter at the point of maximum tenderness, usually 1½″ below the medial joint line or parallel to the tibial tubercle in the concavity of the tibial plateau.

Needle: 1 or 1½″, 22 gauge

Depth: ½ to 1½″ down (or ⅛″ above the periosteum of the tibia)

Volume: 1 to 2 ml of anesthesic plus ½ ml of D80

Note: NEVER inject under pressure.

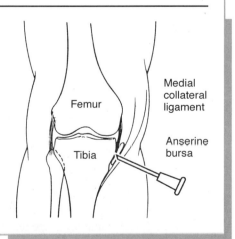

Figure 9–6.   Anserine bursa injection

DESCRIPTION. Anserine bursitis is an inflammation of the bursal sac located between the attachment of the medial collateral ligament (MCL) at the medial tibial plateau and the conjoined tendon formed by the gracilis, sartorius, and semitendinosus tendons. Although it can result from direct trauma, it more commonly develops as a consequence of an abnormal gait. Any loss of the normal mechanical relationships between the knee, hip, and pelvis causes an abnormal pull at the insertion point of the three tendons (the gracilis originates at the pubis, the sartorius from the ilium, and the semitendinosus from the ischium). The increased friction and pressure resulting from this gait disturbance cause anserine bursitis. It frequently accompanies osteoarthritis of the knee, chronic knee effusion, or any other intrinsic knee condition.

SYMPTOMS. The patient complains of knee pain that is often localized to a well-defined area of the inner knee. The patient often points to the area with one finger when describing the local irritation.

"I have a very sharp knee pain right here (pointing to the inner aspect of the knee)."
"I can't sleep on my side. When my knees touch, I get this really sharp pain on the inside of my knee."
"I don't know what happened. I didn't have an injury. I slowly developed this sharp pain inside my knee."
"The inside of my knee looks a little swollen and is very tender to the touch."
"I sleep with a pillow between my legs because my knee is tender."
"I was hit with a line drive when I was playing baseball. The ball hit me in the inside of my knee. The pain was so sharp I couldn't walk for several days."

EXAM. Each patient is examined for tenderness at the medial tibial plateau along with a thorough examination of the knee and an analysis of the patient's gait.

EXAM SUMMARY ● ● ● ● ● ● ● ● ● ● ● ● ● ● ● ●

1. Local tenderness in the concavity of the medial tibial plateau directly over the tibial tubercle in the midline
2. Painless valgus stress testing of the medial collateral ligament
3. Intrinsic knee joint abnormalities or abnormal gait
4. Successful anesthetic block at the bursa

(1) Local tenderness is present 1 to 1 1/4" below the medial joint line parallel to the tibial tubercle. The quarter-sized area is located in the midline in the concavity of the medial tibial plateau. (2) Valgus stress testing of the MCL does not aggravate the pain; that is, the signs of an MCL strain are absent. (3) The knee and lower extremities are examined for any primary musculoskeletal process that would affect the gait.

X-RAYS. X-rays of the knee are not necessary for the diagnosis. No specific changes are seen either in the soft tissues or along the medial tibial plateau. However, x-rays of the knee are strongly recommended to assess the degree of associated osteoarthritis or rheumatoid arthritis (the most common causes of knee effusions).

SPECIAL TESTING. Plain x-rays, arthrocentesis, or an MRI should be used to define the underlying cause.

DIAGNOSIS. The diagnosis is based on localized medial tibial plateau tenderness, the absence of signs indicating a medial collateral ligament strain, and pain relief with local anesthetic. Regional anesthesic block placed within the bursal sac is used to differentiate the symptoms of bursitis from those of medial-compartment osteoarthritis, patellofemoral syndrome, and medial meniscus tear.

TREATMENT.   The goals of treatment are to reduce the pain and swelling in the bursa and to identify and treat any underlying cause of abnormal gait. Restriction, protection, and ice are the treatments of choice for acute bursitis. When bursitis is the primary cause of knee pain, corticosteroid injection is the preferred initial treatment. When bursitis complicates one of the articular disorders of the knee or ankle, treatment should focus on the primary condition.

Step 1: Obtain plain x-rays of the knee, including the sunrise view, assess quadriceps tone, evaluate the gait, and examine the knee for an underlying cause (e.g., knee effusion, osteoarthritis, and so forth).
Recommend elimination of squatting and direct pressure (pillow between the knees at night).
Advise the patient to avoid crossing the legs.
Limit repetitious bending.
Suggest ice applications for acute symptoms.
Prescribe an NSAID (e.g., ibuprofen [Advil, Motrin]) but note that an oral medication may not concentrate sufficiently in this relatively isolated structure.

Step 2 (6 to 8 weeks for persistent cases): Perform an injection of D80.
Repeat the injection of D80 in 4 to 6 weeks if symptoms and signs have not been reduced by 50%.
Continue to investigate for a primary cause.

Step 3 (8 to 10 weeks after improvement): Begin straight-leg–raising exercises with weights (p. 276).
Suggest cautious squatting, kneeling, and repetitive knee flexion until symptoms have been controlled.

PHYSICAL THERAPY.   Physical therapy does not play a direct role in the treatment of anserine bursitis. General toning exercises of the quadriceps and hamstring muscles are used in the recovery.

Ice over the bursa will effectively control pain and some of the swelling. *Phonophoresis* with a hydrocortisone gel may provide temporary relief in asthenic individuals. *General care of the knee* is recommended, with emphasis on toning the quadriceps femoris and the hamstring muscles through straight-leg–raising exercises.

PHYSICAL THERAPY SUMMARY   • • • • • • • • • • • • • • •

1.   Ice applied to the medial tibial plateau
2.   Phonophoresis with a hydrocortisone gel in asthenic individuals
3.   General care of the knee (p. 276).

INJECTION.   Local injection is used (1) to confirm the diagnosis, (2) to treat primary bursitis, and (3) to treat bursitis that persists after the primary gait disturbance has been addressed.

Positioning: The patient is to be in the prone position with the leg extended and externally rotated.

Surface Anatomy and the Point of Entry: The tibial tubercle, medial joint line, and midline of the medial lower leg are identified and marked. The point of entry is in the midline, directly across from the tibial tubercle, or approximately 1 1/2″ below the medial joint line.

Angle of Entry and Depth: The needle is inserted perpendicular to the skin and is directed slightly upward toward the concavity of the medial tibial plateau. The injection depth is always 1/8″ above the periosteum of the tibia or 1/2 to 1 1/2″ deep.

Anesthesia: Ethyl chloride is sprayed on the skin. Local anesthetic is placed at the tissue plane of the tendon and 1/8″ above the periosteum of the tibia (both 1/2 ml).

Technique: A 22-gauge needle is passed through the subcutaneous fat until the subtle resistance of the conjoined tendon is felt. Anesthesia can be injected here for comfort. Then the needle is gently passed an additional 3/8″ to the firm periosteum of the tibia and immediately withdrawn 1/8″ to avoid injection into the medial collateral ligament. The bursa is located between the MCL and the tendon, and anesthesia and corticosteroid are injected here. Injection should be free-flowing, with little resistance. Pressure on injection usually suggests improper position (too deep!).

INJECTION AFTERCARE

1) *Rest* for 3 days, avoiding all direct pressure, squatting, kneeling, repetitive bending, and unnecessary standing and walking.

2) *Ice* (15 minutes every 4 to 6 hours) and *Tylenol ES* (1000 mg twice a day) for soreness.

3) *Protect* the knee for 3 to 4 weeks by limiting repetitive bending, squatting, and kneeling.

4) Begin *straight-leg–raising exercises* for the quadriceps muscle on day 4.

5) Repeat *injection* at 6 weeks with corticosteroid if pain recurs or persists.

6) Request a *consultation* with a surgical orthopedist if two consecutive aspirations and injections fail to eliminate the swelling and the patient still complains of weightbearing pain.

SURGICAL PROCEDURE.   Bursectomy is rarely required (fewer than 1% of cases).

PROGNOSIS.   The completeness and length of response to treatment depend on restoring normal gait. If bursitis recurs at an early interval (4 to 8 weeks) or if response to injection is limited, a more thorough evaluation of gait should be undertaken!

DESCRIPTION.   A Baker cyst is an abnormal collection of synovial fluid in the fatty layers of the popliteal fossa. It must be distinguished from the more common dilated semimembranosus bursa, which gradually enlarges as a result of the hydraulic pressure of repetitive flexing of the knee. Both are located on the medial side of the popliteal fossa, and both become enlarged as a result of an overproduction of synovial fluid. However, only the Baker cyst is a separate anatomic structure. Fluid that escapes from the normal confines of the synovial lining causes a fibrotic reaction in the subcutaneous tissue and cyst formation.

SYMPTOMS.   The patient complains of tightness behind the knee or pain down the back of the leg (the latter symptom is suggestive of cyst rupture). The patient often rubs the back of the knee when describing the condition.

"My doctor told me that I have a cyst behind my knee."
"I felt a lump behind my knee."
"When I bend my knee back, it feels like an egg is behind my knee."
"My knee seems swollen and tight."
"My regular doctor told me I have bad circulation. The doctor in the emergency room thought I had a

Baker Cyst

Enter over the center of the cyst with the needle held vertically.

Needle: 1½", 18 gauge

Depth: ¾" to 1¼"

Volume: 1 to 2 ml of anesthetic plus 1 ml of K40

Note: Use continuous aspiration pressure while advancing the needle; once the cyst has been entered, slowly advance the needle to the mild tissue resistance of the back of the cyst wall.

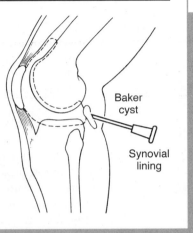

Figure 9–7. Baker cyst aspiration and injection

blood clot in my leg. I'm really confused. I've had all these tests and I still don't know why I have this pain in my leg."

EXAM. Each patient is examined for a palpable, cystic mass in the medial aspect of the popliteal fossa and is given a thorough examination of the knee to determine the cause of synovial fluid overproduction.

(1) With the patient in the prone position and the leg fully extended, an oblong cystic mass is palpable and visible in the medial popliteal fossa. (2) Large cysts may impair knee flexion by as much as 10 to 15 degrees. (3) Signs of a knee effusion may be present (p. 143). (4) Signs of vascular insufficiency (suggesting popliteal aneurysm) and signs of deep venous thrombosis of the popliteal veins (pain in the posterior calf) are absent.

EXAM SUMMARY

1. A cystic mass in the popliteal fossa
2. Impaired knee flexion when the cyst is large
3. Evidence of a current or past chronic knee effusion
4. No evidence of peripheral vascular insufficiency or deep venous thrombosis

X-RAYS. X-rays of the knee are not necessary for this specific diagnosis. Plain films of the popliteal fossa are normal. However, x-rays of the knee are recommended to assess the degree of osteoarthritis or rheumatoid arthritis (the more common causes of knee effusions).

SPECIAL TESTING. Diagnostic ultrasound can be used to define the size and extent of the cyst. However, this test is of questionable utility if the cyst is not obviously palpable (small cysts discovered by ultrasound rarely interfere with knee function). Arthrography may reveal the sinus tract originating from the synovial cavity. This test may be helpful in planning the correct surgical exposure.

DIAGNOSIS.   A tentative diagnosis is based on the presence of a palpable, popliteal mass or on the demonstration of a fluid-filled cyst on ultrasonography. A definitive diagnosis, however, requires aspiration of the characteristic clear, nonbloody, highly tenacious fluid.

TREATMENT.   The goals of treatment are to aspirate the abnormal accumulation of fluid, to correct any underlying cause of chronic knee effusion, and to determine the need for surgery. In general, small cysts should be observed. The treatment of choice for large cysts that interfere with full function of the knee is local aspiration and corticosteroid injection.

Step 1: Evaluate and treat any underlying cause of chronic knee effusion (e.g., rheuma-
toid arthritis, osteoarthritis, and so forth), assess the strength of the quadri-
ceps, and measure the range of motion of the knee.
Educate the patient: "The Baker cyst can resolve on its own over time."
Advise the patient to restrict squatting, kneeling, and repetitious bending.
Encourage straight-leg–raising exercises with weights (p. 276).
Consider a neoprene pull-on knee brace (p. 297).

Step 2 (4 to 6 weeks for follow-up treatment): Repeat the aspiration (remove as much fluid as possible).
Continue the use of the neoprene brace (p. 297).
Educate the patient: "These types of cysts frequently recur regardless of which treatment is used."

Step 3 (8 to 10 weeks for persistent cases): Reaspirate and inject with K40.
Repeat the injection in 4 to 6 weeks if the size of the cyst has not decreased by 50%.

Step 4 (3 to 6 months for chronic cases): If improved, perform straight-leg–raising exer-
cises with weights (p. 276).
Advise the patient to avoid repetitive flexion and squatting.
Consider surgical removal if the patient is a surgical candidate, if all causes of excessive fluid production have been treated optimally, and if the cyst is interfering with the normal function of the knee.

PHYSICAL THERAPY.   Physical therapy plays a minor role in the treatment of a Baker cyst. General care of the knee is recommended, with emphasis on toning the quadriceps femoris and hamstring muscles by doing straight-leg–raising exercises.

INJECTION.   Local injection is used to confirm the diagnosis (by simple aspiration) and to treat large cysts that compromise full flexion of the knee.

Positioning: The patient is to be in the supine position with the leg fully extended.

Surface Anatomy and the Point of Entry: The outline of the cyst is marked; it is typically
an oblong structure located medially in the popliteal fossa and extending
inferiorly. The point of entry is directly over the center of the cyst.

Angle of Entry and Depth: The needle is inserted perpendicular to the skin and is
advanced through the subcutaneous tissue to the subtle tissue resistance of
the cyst wall (3/4 to 1 1/4″ below the skin surface).

Anesthesia: Ethyl chloride is sprayed on the skin. Using a 22-gauge needle, local
anesthesia is placed intradermally, subcutaneously, and just outside the cyst
wall (1/2 ml).

Technique: An 18-gauge needle attached to a 20-ml syringe is held vertically and
passed down to the subtle resistance of the cyst wall. *Note:* the neurovascular
bundle is deep to the cyst; only skin and subcutaneous tissue overlie the cyst

cavity! Continuous negative pressure is used while advancing. The outer wall is often quite thick and a giving-way or popping sensation is often felt as the cyst is entered. After the cyst is punctured, the needle is advanced until the subtle tissue resistance of the back wall is felt or fluid can no longer be easily aspirated. At this point the needle is withdrawn 1/8 to 3/8″. This needle position will assure optimal aspiration of the fluid as the cyst collapses. Manual pressure is applied to either side of the needle to assist in fluid recovery. With the needle left in place, 1 ml of K40 is injected into the cyst.

INJECTION AFTERCARE

1) *Rest* for 3 days, avoiding all squatting, kneeling, and repetitive bending.

2) *Ice* (15 minutes every 4 to 6 hours) and *Tylenol ES* (1000 mg twice a day) for soreness.

3) *Protect* the knee for 3 to 4 weeks by limiting repetitive bending, squatting, kneeling, impact, and prolonged standing.

4) Maximize the treatment of the associated conditions affecting the knee (osteo-arthritis, rheumatoid arthritis, and so forth).

5) Begin *straight-leg–raising exercises* for the quadriceps muscle on day 4.

6) Repeat *aspiration and injection* with corticosteroid at 6 weeks if pain recurs or persists (at the cyst or intra-articularly).

7) Request a *consultation* with a surgical orthopedist if two consecutive aspirations and injections fail to eliminate the swelling, and the patient still complains of pressure and swelling in the popliteal fossa.

SURGICAL PROCEDURE.   Bursectomy is indicated when full flexion of the knee is interfered with and two consecutive injections fail to reduce the cyst's overall size.

PROGNOSIS.   Aspiration and injection with corticosteroids can provide sympto-matic relief for months. Like all ganglia, however, the recurrence rate is high, espe-cially if an underlying chronic knee effusion persists. Baker cysts that interfere with the function of the knee can be referred for surgical removal. Unfortunately, as with medical therapy, recurrence does happen after surgical excision.

Medial Collateral Ligament Sprain

Enter at the midline over the tibial plateau just below the joint line.

Needle: ⅝″, 25 gauge or 1½″, 22 gauge

Depth: ½″ (thin patients) to ¾″ or ⅛″ above the perios-teum of the tibia

Volume: 1 to 2 ml of anesthetic plus ½ ml of D80

Note: NEVER inject between the MCL and the bone; always brace after injection!

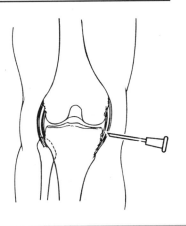

Figure 9–8.   Medial collateral ligament injection

DESCRIPTION.   A medial collateral ligament strain is an irritation, inflammation, or partial separation of the inner "hinge" ligament of the knee. Strains are classified as first, second, or third degree on the basis of the amount of motion of valgus stress testing. Ligaments that are irritated and inflamed but otherwise intact are classified as first-degree strains. Ligaments that are partially torn are classified as second-degree separations. Ligaments that are completely disrupted with gross instability of the knee are classified as third-degree separations.

SYMPTOMS.   The patient complains of knee pain along the inner aspect of the knee joint and has difficulty walking, pivoting, and twisting. The patient often points to or rubs along the joint line down to the tibial plateau insertion site when describing the condition.

"I was playing touch football, and I was tackled from the right side, causing immediate pain along the inner part of my knee."
"I was getting out of the bathtub when my leg caught, my body twisted, and my leg was wrenched. Ever since, I have had pain and sensitivity along the inside of my knee."
"I sprained my knee when I tripped on the rug."
"Every time I twist my leg, I get this sharp pain along the side of my knee."
"I can't even turn over in bed. My leg gets snagged up in the sheets, and any amount of twisting just kills me."
"My knee has been swollen for months, but now it feels different. It feels loose and sloppy."

EXAM.   Each patient is examined for the degree of irritation, inflammation, and laxity of the medial collateral ligament, and an assessment of overall knee stability is made.

EXAM SUMMARY   • • • • • • • • • • • • • • • •

1.   An inch-long band of local tenderness located between the medial joint line and the insertion on the tibia
2.   Pain aggravated by valgus stress testing
3.   Laxity of the medial collateral ligament (with higher degrees of rupture)
4.   Associated knee effusion, anterior cruciate ligament tear, or medial meniscal tear

(1) Tenderness is located from the medial joint line down the insertion of the medial collateral ligament on the tibial plateau. The tenderness is usually about 1" long and parallels the length of the ligament. (2) Valgus stress testing, applied with the leg in the extended position and at thirty degrees of flexion, causes acute pain and (3) may demonstrate laxity. In addition, medial knee pain may be aggravated by forcibly externally rotating the tibia on the femur with the knee bent at 90 degrees. (4) The remaining examination of the knee may show effusion, laxity, or disruption of the anterior cruciate ligament (ACL) or a medial meniscal tear. Trauma severe enough to cause a third-degree separation is often enough to disrupt other supporting tissues of the knee.

X-RAYS.   X-rays of the knee are not necessary for the diagnosis. Routine views are usually normal. Avulsion fractures are unusual. Calcification of the ligament can occur months to years later. A 1 to 1 1/4" crescent-shaped calcification along the medial joint line is referred to as Pellegrini-Stieda syndrome. This radiographic finding is unique but does not correlate directly with clinical findings.

SPECIAL TESTING.   An MRI is indicated when other injuries are suspected. Tears of the joint capsule, the ACL, the meniscal cartilage, or the articular cartilage (osteo-chondritis dissecans) are more likely with second- or third-degree MCL tears.

DIAGNOSIS. The diagnosis is based on a history of a line of pain crossing the medial joint line and an exam showing local tenderness along the medial knee that is consistently aggravated by valgus stress testing. A regional anesthetic block is rarely used to differentiate this local periarticular process from an intra-articular condition.

TREATMENT. The goals of treatment are to allow the ligament to reattach to its bony origins, to strengthen the muscular support to the knee, and to avoid activities that would reinjure the ligament. Immobilization combined with crutches and physical therapy exercises are the initial treatments of choice.

Step 1: Determine the stage of the condition, assess for secondary injuries, estimate the quadriceps strength, and establish a baseline level of function (can walk, can limp, cannot bear weight, and so forth).
Advise walking with crutches for the first 7 days of the acute injury.
Prescribe a Velcro straight-leg knee immobilizer with metal stays to be worn continuously during the day.
Recommend ice applications at the joint line.
Prescribe an NSAID (e.g., ibuprofen [Advil, Motrin]) to control the pain.
Advise sleeping with the leg straight and with loose covers.
Restrict activities of daily living for the first 2 to 4 weeks; no sports.

Step 2 (2 to 4 weeks for persistent cases): Recommend straight-leg–raising exercises without weights (as soon as the acute pain subsides).
Advise continuing use of the brace during activities.
Educate the patient: "This ligament injury can take months to heal."

Step 3 (6 to 8 weeks for persistent cases): Perform a local injection of D80 coupled with continuous bracing for the next 3 to 4 weeks.
Advise on a graduated return to normal activities and a graduated exercise program.
Perform straight-leg–raising exercises with weights.
Strongly encourage the use of a brace during sports and the avoidance of pivoting and twisting.

PHYSICAL THERAPY. Physical therapy plays a minor role in the active treatment of medial collateral ligament strain but a major role in rehabilitation.

PHYSICAL THERAPY SUMMARY ● ● ● ● ● ● ● ● ● ● ● ● ● ●

1. Ice for the acute pain and swelling
2. Straight-leg–raising exercises without weights (while in the brace), isometrically performed
3. Straight-leg–raising exercises with weights in the recovery/rehabilitation phase
4. Cautious return to sports, use of exercise equipment, and so forth

Acute Period. Ice, elevation, crutches, and limited activities are advised during the first 7 to 14 days. Application of *ice* over the medial tibial plateau is an effective local analgesic. Activity restrictions are necessary to allow the injured ligament to reattach to the bone.

Recovery. After 7 to 10 days, exercises are begun to strengthen the supporting structures of the knee. While continuing with the knee brace, *straight-leg–raising exercises* are performed daily. The leg is kept perfectly straight to avoid placing stress on the ligament.

Rehabilitation. As the ligament strengthens, *weighted straight-leg–raising exercises* can be started to enhance the tone of the quadriceps and hamstring muscles (p. 276). *Active exercising and sports,* especially on equipment, must be delayed until the quadriceps muscle tone is restored to the strength and tone of the contralateral muscle. A knee brace should be worn during the first several weeks of retraining. Exercises and equipment that place torque through the knee must be avoided. Fast walking, swimming (kicking with the knees held straight), and NordicTrack-like equipment are preferred.

INJECTION. Immobilization combined with physical therapy strengthening exercises is the treatment of choice. Local corticosteroid injection is indicated if symptoms persist despite adequate restrictions and immobilization.

Positioning: The patient is to be in the prone position with the leg extended and externally rotated.

Surface Anatomy and the Point of Entry: The medial collateral ligament is located in the midplane, originating at the midmedial femoral condyle and inserting on the midmedial tibial plateau. The point of entry is just below the medial joint line on the tibia (the joint line is located parallel to the lower third of the patella when the leg is in the extended position).

Angle of Entry and Depth: The needle is inserted in the midplane on the tibial side of the medial joint line, perpendicular to the skin. The depth is 1/8″ above the periosteum of the tibia (1/2 to 3/4″ from the skin).

Anesthesia: Ethyl chloride is sprayed on the skin. Local anesthesia is placed subcutaneously and 1/8″ above the tibial periosteum (1/2 ml).

Technique: The tibial plateau is identified, just below the medial joint line. A 25-gauge needle is inserted, held perpendicular to the skin and advanced down to the firm resistance of the periosteum of the tibia. Once the bone has been encountered, the needle is withdrawn 1/8″ to ensure that the injection is above the MCL attachment (err on the superficial side rather than going too deep; deep injections may lift the ligament off the bone). Do not inject if firm or hard pressure is encountered. After local anesthesia, retest local tenderness and perform valgus stress testing. If these signs are significantly reduced, then the same area is injected with 1/2 ml of D80. Massage the medication in for 5 minutes.

INJECTION AFTERCARE

1) *Rest* for 3 days, avoiding all twisting, squatting, kneeling, and repetitive bending.

2) Use crutches with touch-down weightbearing for the first few days.

3) Wear the Velcro straight-leg immobilizer continuously during the day.

4) *Ice* (15 minutes every 4 to 6 hours) and *Tylenol ES* (1000 mg twice a day) for soreness.

5) *Protect* the knee for 3 to 4 weeks by avoiding all twisting and pivoting and limiting repetitive bending, squatting, and kneeling.

6) Begin *straight-leg–raising exercises* for the quadriceps muscle on day 4 (perform these in the brace for the first week or two).

7) Repeat the *injection* with corticosteroid at 6 weeks if pain recurs or persists.

8) Request a *consultation* with a surgical orthopedist if two consecutive injections fail and the patient still complains of pain with pivoting and twisting (internal derangement?).

SURGICAL PROCEDURE. Primary repair of second- and third-degree tears is the surgical treatment of choice.

PROGNOSIS.   First-degree sprains heal completely 90% of the time. However, healing may take several months in some cases. Second-degree tears with greater tissue disruption heal less predictably. Third-degree tears rarely confront the primary physician. These injuries are often triaged from the emergency room directly to the orthopedic surgeon.

DESCRIPTION.   A torn meniscus is a disruption of the fibrocartilage pads located between the femoral condyles and the tibial plateaus. Tears are classified as partial or complex; anterior, lateral, or posterior; traumatic or degenerative; and horizontal, vertical, radial, parrot-beak, or bucket-handle. Because of the strategic location and inherent shock-absorbing properties of the meniscus, significant tears lead to loss of smooth motion of the knee—the classic locking phenomenon, knee effusion, and premature osteoarthritis.

SYMPTOMS.   The patient complains of popping, locking, and giving out or has a vague sense that the knee is not moving properly. Athletic patients attempt to demonstrate the catching or locking phenomenon when describing their symptoms.

"My knee locks up whenever I get it in certain bent positions."
"My knee catches."
"My knee locks up on me when I bend down. When I stand up, it won't straighten right away. When it pops, I feel a bunch of pain and then it releases. It's always right here (pointing to the inner knee)."
"I can't squat anymore."
"If I twist just right, I get this real sharp pain."
"I was getting out of the car. My leg was twisted. I tried to shift my weight when I felt this loud pop and immediate sharp pain inside my knee."
"I can't put my finger on it, but whenever I try to shift my weight, the pain inside my knee practically kills me."

EXAM.   Each patient is examined for loss of smooth motion, for the presence of a joint effusion, and for specific meniscal signs.

EXAM SUMMARY   • • • • • • • • • • • • • •

1.   Loss of smooth motion of the knee, passively performed
2.   Inability to squat or kneel
3.   Palpable popping on the joint line (McMurray maneuver)
4.   Joint effusion

---

(1) Patients with certain types of meniscal tears can have a completely normal knee exam. Partial tears, horizontal tears, and anterior tears may not produce abnormal knee signs because of their size and anatomic location. These types of tears do not interfere with the normal mechanics of the knee and thus are less likely to compromise function or cause mechanical locking. (2) Screening tests for significant meniscal tears should start with an assessment of general knee function. The knee can be assessed by observing gait, passive and active flexion and extension, squatting, and duck waddling. The latter is virtually impossible with large, complex, vertical, or bucket-handle tears. (3) The McMurray test and the Apley grinding test are relatively specific for meniscal tears; however, their sensitivity is poor. These tests have a false-negative rate of 20 to 25%. The McMurray maneuver should be performed several times. The knee is fully flexed. The tibia is internally rotated (relative to the femur) to trap the lateral meniscus and externally rotated to trap the medial meniscus. A

MENISCAL TEAR OF THE KNEE

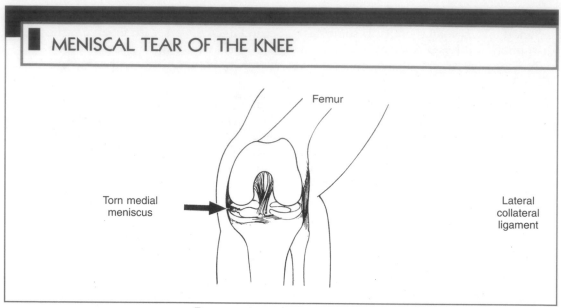

Figure 9–9.   Medial meniscus

popping sensation under the examiner's fingers held firmly along the joint line is considered abnormal. (4) Large or complex tears and tears associated with degenerative arthritis often have an associated joint effusion. Signs of underlying osteoarthritis may be present, either as a cause of the degenerative meniscus or as a result of a long-standing meniscal tear.

X-RAYS.   X-rays of the knee (including the sunrise, tunnel, posteroanterior, and lateral views) are recommended. Plain films of the knee may show degenerative change, calcification of the meniscus, or calcified loose bodies. The tunnel view demonstrates the intercondylar notch and may show a sequestered loose body!

SPECIAL TESTING.   An MRI will define the extent and type of meniscal tear. Note that the MRI must be interpreted cautiously. The images obtained from an MRI provide information that may or may not be clinically relevant or useful. Mucinoid degenerative change (increased signal arising from the center of the meniscus) is a common finding. This is a normal part of the aging process of the meniscus and should not be misinterpreted as a traumatic meniscal tear. Arthroscopy is the definitive diagnostic and therapeutic test.

DIAGNOSIS.   A tentative diagnosis is based on a history of mechanical catching or locking along with corroborative signs on exam. The diagnosis is confirmed by an MRI or, preferably, by arthroscopy. Note that the decision to proceed to an MRI or arthroscopy should be based on the patient's age, the patient's operative candidacy, and the need to proceed with surgery. The surgical decision should be based on frequency of symptoms (daily), the general function of the knee (unable to squat, unstable knee, and so forth), the type of tear (complex tear extending to the articular surfaces), its location (correlating with the patient's symptoms), and the likelihood that leaving it in place might lead to further articular cartilage damage.

TREATMENT.   The goals of treatment are to define the type and extent of the tear, to strengthen the muscular support of the knee, and to determine the need for surgery. Meniscal tears that are small, cause infrequent symptoms, and do not interfere with the general function of the knee should be observed. Large, complex tears associated with persistent knee effusion should be referred for surgical repair or removal.

Step 1: Assess the general function of the knee, determine the frequency of locking, and order plain x-rays.

Restrict activities and all sports.

Recommend applications of ice with leg elevation.

Strongly encourage the use of crutches for the acute and severe case.

Begin straight-leg–raising exercises without weights as the pain begins to wane (p. 276).

Prescribe a patellar restraining brace if quadriceps tone is poor and giving-out is frequent.

Step 2 (2 to 4 weeks for persistent cases): Aspirate persistent knee effusions for diagnostic studies and to relieve pain.

Order an MRI if mechanical symptoms and effusion persist.

Step 3 (4 to 6 weeks for persistent cases): Consider consultation with an orthopedic surgeon for persistent effusion, frequent locking, and disabling symptoms.

Educate the patient: "Arthritis can result if severely damaged cartilage remains in the joint. However, removal of a large part of the "shock-absorber" cartilage may lead to premature arthritis."

PHYSICAL THERAPY.   Physical therapy does not play a significant role in the active treatment of a surgical meniscal tear but is very important in the preoperative preparation and the postoperative rehabilitation process. *General care of the knee* is always recommended, with particular emphasis on strengthening the quadriceps and hamstring muscles that have been weakened by disuse (p. 276).

For nonsurgical meniscal tears, even greater emphasis is placed on toning the thigh muscles. *Quadriceps and hamstring toning exercises* provide greater stability to the knee, allow the joint surfaces to better approximate, and increase the knee's endurance. In addition, these treatments combine to reduce the knee's susceptibility to future injury.

PHYSICAL THERAPY SUMMARY   ● ● ● ● ● ● ● ● ● ● ● ● ● ● ●

1. Ice and elevation for acute symptoms
2. Straight-leg–raising exercises, performed isometrically
3. Quadriceps and hamstring toning on apparatus (initially, only to 30 to 45 degrees)
4. Gradual resumption of activities

INJECTION.   For large meniscal tears that interfere with the normal smooth motion of the knee, arthroscopy with débridement is the treatment of choice. However, aspiration of the knee can be used as an interim treatment and is recommended to rapidly reduce the pressure symptoms of the acute, tense, bloody effusion. In addition, local corticosteroid injection is recommended in the select group of patients with osteoarthritis complicated by a degenerative meniscal tear (see the technique of knee aspiration, p. 143).

SURGICAL PROCEDURE.   Meniscectomy, partial or complete.

PROGNOSIS.   The management of meniscal tears depends on the type of tear (e.g., intrasubstance, horizontal, or vertical), the presence of significant mechanical symptoms, and the presence of persistent knee effusion. Intrasubstance and horizontal tears can be managed medically with rest, restriction, exercises, and aspiration. Vertical tears (in contact with articular cartilage), tears associated with large, persistent effusions, and tears with frequently disabling symptoms should be evaluated by arthroscopy. Partial or complete meniscectomy is determined at the time of operation.

chapter 10

Ankle

Ankle Sprain

Enter ½" anterior to the lateral malleolus for the talofibular ligament and ½" below the tip of the lateral malleolus for the fibulocalcaneal ligament.

Needle: ⅝", 25 gauge

Depth: ½ to ⅝"

Volume: 1 to 2 ml of anesthetic plus ½ ml of D80

Note: Confirm the placement with local anesthetic first; immobilize for 1 to 4 weeks, depending on the severity.

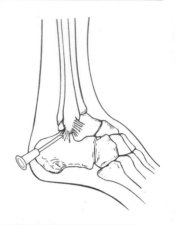

Figure 10–1.   Fibulocalcaneal ligament injection

DESCRIPTION.   An ankle sprain is a partial tear of the supporting ligaments of the ankle joint. Inversion injuries cause the fibulocalcaneal or the fibulotalar ligaments to pull away from their normal bony attachments. Sprains are classified as acute, recurrent, or chronic. Ligaments that do not heal properly and do not reattach to their bony origins can cause significant ankle instability which, in turn, can lead to osteochondritis dissecans or osteoarthritis.

SYMPTOMS.   The patient complains of ankle pain, ankle swelling and bruising, or instability of the ankle (in the recurrent or chronic case).

"I stepped off a high curb, higher than I thought, and came down on the side of my foot. My ankle immediately swelled, and I couldn't put any weight on it."
"I tried to turn a corner while running, and my ankle suddenly gave out."
"I jumped up and landed on the side of my foot. Ever since, I have had sharp pain along the outside."
"I injured my ankle years ago, and it has been weak ever since."
"Four weeks ago I sprained my ankle. I had this huge black-and-blue spot that went away. My ankle still feels weak."
"Every time I try to play basketball my ankle gives out. I wear high-top shoes, but I still can't run or jump very well."

EXAM.   Each patient is examined for irritation, inflammation, and laxity of the individual lateral ankle ligaments, and an assessment is made of general ankle alignment and function.

EXAM SUMMARY   • • • • • • • • • • • • • • •

1. Tenderness, swelling, or bruising anterior and inferior to the lateral malleolus
2. Pain aggravated by forced inversion of the foot
3. No pain with resisted plantar flexion and eversion, isometrically performed
4. Full range of motion of the ankle (in the nonacute case)
5. Ankle instability (positive drawer sign or talar knock sign) documented in the recovery phase

(1) Minor ankle sprains are tender anterior and inferior to the lateral malleolus. Moderate to severe ankle sprains have tenderness combined with swelling and bruising. The acute and severe sprain may be so intensely sore that the remaining portions of the exam are not possible. (2) As the acute symptoms resolve, forced inversion of the ankle aggravates the pain. This should improve gradually as the condition resolves. (3) Isometric testing of the peroneus tendons may demonstrate pain inferior to the lateral malleolus (active tendinitis) or may demonstrate pain and tenderness at the insertion at the base of the fifth metatarsal (avulsion fracture). (4) The range of motion of the ankle should be normal once the acute symptoms have resolved. (5) Long-standing recurrent or chronic cases may show instability of the ankle. An anterior or posterior drawer sign may be present. Rocking the ankle back and forth passively may produce a knocking, the talar knock sign. The latter usually indicates a separation of the interosseous membrane between the tibia and the fibula. Lastly, long-standing ankle instability may lead to signs of limited range of motion, crepitation, and pain at the extremes of motion—that is, osteoarthritis of the ankle.

X-RAYS. X-rays of the ankle (including the routine PA, mortise, and lateral views) are ordered to evaluate the ankle joint, the subtalar joint, and the malleoli. In addition, the special PA oblique and subtalar views are used to further assess the integrity of the joints and to exclude an avulsion fracture at the lateral malleolus or at the base of the fifth metatarsal, the attachment of the peroneus tendon. Most x-rays are normal.

SPECIAL TESTING. Patients with persistent localized findings despite immobilization, recovery-oriented physical therapy exercises, and time may benefit from an MRI. Osteochondritis dissecans of the talar dome or early arthritic changes may be seen.

DIAGNOSIS. The diagnosis is based on the history of inversion injury coupled with the obvious physical findings. Plain x-rays are used to exclude avulsion or complete fracture of the lateral malleolus or the base of the fifth metatarsal. Rarely, regional anesthetic block is indicated to differentiate the symptoms and signs of ankle sprain from peroneus tenosynovitis, subtalar arthritis, and so forth.

TREATMENT. The goals of treatment are to allow the lateral ligaments of the ankle to reattach to their bony insertions, to strengthen the tendons that cross the ankle, and to prevent recurrent ankle sprains. Limited weightbearing and immobilization of the ankle are the treatments of choice for acute ankle sprain.

Step 1: Examine the patient, perform plain x-rays of the ankle, and assess the severity of the injury.
Strongly advise on limited weightbearing.
Prescribe immobilization with an Ace wrap and crutches, overlap-taping, an air cast, an Unna boot, or a short-leg walking cast, depending on the severity of the injury. Note that because of the 10 to 20% rate of recurrent ankle sprain (nonanatomically or poorly healing ligaments), it is important to emphasize immobilization that prevents inversion and eversion.

Step 2 (1- to 3-week follow-up evaluation): Perform gentle stretching exercises beginning with dorsiflexion and plantar flexion.
Begin isometric toning exercises of eversion once flexibility has significantly improved.
Advise the patient to wear high-top shoes or a Velcro ankle brace (p. 300).
Recommend limiting stop-and-go sports, basketball, running, and impact aerobics.
Educate the patient: "Healing is measured in months rather than weeks."

Step 3 (6 to 8 weeks for persistent cases): Perform a local injection of D80 and combine it with a short-leg walking cast.
Repeat the injection in 4 to 6 weeks if symptoms have not been reduced by 50%.

Reemphasize the need to perform daily stretching and toning exercises.
Order an MRI of the ankle for persistent swelling, intractable pain, or instability.
Consider referral to a surgical orthopedist if symptoms and instability persist.

PHYSICAL THERAPY.   Physical therapy plays an essential role in the active treatment and rehabilitation of ankle sprain.

PHYSICAL THERAPY SUMMARY

1. Ice and elevation for the acute pain and swelling
2. Heating and ankle stretching for postimmobilization rehabilitation
3. Toning exercises in eversion, isometrically performed

Acute Period.   Ice and elevation are used in the first few days to effectively reduce the acute pain and swelling. Treatments lasting 15 to 20 minutes several times a day will reduce tissue distortion due to bleeding and swelling.

Recovery Rehabilitation.   After the acute pain and swelling have subsided, exercises are performed to restore normal range of motion and to strengthen the ankle joint. *Stretching exercises* of the ankle joint are performed after immobilization, especially with fixed casting. Dorsiflexion and plantar flexion stretching are performed initially, followed by gentle inversion and eversion. The ankle is heated prior to stretching. Sets of 20 passive stretches in each direction are performed daily. *Isometric exercises* are used to strengthen and stabilize the ankle joint and are the most effective means of preventing further injuries. Toning exercises are necessary to overcome the weakness of a tear or of severe separation of the ligaments. Both types of recovery exercises are necessary prior to resumption of normal activities.

INJECTION.   Immobilization combined with physical therapy (strengthening exercises) are the treatments of choice. It is uncommon to perform local corticosteroid injection. Injection is reserved for patients with persistent inflammation despite immobilization (first-degree sprains only).

Positioning: The patient is in the supine position. The ankle is kept in a neutral position.

Surface Anatomy and the Point of Entry: The tip of the lateral malleolus and the point of maximum tenderness are identified and marked. The point of entry is 1/2" anterior or inferior to the lateral malleolus (the fibulotalar and fibulocalcaneal ligaments, respectively).

Angle of Entry and Depth: The needle is inserted directly over the point of maximum tenderness, perpendicular to the skin. The depth is 1/2 to 5/8" beneath the skin.

Anesthesia: Ethyl chloride is sprayed on the skin. Local anesthesia is placed subcutaneously and at the firm resistance of the lateral ligament, 1/4 to 1/2" beneath the skin (1/2 ml).

Technique: All medication injections should be placed atop the ligament—between the subcutaneous tissue and the ligament. This tissue plane can be easily identified by advancing the needle gradually until the firm resistance of the ligament is appreciated or until the tip of the needle stays in place when skin traction is applied (if the needle is above the ligament, the needle will move with the skin and subcutaneous tissue when traction is applied!). After local anesthesia, the ankle is reexamined for instability and pain relief. If the anterior drawer and talar knock signs are negative and local palpation and passive inversion are no longer painful, 1/2 ml of D80 is injected.

INJECTION AFTERCARE

1) *Rest* for 3 days, avoiding all unnecessary weightbearing.

2) Use crutches with touch-down–weightbearing for the first few days in severe cases.

3) Recommend immobilization with lace-up, high-top shoes, an air cast, or a short-leg walking cast for 1 to 4 weeks, depending on the severity of the original injury.

4) *Ice* (15 minutes every 4 to 6 hours) and *Tylenol ES* (1000 mg twice a day) for soreness.

5) *Protect* the ankle for 3 to 4 weeks by avoiding all twisting and pivoting and limiting unnecessary walking and standing.

6) Begin *isometric toning exercises* of ankle eversion and inversion at 3 to 4 weeks.

7) Repeat the *injection* at 6 weeks with corticosteroid if pain recurs or persists.

8) Order an *MRI* for persistent instability or intractable pain.

9) Request a *consultation* with a surgical orthopedist if two consecutive injections fail and the patient still complains of pain when pivoting and twisting.

SURGICAL PROCEDURE.   Instability of the ankle is the principal indication for primary repair of the damaged ligament.

PROGNOSIS.   The majority of sprained ankles heal without residual effects. However, ankle sprains associated with severe swelling, bruising, and instability must be managed carefully to avoid the 10 to 20% chance of persistent ankle instability and recurrent ankle sprain. Inadequate activity restriction, immobilization, or physical therapy rehabilitation exercising can lead to nonanatomic healing, weakness of the supporting ligaments, recurrent ankle sprains and, ultimately, osteoarthritis of the joint in later years. In order to avoid the consequences of incomplete healing (recurrent ankle sprain and instability), treatment should emphasize strict immobilization, physical therapy toning exercises, and very gradual resumption of activity. This management strategy will ensure optimal protection for the patients who are at the greatest risk for postrecovery instability.

Most sprained ankles respond to immobilization. Local corticosteroid injection and surgery are rarely necessary. Surgery is reserved for the patient with an unstable joint (positive drawer sign, a positive talar knock sign, or inversion instability). Fewer than 2% would qualify for surgical intervention.

DESCRIPTION.   Aspiration and synovial fluid analysis of the tibiotalar joint are necessary to distinguish among the variety of causes of ankle effusion, which include traumatic bloody effusions, noninflammatory effusions due to osteoarthritis, inflammatory effusions due to rheumatoid disease, and the rare case of septic arthritis.

SYMPTOMS.   The patient complains of swelling in front of or along the sides of the ankle and stiffness or pain in the ankle. Patients often gaze at the ankle and ask the provider if the ankle appears swollen while they are describing the condition.

"I think my ankle is swollen."
"My ankle feels tight inside."
"I can't find a pair of shoes that fit."
"I didn't fall, but my ankle feels like it did when I broke it years ago."

EXAM.   Each patient is examined for joint effusion, local joint line tenderness, and range of motion of the tibiotalar joint.

Arthrocentesis of the Ankle

The ankle can be entered anteromedially just medial to the extensor hallicis longus or anterolaterally just lateral to the extensor digiti minimi.

Needle: 1½", 22 gauge

Depth: 1 to 1¼" through either the tibionavicular ligament or the fibulonavicular ligament

Volume: 2 to 3 ml of anesthetic plus ½ ml of K40

Note: If bone is encountered, withdraw back through the ligament, redirect with skin traction either toward the midline or inferiorly, and advance again.

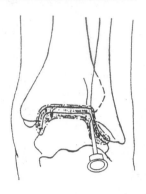

Figure 10–2.   Arthrocentesis and injection of the ankle

EXAM SUMMARY

1. Anterior swelling or general fullness to the ankle
2. Anterior joint line tenderness
3. Loss of or painful plantar flexion or dorsiflexion
4. A characteristic aspirate or confirmation with local anesthetic block

(1) The detection of an effusion of the ankle joint can be elusive. Small effusions cause mild general fullness of the anterior ankle (which is very difficult to differentiate from lower extremity edema). Moderate to large effusions should be ballotable. With finger pressure placed behind both malleoli and both thumbs placed anteriorly, fluid should be palpable as a softness or sponge-like quality when alternating pressure is applied on either side of the extensor tendons. (2) Tenderness is present along the anterior joint line (a line drawn between the two points, 1/2" above the tip of the malleolus and 3/4" above the tip of the lateral malleolus). (3) Acute synovitis causes endpoint stiffness, endpoint pain, or absolute loss of plantar flexion or dorsiflexion. (4) Aspiration of joint fluid or a beneficial response to intra-articular injection is necessary to confirm the involvement of the joint.

X-RAYS.   Plain x-rays of the ankle (PA, lateral, and oblique) are strongly recommended. Osteoarthritic narrowing between the tibia and talus with accompanying medial or lateral osteophytes is best appreciated on the lateral and PA projections. The width of the articular cartilage averages 2 to 3 mm.

SPECIAL TESTING.   Synovial fluid analysis should be performed. An MRI is indicated to exclude osteochondritis of the talar dome or loose body.

DIAGNOSIS.   The diagnosis is suggested by general fullness and ballotable fluid anteriorly. The diagnosis and determination of specific cause require arthrocentesis and synovial fluid analysis.

TREATMENT.   Diagnostic aspiration and synovial fluid analysis are the procedures of choice for the acute effusion. Ice, elevation, limited weightbearing, and range-of-motion exercises are the treatments of choice.

Step 1: Aspirate the joint for diagnostic studies (Gram stain and culture, uric acid crystal analysis, and cell count and differential); order plain x-rays of the ankle; and measure the baseline range of motion of the ankle, especially dorsiflexion.

Strongly advise on limited weightbearing.

Prescribe immobilization with an Ace wrap, high-top shoes, an air cast, an Unna boot, or a short-leg walking cast, depending on the severity of symptoms and signs; combine this with crutches, as indicated.

Step 2 (1 to 3 days after lab analysis): Evaluate and treat for gout, repeat drainage of hemarthrosis, or perform an intra-articular injection of K40 for the osteoarthritic or inflammatory arthritic flare.

Perform gentle stretching exercises beginning with dorsiflexion and plantar flexion.

Begin isometric toning exercises of eversion once flexibility has significantly improved.

Advise the wearing of high-top shoes or a Velcro ankle brace (p. 300).

Recommend limiting stop-and-go sports, basketball, running, and impact aerobics.

Step 3 (3 to 4 weeks for persistent cases): Repeat local injection of K40 and couple this with limited weightbearing or immobilization.

Reemphasize the need to perform daily Achilles tendon stretching exercises and peroneus tendon toning exercises.

Step 4 (8 to 10 weeks for chronic cases): Consider surgical referral for persistent symptoms that interfere with activities of daily living.

PHYSICAL THERAPY.   Physical therapy plays an important role in the rehabilitation of ankle effusion. During the acute period, ice and elevation are used in the first few days to effectively reduce the acute pain and swelling.

PHYSICAL THERAPY SUMMARY

1. Ice and elevation of the ankle for acute pain and swelling
2. Heat prior to range-of-motion exercises, passively performed
3. Toning exercises in eversion to enhance ankle support, isometrically performed

Recovery Rehabilitation.   After the acute pain and swelling have subsided, exercises are performed to restore normal range of motion and to strengthen the ankle joint. *Stretching exercises* of the ankle joint are performed after heating the joint for 15 to 20 minutes. Emphasis is placed on restoring dorsiflexion and plantar flexion first. Eversion and inversion are often restored naturally after the return to regular activities. Sets of 20 passive stretches in each direction are performed daily.

Eversion and inversion toning exercises, isometrically performed, are used to strengthen and stabilize the ankle joint. Emphasis is placed on enhancing the tone of the everter tendons, the peroneus longus in particular. Sets of 20 ankle eversions and inversions, each held 5 seconds, are performed daily. Recovery of eversion and inversion strength is necessary prior to resuming normal activities.

INJECTION.   Ice, elevation, and limited weightbearing are always indicated for the recurrent arthritic flare. Diagnostic aspiration is mandatory if septic arthritis is suspected. Local corticosteroid injection is indicated for large or persistent nonseptic effusions.

Positioning: The patient is to be in the prone position and the ankle is held in 15 to 20 degrees of plantar flexion (this tightens the anterior capsule).

Surface Anatomy and the Point of Entry: A horizontal line is drawn 1/2″ above the medial malleolar tip and 3/4″ above the lateral malleolar tip. The point of entry is at the intersection of this line and just lateral to the extensor digit minimi (anterolateral approach) or, alternatively, just medial to the extensor hallicis longus (anteromedially).

Angle of Entry and Depth: The needle is inserted perpendicular to the skin and angled toward the center of the joint. The depth is 1 to 1 1/4″ beneath the skin.

Anesthesia: Ethyl chloride is sprayed on the skin. Local anesthesia is placed subcutaneously, at the firm resistance of the extensor retinaculum, and intra-articularly (1/2 ml).

Technique: The *anterolateral* approach is preferred because the lateral synovial cavity is larger, and there are fewer obstructing structures. Following anesthesia placement in the superficial tissues, the 22-gauge needle is slowly advanced to the firm resistance of the extensor retinaculum. If bone is encountered at a superficial level (1/2″), the needle is redirected more inferiorly or medially. The joint is entered. If active infection is excluded by fluid inspection or fluid analysis, 1/2 ml of K40 is injected intra-articularly.

INJECTION AFTERCARE

1) *Rest* for 3 days, avoiding all unnecessary weightbearing.

2) Use crutches with touch-down–weightbearing for the first few days in severe cases.

3) Recommend immobilization with lace-up, high-top shoes, an air cast, or a short-leg walking cast for 1 to 4 weeks, depending on the severity of the arthritis and swelling.

4) *Ice* (15 minutes every 4 to 6 hours) and *Tylenol ES* (1000 mg twice a day) for soreness.

5) *Protect* the ankle for 3 to 4 weeks by avoiding all twisting and pivoting and limiting unnecessary walking and standing.

6) Begin *passive stretching* of the ankle in flexion and extension after the pain and swelling have significantly improved.

7) Begin *isometric toning exercises* of ankle eversion and inversion at 3 to 4 weeks.

8) Repeat *injection* at 6 weeks with corticosteroid if swelling recurs or persists.

9) Request an MRI and a *consultation* with a surgical orthopedist if two consecutive injections fail and the patient still complains of weightbearing pain (loose bodies, osteochondritis dissecans, and so forth).

SURGICAL PROCEDURE.   Débridement or arthrodesis.

PROGNOSIS.   Ankle effusions, whether the result of injury, osteoarthritis, or rheumatoid disease, are difficult to manage. To be effective, aspiration and drainage, with or without intra-articular injection of corticosteroid, must be combined with limitations on weightbearing and restriction of activities. Immobilization is often necessary in the advanced case. Patients with refractory effusion and limitations in performing the activities of daily living should be referred for possible arthrodesis.

DESCRIPTION.   Achilles tendinitis is an inflammation of the musculotendinous junction of the Achilles tendon. Repetitive irritation and persistent inflammation lead to microtearing. Runners, patients with short Achilles tendons, and patients with Reiter syndrome are at particular risk. Dramatic changes in the level of activity, incomplete warm-ups prior to sports, and inadequate stretching of the tendon predispose to irritation. Persistent or untreated tendinitis may be complicated by acute rupture (in up to 10% of cases) or chronic tendinitis.

Achilles Tendinitis

This is a peritendinous injection; enter along the outer edge of the tendon, approximately 1½" above the calcaneus.

Needle: 1½", 22 gauge

Depth: superficial—⅜" to ½"

Volume: 2 to 3 ml of anesthetic plus ½ ml of D80 on either side of the tendon

Note: Do not enter the tendon; minimal pressure is needed when injecting. Immobilize with an air-cast or short-leg walking cast for 3 to 4 weeks.

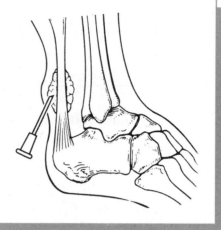

Figure 10–3. Peritendinous injection for Achilles tendinitis

SYMPTOMS. The patient complains of pain behind the ankle with walking, standing, or weightbearing sports activities. The patient often points to the back of the heel when describing the condition.

"I have to stop running after 2 miles because the back of my ankle begins to hurt."
"I get sharp pain through my ankle and up the back of my leg whenever I jump."
"My shoes feel like they're rubbing against the bone."
"I've had to shorten my jogging stride because my cords hurt."
"My Achilles tendon is larger on the right side."
"If I try to do my leg stretches, I get a sharp pain up the back of my leg."
"I was playing basketball when I got this sudden shock of pain right behind my ankle. I looked back to see who might have kicked me, but no one was there. Every step I take now causes pain behind my ankle."

EXAM. Each patient is examined for Achilles tendon irritation, for paratendinous thickening at the musculotendinous junction, and for signs of tendon rupture.

EXAM SUMMARY   ● ● ● ● ● ● ● ● ● ● ● ● ● ●

1. Tenderness and "cobblestone" thickening 1 1/2" above the calcaneus
2. Pain aggravated by resisting plantar flexion, isometrically performed
3. Pain aggravated by stretching in dorsiflexion, passively performed
4. Range of motion of the ankle that is otherwise normal
5. Strength and tendon integrity that are intact

(1) The Achilles tendon is enlarged at the musculotendinous junction. The thickening is 1 to 1 1/2" above the calcaneal insertion, fusiform in shape, and cobblestone-like to the touch. The entire area is sensitive to pressure, especially with side compression. (2) The pain is aggravated by resisting active plantar flexion isometrically and (3) by passive stretching in dorsiflexion. (4) The range of motion of the ankle is

preserved, although pain may limit the ability to measure dorsiflexion accurately. (5) Palpation of the length of the tendon demonstrates that it is free of defects. The strength of the calf muscles is preserved.

X-RAYS.   Plain x-rays of the ankle and lower extremity bony structures are normal. Calcification does not occur at the musculotendinous junction; incidental calcification of the calcaneal insertion of the tendon commonly occurs, but it does not correlate with signs of tendinitis.

SPECIAL TESTING.   An MRI is often used for preoperative staging. Peritendinous swelling, degenerative change, and macrotears of the tendon can be demonstrated.

DIAGNOSIS.   The diagnosis is based on the abnormalities found on physical examination. An MRI is used to distinguish the microtorn tendon with inflammatory reaction from the partial- or full-thickness tendon rupture. Alternatively, regional anesthetic block followed by careful palpation and stress testing may disclose subtle weakness or difficult-to-feel tendon separations.

TREATMENT.   The goals of treatment are to allow the microtorn tendon to heal, to reduce the peritendinous swelling and thickening, to prevent frank rupture of the tendon, and to gradually stretch out the muscle and tendon to prevent recurrent tendinitis. Treatment must be individualized. Passive stretching and limited weight-bearing are the treatments of choice for mild tendinitis. Immobilization with an air cast or a short-leg walking cast is the treatment of choice for moderate to severe involvement.

Step 1: Educate the patient on the importance of rest and reduced weightbearing.
Strongly recommend the use of crutches for 7 to 10 days if symptoms are hyperacute.
Recommend applications of ice for acute swelling and pain.
Advise on shortening the walking stride.
Prescribe padded heel cups or a heel lift (p. 303).
Recommend New-Skin, moleskin, or double socks to reduce friction over the tendon thickening (p. 300).
Recommend v-notched tennis shoes.

Step 2 (3 to 6 weeks for persistent cases): Prescribe an NSAID (e.g., ibuprofen [Advil, Motrin]) at full dosage for 3 to 4 weeks and discuss its partial effectiveness due to poor penetration into these avascular tissues.
Prescribe a Velcro ankle brace or an air cast (pp. 300 to 301).

Step 3 (6 to 8 weeks for persistent cases): Perform a local injection of D80 and combine it with an air cast or a short-leg walking cast ("in equinous" position).

Step 4 (10 to 12 weeks for chronic cases): Prescribe daily Achilles tendon stretching exercises (p. 279).
Recommend following the stretching exercises with toning exercises (p. 280).
Recommend high-top tennis shoes.
Advise on resuming activities very gradually (increasing time or distance by 10% each week; alternating running days with weight training, and so forth).
Recommend continued reduction of friction over the back of the heel.
Limit high-impact sports, jumping, and long-distance running.
Consider a surgical consultation for persistent pain and swelling despite adequate immobilization and local injection.

PHYSICAL THERAPY.   Physical therapy plays an important role in the treatment and rehabilitation of Achilles tendinitis.

PHYSICAL THERAPY SUMMARY   • • • • • • • • • • • • • • •

1. Ice for acute swelling and pain
2. Phonophoresis with a hydrocortisone gel
3. Stretching exercises in dorsiflexion, passively performed
4. Active stretching exercises in dorsiflexion
5. Toning exercises in plantar flexion, isometrically performed

Acute Period.   Ice and phonophoresis are used in the first few weeks to reduce the acute pain and swelling. *Ice* and *phonophoresis* applied directly to the musculotendinous junction provide short-term relief of pain and swelling. *Gentle passive stretching* in dorsiflexion is always recommended after the acute symptoms abate. A foreshortened, inflexible tendon is susceptible to continued irritation! Stretching applied with hand pressure or very gentle wall stretches should be performed daily (p. 279). Mild discomfort in the calf is normal, but acute or sharp pain in the tendon area must be avoided. This stretching is performed after heating.

Recovery/Rehabilitation.   Complete healing requires continued daily stretching of the tendon. Prevention of recurrent tendinitis requires stretching and toning exercises. *Passive stretching exercises* are continued in the recovery period. Vigorous stretching exercises to achieve 30 degrees of dorsiflexion without experiencing pain are started 3 to 4 weeks after the acute symptoms have resolved. Once full dorsiflexion has been obtained, *isometric toning exercises* are begun. These exercises should be performed daily using a TheraBand, oversized rubber bands, or a bungee cord. Sets of 20 are performed with the ankle kept in a neutral position. As strength and tone increase, weightbearing active toning exercises can be performed (p. 280). With increasing strength, full weightbearing activities can be resumed.

INJECTION.   The role of local injection remains controversial. Local corticosteroid injection can effectively reduce the chronic peritendinous inflammation and thickening. However, the benefits of injection must be balanced against the risk of tendon rupture. To reduce this risk, it is strongly advised that injection be combined with rigid immobilization.

Positioning: The patient is to be in the prone position with the foot hanging over the end of the exam table. The ankle is kept in a neutral position.

Surface Anatomy and the Point of Entry: The peritendinous thickening surrounding the tendon is identified. The two points of entry are on each side of the thickening.

Angle of Entry and Depth: The needle is inserted alongside the tendon in the peritendinous thickening at an angle paralleling the tendon. The depth is 3/8 to 1/2" from the surface.

Anesthesia: Ethyl chloride is sprayed on the skin. Local anesthesia is placed subcutaneously (1/2 ml) and within the peritendinous thickening (1/2 ml on each side).

Technique: A peritendinous injection is performed; both the anesthetic and the corticosteroid are injected in a 1"-long linear track within the peritendinous thickening. Note: NEVER inject into the body of the tendon! The optimal injection is accomplished by entering at the most inferior portion of the peritendinous thickening, advancing the needle to the most superior point of the thickening, and then slowly withdrawing the needle inferiorly, leaving a track of medication parallel to the tendon. If local tenderness is significantly relieved and dorsiflexion strength is unquestionably normal, then 1/2 ml of D80 is injected similarly. The procedure is repeated on the opposite side of the tendon.

INJECTION AFTERCARE

1) Strongly recommend immobilization in a short-leg walking cast or air cast for 3 to 4 weeks: "A cast is necessary to protect the tendon from rupture following injection!"

2) Recommend the use of crutches with touch-down weightbearing for the first few days if an air cast has been chosen.

3) *Tylenol ES* (1000 mg twice a day) for soreness.

4) Begin *passive stretching* of the ankle in flexion and extension after the cast is removed, first by hand and then with gentle wall stretches.

5) Keep the stride short while in the recovery phase.

6) Use high-top shoes with padding over the tendon (double socks, felt ring, or molefoam).

7) Begin *isometric toning exercises* of ankle eversion and inversion after flexibility has been partially restored.

8) Request an *MRI* and a *consultation* with a surgical orthopedist if injection combined with immobilization fail.

SURGICAL PROCEDURE.   Achilles tendon stripping or primary repair.

PROGNOSIS.   Achilles tendinitis can be dishearteningly persistent or recurrent, probably owing to the variability in tendon disruption (microtears to full-thickness tears) and degrees of inflammation. Treatment must be individualized based on the degree of thickening, the length of time symptoms have been present, the risk of tear, and the acceptance of treatment by the patient. Simple rest, reduction in the activities of daily living and sports, and stretching exercises are a prudent starting point for mild disease. However, the decision to treat with rigid immobilization or local injection should not be postponed for moderate to severe disease. Chronic inflammation around and through the tendon contributes in a major way to spontaneous tendon rupture. Significant degrees of tendon inflammation must be treated in a timely fashion. Local injection should be strongly considered at 2 to 3 months if tendon thickening is dramatic.

All spontaneous tendon ruptures and most cases of persistent tendinitis should be seen by an orthopedic surgeon. Primary tendon repair can be combined with surgical stripping of the peritendinous tissue or sharp dissection of the mucinoid degeneration.

DESCRIPTION.   Pre-Achilles bursitis is an inflammation of the bursal sac located between the calcaneal insertion of the Achilles tendon and the overlying skin. Its function is to reduce the friction between the skin and the tendon. Although frequently misdiagnosed as Achilles tendinitis, it is distinctly different in pathology, location, and response to treatment. Specifically, pre-Achilles bursitis is rarely disabling and does not contribute directly to tendon rupture.

SYMPTOMS.   The patient has pain and localized swelling behind the heel. The patient attempts to rotate the foot to demonstrate the swelling or rubs along the posterior heel when describing the condition.

"I can't find a comfortable pair of shoes. I can't stand any pressure over the back of my heel."
"There's a lump over the back of my heel."
"My doctor tells me that I have a calcium deposit over the back of my heel. He referred me to you because he didn't know how to treat it."
"The back of my heel hurts."

EXAM.   Local bursal tenderness and swelling are examined in each patient.

Pre-Achilles Bursitis

Enter over the posterior-superior calcaneus in the midline.

Needle: ⅝", 25 gauge

Depth: ¼ to ⅜"

Volume: ½ to 1 ml of anesthetic plus ½ ml of D80

Note: The injection should be superficial to the tendon.

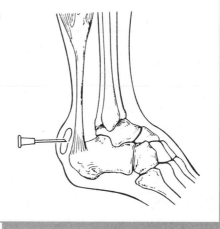

Figure 10—4.   Pre-Achilles bursa injection

EXAM SUMMARY

1. Local tenderness and swelling directly over the posterior calcaneus
2. Minimal pain with stretching of the ankle in dorsiflexion, passively performed
3. Painless resisted plantar flexion of the ankle, performed isometrically
4. Normal range of motion of the ankle

(1) Local tenderness and swelling are present directly over the posterior calcaneus. The quarter-sized area of inflammation is 1" superior to the heel pad, in the midline. (2) Signs of Achilles tendinitis are absent. Passive stretching of the tendon in dorsiflexion and (3) actively resisted plantar flexion are minimally aggravating. (4) The range of motion of the ankle is normal.

X-RAYS. Plain x-rays of the ankle are often ordered but are not necessary for the diagnosis. The lateral view may show calcification arising at the posterior calcaneus. In most cases, the presence of the calcification does **not** influence either the clinical decision-making or the long-term outcome. However, calcific deposits approaching 1 cm in length are large enough to cause pressure and affect walking.

SPECIAL TESTING. None.

DIAGNOSIS. The diagnosis is based on the findings of swelling and tenderness on physical examination. A regional anesthetic block is rarely necessary to distinguish superficial involvement of the bursa from any involvement of the underlying calcaneus (stress fracture, epiphysitis, or subtalar arthritis).

TREATMENT. The goals of treatment are to reduce the friction over the heel, to reduce the bursal inflammation, and to prevent recurrent bursitis by means of stretching exercises. Measures to reduce friction over the back of the heel (a large felt ring, moleskin, New-Skin, v-notched tennis shoes, or padded heel cups) are the treatments of choice.

Step 1: Prescribe padded heel cups, moleskin, double socks, or adhesive New-Skin (p. 300) to reduce heel friction.

Suggest the use of a large felt ring (p. 305).
Recommend the wearing of fleece heel pads while lying in bed.
Advise avoiding shoes with rigid backs.
Recommend v-notched tennis shoes.
Advise on shortening the walking and running stride.
Recommend Achilles tendon stretching exercises (p. 279).

Step 2 (3 to 6 weeks for persistent cases): Perform a local injection of D80.
Reemphasize Step 1.

Step 3 (8 to 10 weeks for persistent cases): Repeat the injection at 4 to 6 weeks if symptoms are not relieved by at least 50%.
Encourage the patient to combine the second injection with a walking cast.

Step 4 (2 to 3 months for chronic cases): Consider an orthopedic consultation for large calcifications or chronic inflammation.

PHYSICAL THERAPY. Physical therapy plays a minor role compared with measures to reduce friction, local injection, and immobilization. Ice is a very effective analgesic, as the bursa is located in the superficial tissues, 1/4 to 3/8″ below the skin surface. Stretching exercises of the Achilles tendon are generally helpful (p. 279).

INJECTION. Local injection with anesthetic is often used to confirm the diagnosis and can be combined with corticosteroid to effectively arrest the local inflammation. Injection and fixed immobilization (air or walking cast) can be combined to improve the outcome in the severe or recurrent case.

Positioning: The patient is to be prone, with the foot hanging over the edge of the table. The ankle is kept in a neutral position.

Surface Anatomy and the Point of Entry: The insertion of the Achilles tendon on the calcaneus is identified. The point of entry is in the midline, directly over the superior portion of the tendon attachment.

Angle of Entry and Depth: The angle of entry is perpendicular to the skin. The needle is advanced down to the firm to hard resistance of the tendon insertion (1/4 to 3/8″ below the skin).

Anesthesia: Ethyl chloride is sprayed on the skin. Local anesthesia is placed in the subcutaneous tissue (1/4 ml) and just posterior to the tendon (1/4 to 1/2 ml).

Technique: A *special pressure technique* is used to identify the bursal sac accurately. The skin is puckered in the midline to facilitate entry of the needle. The needle is advanced down to the firm to hard tissue resistance of the tendon (felt with the needle tip as increased tissue resistance or as increased pressure when attempting to inject anesthetic). With a constant, moderate injection pressure, the needle is very slowly withdrawn until the anesthetic flows easily. The proper placement should create a visible bulge the size of a dime. Note: The bursa will accept only a small volume! Use the least possible amount of anesthetic to confirm the diagnosis. Then reexamine the patient. If the local tenderness is significantly relieved, then 1/2 ml of D80 is injected. *Caution:* Firm to hard pressure on injection suggests an intratendinous injection!

INJECTION AFTERCARE

1) *Rest* for 3 days, avoiding all unnecessary weightbearing.

2) Recommend lace-up, high-top shoes with generous heel padding (double socks, felt ring, or mole-foam).

3) *Ice* (15 minutes every 4 to 6 hours) and *Tylenol ES* (1000 mg twice a day) for soreness.

4) *Protect* the ankle for 3 to 4 weeks by avoiding all unnecessary walking and standing.

5) Recommend shortening the stride: *"Take extra time when walking to and from work!"*

6) Begin *passive stretching* of the ankle in flexion and extension after the pain and swelling have resolved.

7) Repeat *injection* at 6 weeks with corticosteroid if swelling recurs or persists.

8) Request *plain x-rays* and a *consultation* with a surgical orthopedist or podiatrist if two consecutive injections fail and the patient still complains of posterior heel pain.

SURGICAL PROCEDURE.   Calcaneal calcification excision is necessary when the length of the calcification is longer than 1 cm.

PROGNOSIS.   This lower extremity bursa is sensitive to pressure and friction from shoes and may be difficult to heal. Retreatment is not unusual. Emphasis has to be placed on protection and prevention. Bursectomy is rarely suggested.

Retrocalcaneal Bursitis

Enter from the lateral side of the Achilles tendon, 1" above the calcaneus.

Needle: 1½", 22 gauge

Depth: ¾ to 1" (½" above the tibia/talus)

Volume: ½ ml of D80

Note: Place the medication adjacent to the talus rather than the Achilles tendon.

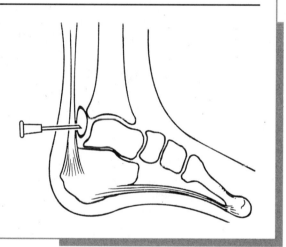

Figure 10–5.   Retrocalcaneal bursa injection

DESCRIPTION.   Retrocalcaneal bursitis is an inflammation of the bursal sac located between the Achilles tendon and the posterior aspect of the ankle. The bursa lubricates the tendon and the talus bone when the foot is in extreme plantar flexion. Retrocalcaneal bursitis is an uncommon problem.

SYMPTOMS.   The patient has ankle pain behind the ankle and painful walking. The patient often takes two fingers and rubs along either side of the Achilles tendon.

"The back of my ankle hurts whenever I go upstairs too fast."
"My knee has been swollen, and I've been limping. Now I have a pain in the back of my ankle."
"I can't see any swelling. My ankle still moves okay, but I'm having this pain behind my ankle."

EXAM.   Each patient is examined for local tenderness and swelling in the soft tissues behind the ankle and an evaluation is made of Achilles tendon flexibility.

1. Local tenderness and swelling in the space between the Achilles tendon and the ankle
2. Pain aggravated by ankle plantar flexion, passively performed
3. Painless resisted ankle eversion, inversion, and plantar flexion, isometrically performed
4. Normal range of motion of the ankle

(1) Local tenderness and swelling are present in the soft-tissue space between the Achilles tendon and the posterior ankle. Pressure applied to the soft tissues just posterior to the talus is painful. Severe cases may swell dramatically, filling in the space between the talus and the Achilles tendon. (2) Pain is aggravated by forcing the ankle into extreme plantar flexion, thus compressing the bursa. (3) The bursa is unaffected by isometric testing of the tendons that cross the ankle. Resisted ankle dorsiflexion, plantar flexion, inversion, and eversion are painless. (4) The range of motion of the ankle is normal.

X-RAYS.   X-rays of the ankle are not necessary for the diagnosis. Calcification does not occur. Ankle films or a radionuclide bone scan may be necessary in a long-distance runner to exclude a stress fracture of the calcaneus.

SPECIAL TESTING.   None.

DIAGNOSIS.   A presumptive diagnosis is based on the characteristic findings on physical examination. The diagnosis is confirmed by a regional anesthetic block placed in the bursa adjacent to the talus.

TREATMENT.   The goals of treatment are to reduce the swelling and inflammation in the bursa and to prevent a recurrence by recommending Achilles tendon stretching exercises. Restrictions placed at the ankle and local corticosteroid injection are the treatments of choice.

Step 1: Advise restriction of repetitive ankle motion (e.g., limit stair-climbing, walk on flat surfaces, no jumping or jogging).
Advise the patient to avoid high heels.
Suggest shortening the stride when walking.
Prescribe padded heel cups (p. 303).

Step 2 (3 to 6 weeks for persistent cases): Prescribe an NSAID (e.g., ibuprofen [Advil, Motrin]) and note that it may have limited benefit because of poor tissue penetration.
Suggest high-top shoes or apply a Velcro ankle brace (p. 300).
Perform a local injection of K40.

Step 3 (8 to 10 weeks for persistent cases): Repeat the injection in 4 to 6 weeks if symptoms have not decreased by 50%.

Step 4 (12 to 14 weeks): Recommend stretching exercises for the Achilles tendon (p. 279).
Advise gradual resumption of regular activities.

PHYSICAL THERAPY.   Physical therapy does play a minor role in the treatment of retrocalcaneal bursitis. Ice and elevation are always recommended for pain and swelling. Recommendations are made for the general care of the ankle. No other treatments are specific for this isolated bursitis.

INJECTION.   Local injection with anesthetic is used to confirm the diagnosis and to differentiate this soft-tissue condition from ankle arthritis, calcaneal bony lesions, tarsal tunnel, and so forth. Local corticosteroid injection is the preferred anti-inflammatory treatment.

Positioning: The patient is prone, with the foot hanging over the end of the exam table. The ankle is kept in a neutral position.

Surface Anatomy and the Point of Entry: The Achilles tendon, the superior portion of the calcaneus, and the posterior aspect of the ankle are identified and marked. The point of entry is lateral to the Achilles tendon, 1" above the calcaneus.

Angle of Entry and Depth: The needle is angled from the lateral aspect of the Achilles tendon toward the center and midline of the talus. The depth is approximately 1".

Anesthesia: Ethyl chloride is sprayed on the skin. Local anesthesia is placed in the subcutaneous tissue (1/2 ml) and just posterior to the talus (1/2 ml).

Technique: A *lateral approach* is used to avoid the neurovascular bundle of the foot, the posterior tibialis artery and nerve. The needle is advanced down to the hard resistance of the talus. Local anesthesia is injected just posterior to the talus, and the patient is reexamined. If the local tenderness and pain with forced plantarflexion are relieved, 1/2 ml of K40 is injected.

INJECTION AFTERCARE

1) *Rest* for 3 days, avoiding all unnecessary weightbearing.
2) Recommend lace-up high-top shoes.
3) *Ice* (15 minutes every 4 to 6 hours) and *Tylenol ES* (1000 mg twice a day) for soreness.
4) *Protect* the ankle for 3 to 4 weeks by avoiding all unnecessary walking and standing.
5) Recommend shortening the stride: *"Take extra time when walking to and from work!"*
6) Begin *passive stretching* of the ankle in flexion and extension at 3 to 4 weeks.
7) Repeat the *injection* at 6 weeks with corticosteroid if pain recurs or persists.
8) Request *plain x-rays* of the ankle (look for subtle changes in the tibiotalar joint) and a *consultation* with a surgical orthopedist or podiatrist if two consecutive injections fail and the patient still complains of posterior heel pain.

SURGICAL PROCEDURE.   None.

PROGNOSIS.   Retrocalcaneal bursitis is an uncommon condition. Local corticosteroid injection is a very effective treatment. Stretching and strengthening exercises of the Achilles tendon will decrease the likelihood of a recurrence. If symptoms and signs persist, subtle abnormalities of the ankle joint (pronation, arthritis, tarsal coalition), the talus (subtalar arthritis, talar dome osteochondritis dissecans), or the calcaneus (bony lesions) need to be excluded. Bursectomy is not performed.

DESCRIPTION.   Posterior tibialis tenosynovitis is an inflammation of the tendon as it courses around the medial malleolus. It lies in a tenosynovial sheath that provides lubrication to reduce friction as it curves under the bone. Ankle pronation, pes planus, ankle arthritis, and excessive body weight are predisposing factors to active tenosynovitis. In cases of severe pronation, tenosynovitis may be accompanied by the entrapment of the posterior tibial nerve, tarsal tunnel syndrome.

SYMPTOMS.   The patient complains of pain and swelling on the inner aspect of the ankle and painful walking. The patient points to the area of irritation when describing the symptoms.

Posterior Tibialis Tenosynovitis

Enter just below the posterior edge of medial malleolus.

Needle: ⅝", 25 gauge

Depth: ⅜ to ½"

Volume: 1 to 2 ml of anesthetic plus ½ ml of D80

Note: Keep the bevel of the needle parallel to the tendon.

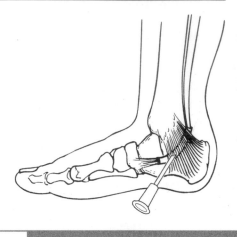

Figure 10–6.   Posterior tibialis tendon injection

"I have this sharp pain around the inside of my ankle whenever I step."
"There's swelling around the back of my ankle" (pointing to the inner aspect of the ankle).
"Tight shoes have rubbed the inside of my ankle raw. . . . It must be inside because the skin looks normal."

EXAM.   Each patient is examined for inflammation and swelling of the tendon sheath and an assessment is made of ankle range of motion and alignment.

EXAM SUMMARY

1. Local tenderness and swelling just inferior and posterior to the medial malleolus
2. Pain aggravated by resisting ankle inversion and plantar flexion, isometrically performed
3. Pain possibly aggravated by stretching in eversion, passively performed
4. Normal range of motion of the ankle
5. Associated conditions, including ankle pronation, pes planus, or pes cavus

(1) Local tenderness and swelling are located in a crescent-shaped area inferior and posterior to the medial malleolus. The swelling may be so dramatic as to fill in the dimpling below the inferior tip of the malleolus. (2) The pain is consistently aggravated by resisting the action of the tendon isometrically. Inversion is usually more painful than resisting plantar flexion. (3) The pain may be aggravated by forced eversion of the ankle, passively performed. (4) The range of motion of the ankle is normal in an uncomplicated case. (5) Pes planus, pes cavus, or ankle pronation may be present.

X-RAYS.   X-rays are not necessary for the diagnosis. Calcification does not occur. Ankle views are normal unless there is a concomitant arthritic process.

SPECIAL TESTING.   None.

DIAGNOSIS.   A presumptive diagnosis is based on a history of medial ankle pain and an examination demonstrating local tenosynovial tenderness and isometric pain that is confirmed by local anesthetic block. The latter is necessary to distinguish tenosynovitis from the pain arising from the ankle joint or tarsal tunnel.

TREATMENT.   The goals of treatment are to reduce the inflammation in the tendon sheath and to correct any underlying abnormalities of the ankle joint or ankle alignment. The initial treatment of choice involves correction of ankle pronation, pes planus, or pes cavus, or management of ankle arthritis.

Step 1: Evaluate and correct ankle pronation (high-top shoes, arch supports, or a medial wedge), pes planus (arch supports), or metatarsalgia (padded insoles).
Advise the patient to limit standing and walking.
Recommend ice applications to reduce pain and swelling.
Prescribe a Velcro pull-on ankle brace (p. 300).
Prescribe an NSAID (e.g., ibuprofen [Advil, Motrin]) for 4 weeks at full dosage.

Step 2 (6 to 8 weeks for persistent cases): Perform a local injection of D80 and combine it with immobilization (a short-leg walking cast, an air cast, and so forth).
Repeat the injection of D80 if symptoms have not improved by 50%.
Strongly suggest combining the second injection with rigid immobilization if this was not recommended with the first injection.

Step 3 (8 to 10 weeks for recovery): Advise gentle performance of stretching exercises of the ankle in all four directions.
Consider a referral to a podiatrist for custom-made plaster-molded, rigid orthotics.

PHYSICAL THERAPY.   Physical therapy is important in the rehabilitation of posterior tibialis tenosynovitis in the postcast recovery period. Gradual stretching exercise of the ankle (emphasizing dorsiflexion and eversion) are performed daily (p. 279). These exercises are performed in sets of 20 after heating the ankle. They are begun immediately after casting or approximately 4 weeks after local injection.

INJECTION.   Local injection with anesthetic can be used to confirm the diagnosis and to differentiate this soft-tissue condition from subtalar arthritis. Local corticosteroid is indicated for persistent symptoms that fail to respond to correction of ankle alignment, arch abnormalities, and ankle immobilization.

Positioning: The patient is in the prone position. The leg is kept straight and the lower leg is externally rotated.

Surface Anatomy and the Point of Entry: The tip of the medial malleolus is identified. The needle is inserted just behind the posterior edge of the bone.

Angle of Entry and Depth: The needle is inserted perpendicular to the skin and is advanced to the firm resistance of the tendon (3/8") or to the hard resistance of the bone (1/2").

Anesthesia: Ethyl chloride is sprayed on the skin. Local anesthesia is placed in the subcutaneous tissue (1/2 ml) and at the firm resistance of the tendon (1/2 ml)

Technique: An *intratenosynovial* injection is the aim of this technique. It can be performed in two ways. If the firm resistance of the tendon is easily identified as the needle is advanced, the injection can be placed at this site. However, if the tendon is not readily identified, the needle is advanced down to the hard resistance of the bone and then withdrawn 1/8". Note: As the needle is advanced to the bone, the bevel must be kept parallel to the course of the tendon fibers. The pressure of injection will be minimal if the needle is in the tenosynovial sheath. Finally, if the local tenderness and isometric pain with resisted ankle inversion are improved, then 1/2 ml of D80 is injected.

INJECTION AFTERCARE

1) *Rest* for 3 days, avoiding all unnecessary weightbearing.

2) Recommend lace-up high-top shoes, an air cast, or a short-leg walking cast, depending on the severity of the symptoms and signs and the associated conditions (pronation, arthritis, etc.).

3) *Ice* (15 minutes every 4 to 6 hours) and *Tylenol ES* (1000 mg twice a day) for soreness.

4) *Protect* the ankle for 3 to 4 weeks by avoiding all unnecessary walking and standing.

5) Recommend shortening the stride: "Take extra time when walking to and from work!"

6) Begin *passive stretching* of the ankle in flexion and extension at 3 to 4 weeks.

7) Begin *isometric toning exercises* of ankle inversion and eversion once flexibility has been partially restored.

8) Repeat *injection* at 6 weeks with corticosteroid if pain recurs or persists.

9) Request *plain x-rays* of the ankle (look for subtle changes in the tibiotalar joint) and a *consultation* with a surgical orthopedist or podiatrist if two consecutive injections fail and the patient still complains of medial ankle pain and swelling.

SURGICAL PROCEDURE.   None.

PROGNOSIS.   An injection combined with immobilization is usually successful in those cases uncomplicated by pronation, pes planus, and so forth. Recurrent tenosynovitis is often a result of the biomechanical stresses of difficult-to-manage ankle instability, ankle deformity, obesity, or old trauma. Long-term success depends on the correction of these associated conditions. Surgery is usually reserved for tendon rupture, a rare event.

Plantar Fasciitis

Enter in the midline, ¾" distal to the origin of the plantar fascia.

Needle: 1½", 22 gauge

Depth: 1½"

Volume: 1 to 2 ml of anesthetic plus 1 ml of D80

Note: The injection must be at a depth greater than 1" to avoid injecting steroid into the specialized fat of the heel pad.

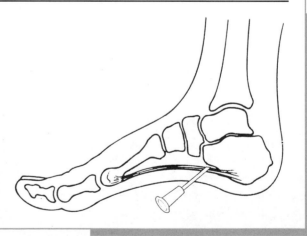

Figure 10–7.   Plantar fascial injection from the plantar approach

DESCRIPTION.   Plantar fasciitis is an inflammation of the origin of the longitudinal ligament, the principal ligament that forms the arch of the foot. Flat feet (pes planus), high arches (pes cavus), turned-in ankles (ankle pronation), and short Achilles tendons predispose to this condition. Obesity, working on concrete, poorly fitted shoes, and prolonged daily standing aggravate the condition. A few cases are purely inflammatory in nature and are associated with Reiter syndrome.

This condition must be distinguished from another common condition presenting with heel pain, heel pad syndrome. This is an irritation of the specialized fat pad that is caused by trauma. The tenderness is located over the entire heel pad and is aggravated by squeezing the pad from side to side. It is a self-limited condition, usually lasting 2 to 3 weeks. Response to heel cups or heel pads is usually dramatic.

SYMPTOMS.   The patient complains of heel pain aggravated by walking and standing. The patient grabs the bottom of the heel and rubs it back and forth when describing the condition.

"Whenever I put pressure down on my heel, I get a severe, sharp pain under my heel."
"The pressure over my heel is so bad that I have started to walk on my tiptoes."
"My flat feet never bothered me until I took this job where I have to stand on concrete all day long."
"I can't wear these kinds of shoes [flats] because my heel will really start to hurt."
"It's like the bottom of my heel is bruised."
"I can't wear high heels any more because my heel hurts."
"I can't do my Jazzercise any more because of my heel."

EXAM.   Each patient is examined for local irritation and inflammation of the origin of the plantar fascia and an evaluation is made of ankle alignment, Achilles tendon flexibility, and the configuration of the arch of the foot.

EXAM SUMMARY

1. Local tenderness at the calcaneal origin of the plantar fascia
2. Pain with calcaneal compression
3. Achilles tendon inflexibility
4. Associated conditions that include ankle pronation, pes planus, and pes cavus
5. Anesthetic block at the origin of the plantar fascia

(1) Local tenderness is present in the midline or slightly medial of midline at the origin of the longitudinal arch of the foot. The dime-sized area of tenderness is located 1 1/4 to 1 1/2″ from the posterior heel. Firm pressure may be needed! (2) Medial to lateral compression of the calcaneus may be mildly painful but rarely more painful than the local tenderness. If the calcaneal compression sign is more painful than the local tenderness, studies should be obtained to exclude a calcaneal stress fracture. (3) Achilles tendon flexibility may be limited, especially in cases over 2 to 3 months in duration. The tendon often shortens as a result of a shortened stride or favoring the foot. Normally, the ankle should dorsiflex 25 to 30 degrees. (4) Ankle pronation, pes planus, or pes cavus may be associated findings. Ankle alignment and arch configuration must be examined in the standing position.

X-RAYS.   Plain x-rays of the ankle are not necessary to make the diagnosis. They are indicated for long-distance runners to exclude a stress fracture of the calcaneus, for patients with calcaneal injuries to exclude a routine fracture, and for patients with chronic symptoms to exclude a large (>1 cm) pressure-aggravated heel spur. Small calcaneal calcifications at the origin of the fascia are exceedingly common (10% of the population—much greater than the incidence of fasciitis); they are a reflection of the chronic inflammatory response. These small heel spurs, protected by the shelf of the calcaneus, are not an indication for surgery.

SPECIAL TESTING.   Nuclear medicine bone scanning is used to exclude a stress fracture in the long-distance runner. A bone scan should be obtained when the calcaneal compression sign is more painful than the local heel tenderness.

DIAGNOSIS.   The diagnosis is based on the history and the characteristic findings on physical examination. A regional anesthetic block at the origin of the plantar fascia can be used to differentiate heel pad syndrome (self-limited irritation to the specialized fat of the heel), calcaneal stress fracture (seen nearly exclusively in runners), and subtalar arthritis.

TREATMENT.   The goals of treatment are to reduce the inflammation in the longitudinal arch and to improve the mechanics of the heel and ankle. Reduced weightbearing combined with padded arch supports is the treatment of choice.

Step 1: Examine the heel, evaluate the configuration of the arch with the patient standing, and confirm the diagnosis with local anesthesia in selected cases.
Recommend cushioning for the heel with heel cups, foam to stand on at work, padded insoles, or double socks (p. 303).
Advise the patient to limit standing and walking.
Recommend padded arch supports (e.g., Spenco, Sorbothane) (p. 304).
Recommend application of ice to the heel.
Recommend Achilles tendon stretching exercises (p. 279).
Suggest massage over the heel with a rubber ball.

Step 2 (3 to 4 weeks for persistent cases): Prescribe an NSAID (e.g., ibuprofen [Advil, Motrin]) and note that the response may be limited.
Reemphasize the use of padding.

Step 3 (6 to 8 weeks for persistent cases): Perform x-rays of the foot (including PA, PA oblique, and lateral views).
Perform a local injection of D80.
Repeat the injection in 4 to 6 weeks if symptoms have not decreased by 50%, and combine injection with immobilization to optimize the outcome.

Step 4 (3 to 4 months for chronic cases): Consider a referral to a podiatrist for custom-made orthotics (p. 304) or surgical débridement.

PHYSICAL THERAPY.   Physical therapy plays a significant role in the active treatment of plantar fasciitis and in its prevention.

PHYSICAL THERAPY SUMMARY ● ● ● ● ● ● ● ● ● ● ● ● ● ● ● ●

1.   Ice for acute pain
2.   Heat and massage of the heel
3.   Achilles tendon stretching, passively performed

Acute Period.   Ice, massage, and padding are used in the first several weeks to reduce pain and swelling. *Ice* placed over the center of the heel provides effective analgesia and may help to reduce swelling. Cold must be applied for 10 to 15 minutes in order to penetrate 3/4 to 1" down to the origin of the fascia. For other patients, *heating and massage* provide more effective analgesia and may help to disperse swelling. Massage can be accomplished by rolling a tennis ball under the heel or using a vibrating foot massage unit.
Recovery/Rehabilitation.   After the acute symptoms have significantly decreased, stretching exercises are begun. The most important treatment for plantar fasciitis is

the *Achilles tendon stretching exercises* (p. 279). Increasing Achilles tendon flexibility lessens the tension over the plantar fascia. The fascia, calcaneus, and Achilles tendon must share the workload of ankle motion. Stiffness in one area will increase the tension and stress in other areas. Passive and active stretching exercises are to be performed daily. The combined use of padded insoles, arch supports, and shoes with good support makes plantar fasciitis less likely to recur.

INJECTION.   Treatment focuses on padding the heel (heel cups, heel cushions, padded insoles), supporting the arch (padded arch supports, shoes with good support), and doing Achilles tendon stretching exercises. Local injection with corticosteroids is indicated for persistent symptoms. Difficult cases may require two injections and rigid immobilization.

Positioning: The patient is to be in the prone position with the foot hanging just off the edge of the exam table.

Surface Anatomy and the Point of Entry: The inferior surface of the calcaneus and the origin of the plantar fascia (approximately 1 to 1 1/2" from the back of the heel) are identified. The point of entry is three quarters **distal** to the origin of the fascia in the midline.

Angle of Entry and Depth: The needle is inserted at a 45-degree angle and is advanced to the firm resistance of the fascia (1") and then to the hard resistance of the bone (1 1/2").

Anesthesia: Ethyl chloride is sprayed on the skin. Local anesthesia is placed in the subcutaneous tissue (1/2 ml), intradermally (1/4 ml), at the firm resistance of the tendon (1/2 ml), and in between the fascia and the calcaneus (1/2 ml).

Technique: In order to inject accurately between the plantar fascia and the calcaneus and hence avoid injecting into the specialized fat of the heel pad, a *plantar approach* is strongly suggested. Generous anesthesia is given at the plantar surface. The needle is then advanced through the low-resistance fat to the subtle to firm resistance of the fascia. A popping or giving-way is often felt when passing through the fascia. *Caution*: The patient may experience pain as the periosteum is touched. If the local tenderness is significantly relieved, a full ml of D80 is injected slowly. *Caution*: The space is small; a rapid injection of medication can be painful!

INJECTION AFTERCARE

1) *Rest* for 3 days, avoiding all unnecessary weightbearing.

2) Recommend immobilization with lace-up high-top shoes, an air cast, or a short-leg walking cast, depending on the severity and associated pronation, arthritis, and so forth.

3) *Ice* (15 minutes every 4 to 6 hours) and *Tylenol ES* (1000 mg twice a day) for soreness.

4) *Protect* the ankle for 3 to 4 weeks by avoiding all unnecessary walking and standing.

5) Recommend shortening the stride: "Take extra time when walking to and from work!"

6) Begin *passive stretching* of the Achilles tendons at 3 to 4 weeks.

7) Repeat *injection* at 6 weeks if pain recurs or persists and combine with immobilization.

8) Request a *consultation* with a surgical orthopedist or podiatrist if two consecutive injections and fixed immobilization fail.

SURGICAL PROCEDURE.   Fascial débridement, calcaneal spur removal.

PROGNOSIS.   Corticosteroid injection combined with padded arch supports and limited weightbearing is successful in approximately 60% of cases. However, the combination of injection with 3 to 4 weeks of rigid immobilization (a short-leg walking cast) increases the response to 90% and provides the additional advantage of maintaining mobility.

Persistent or recurrent fasciitis (approximately 10% of cases) is seen most often in patients with obesity, with abnormal arch and ankle conditions, with calcaneal spurs over 1/2 to 3/4″ in length, or with jobs demanding prolonged standing or walking on concrete surfaces. Surgical débridement of the devitalized tissue or resection of the accompanying bone spur (longer than 1 cm) can be considered in these cases.

chapter 11

Foot

Bunions

Enter over the MTP joint medially at the distal metatarsal head.

Needle: ⅝", 25 gauge

Depth: ¼ to ⅜" (flush against the bone)

Volume: ½ ml of anesthetic plus ¼ ml of K40

Note: The injection is made under the synovial membrane adjacent to the bone, not in between the articular surfaces of the joint.

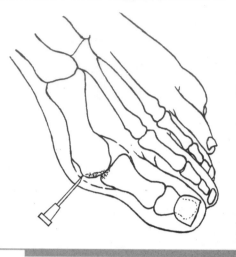

Figure 11–1.   Bunion injection

DESCRIPTION.   "Bunion" is the term used to describe the bony prominence and abnormal angle of the great toe, the hallmark of osteoarthritis of the first metatarsalphalangeal (MTP) joint. Asymmetric pressure over the articular cartilage caused by narrow–toe-box shoes leads to loss of cartilage, angulation of the joint, and gradual subluxation of the extensor tendons. The asymmetrical wear and tear on the joint leads to the typical valgus deformity. The condition develops over many years. Continued pressure over the medial joint line can cause acute arthritic flares or acute adventitial bursitis.

SYMPTOMS.   The patient complains of abnormal-looking toes, problems with shoe wear, and pain in the great toe. The patient often rubs the top and bottom of the toe or simply stares with disgust at the deformity when describing the condition.

"I can't get a pair of shoes to fit comfortably now."
"I get this sharp pain in my big toe whenever I walk too far."
"My toe looks funny."
"Are these bunions? My grandmother had ugly toes too."
"My big toe aches all the time, especially when I bend it."
"I can't walk normally. My big toe doesn't bend very much any more."

EXAM.   Each patient is examined for degree of arthritic change, valgus angulation, and local inflammation. The involvement of the first MTP joint is compared to the involvement of the overlying adventitial bursa.

(1) The MTP joint is tender and enlarged. Tenderness occurs along the medial joint line or over the entire joint if an acute arthritic flare is present. Joint enlargement is due to subluxation, osteophyte formation, and swelling. (2) The typical hallux valgus deformity is characterized by a prominent medial metatarsal head, an abnormal lateral angulation of the proximal phalanges and, in an advanced case, the overlapping of the first and second toes. (3) Passive movement of the joint may cause crepitation. (4) Pain may be present at the extremes of plantarflexion and dorsiflexion, passively performed. (5) The range of motion of the joint may be limited (hallux rigidus).

X-RAYS. Plain x-rays of the foot are recommended to confirm the diagnosis, to calculate the valgus angle, and to assess the degree of arthritic change. Progressive arthritic changes include asymmetric narrowing of the articular cartilage, bony osteophyte formation, subchondral bony sclerosis, and subchondral cyst formation. X-rays are always a prerequisite to surgical consultation.

SPECIAL TESTING. None.

DIAGNOSIS. Advanced cases are easily diagnosed by simple inspection and exam. Moderate cases may require x-rays of the foot for confirmation. A regional anesthetic block is necessary occasionally to differentiate symptoms arising from the MTP joint, the adventitial bursa, or a Morton neuroma.

TREATMENT. The goals of treatment are to reduce the joint inflammation, to prevent arthritic deterioration, and to retard further valgus deformity. Wide–toe-box shoes, toe spacers, and adhesive pads are the treatments of choice.

Step 1: Educate the patient: "This is an arthritis of the big toe. The most common cause is tight-fitting shoes." Strongly encourage the wearing of wide–toe-box shoes.
Demonstrate the use of a cotton or rubber spacer between the first and second toes (p. 306).
Recommend a thick felt ring over the medial joint (p. 305).
Prescribe a bunion shield (p. 304).
Recommend applications of ice over the side and top of the toe for comfort.

Step 2 (4 to 6 weeks for moderate cases): An NSAID (e.g., ibuprofen [Advil, Motrin]) may provide relief in a small percentage of cases.
Reemphasize the importance of loose-fitting shoes.
Perform a local intra-articular injection of K40.
Repeat the injection in 4 to 6 weeks if symptoms have not improved by at least 50%.

Step 3 (8 to 10 weeks for chronic cases): Consider a referral to an orthopedist or podiatrist if symptoms are persistent or if the deformity is great.

PHYSICAL THERAPY. Physical therapy does not play a significant role in the treatment of bunions. Ice and elevation are always recommended for acute arthritic flares. Stretching exercises of the extensor and flexor tendons are important early in the condition before subluxation and deformity become permanent.

INJECTION. Treatment focuses on protecting the joint from pressure against the medial and inferior surfaces. Local corticosteroid injection is used to control the symptoms of an acute inflammatory flare and to provide temporary relief for this progressive arthritic condition.

Positioning: The patient is to be in the supine position with the leg extended and the foot externally rotated.

Surface Anatomy and the Point of Entry: The head of the first metatarsal (the medial prominence) and the medial MTP joint line are palpated and marked. The point of entry is adjacent to the joint line approximately 1/4″ distal to the prominence.

Angle of Entry and Depth: The needle is inserted perpendicular to the skin and is advanced to the hard resistance of the bone (1/4 to 3/8″).

Anesthesia: Ethyl chloride is sprayed on the skin. Local anesthesia is placed in the subcutaneous tissue (1/4 ml) and just outside the synovial membrane at 1/4″ (1/4 ml). All anesthesia should be injected outside the joint. The intra-articular injection is reserved for the corticosteroid, as the joint accepts only small volumes!

Technique: A *medial approach* to the joint's synovial membrane is the safest and easiest approach. After placing the anesthetic just outside the synovial membrane, the first syringe is replaced with a second syringe containing the corticosteroid. Then the needle is advanced down to the periosteum of the bone. If the tip of the needle rests against the metatarsal bone, then the injection will flow under the synovial membrane and into the joint. Gentle pressure is required. Note that the needle is *not* advanced into the center of the joint!

INJECTION AFTERCARE

1) *Rest* for 3 days, avoiding all unnecessary weightbearing.
2) Recommend loose-fitting, wide–toe-box shoes with extra padding (double socks, felt ring, molefoam) combined with a padded insole.
3) Use a toe spacer to improve alignment.
4) *Ice* (15 minutes every 4 to 6 hours) and *Tylenol ES* (1000 mg twice a day) for soreness.
5) *Protect* the great toe for 3 to 4 weeks by avoiding all unnecessary walking and standing.
6) Recommend shortening the stride: "Take extra time when walking to and from work!"
7) Begin *passive stretching* of the great toe in flexion and extension at 3 to 4 weeks.
8) Repeat *injection* with corticosteroid at 6 weeks if pain recurs or persists.
9) Request *plain x-rays* of the foot and a *consultation* with a surgical orthopedist or podiatrist if two consecutive injections fail to control pain and swelling.

SURGICAL TREATMENT. Bunionectomy includes osteotomy, realignment, and extensor tendon release to restore the normal alignment and appearance of the great toe. When the toe deformity (hallux valgus) is dramatic, ambulation is impaired, or arthritic flares have occurred frequently, surgery can be considered. Several surgical procedures are available, all of which strive to improve alignment, reduce medial joint line pressure, and improve function. However, the patient should be advised that no one procedure is better than another and that the toe may lack full range of motion postoperatively. The patient must be willing to take the risk of developing a functionally stiff joint.

PROGNOSIS. The underlying arthritis and deformity gradually worsen over the years. Once this wear-and-tear process begins, it tends to be relentlessly progressive. Prevention and protection cannot be overemphasized. All treatments, including surgery, are palliative.

Adventitial Bursistis of the First MTP

Enter the bursal sac medially over the point of maximum swelling.

Needle: ⅝", 25 gauge

Depth: ¼ to ⅜" (⅛" above the bone)

Volume: 1 ml of anesthetic plus ½ ml of K40

Note: The bursa lies between the subcutaneous fat layer and the synovial membrane.

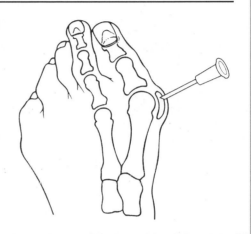

Figure 11–2.   Injection of the bursa over the first MTP joint

DESCRIPTION.   The constant pressure and friction of tight shoes over the medial aspect of the first MTP joint causes a bursal sac to develop. Repetitive pressure and friction cause the bursal sac to become acutely inflamed. The swelling, redness, and tenderness are so dramatic that the condition is often misdiagnosed as acute podagra. However, the inflammation in this bursitis is restricted to the medial aspect of the joint. By contrast, acute gout causes the entire joint to become inflamed.

SYMPTOMS.   The patient complains of toe pain, swelling, and redness over the inner aspect of the toe.

"My big toe is swollen."
"I can't wear my shoes anymore. My big toe rubs on the inner side of my shoe."
"I have had to switch to sandals because my walking shoes rub too much on my big toe."
"I think I have gout."
"I've always had bunions, but now my toe has really begun to swell."

EXAM.   Each patient is examined for the degree of bursal inflammation, underlying arthritic change, and loss of range of motion of the first MTP joint.

EXAM SUMMARY

1. Swelling and pain over the medial aspect of the MTP joint
2. Typical valgus deformity of the MTP joint (bunion deformity)
3. Mild pain when moving the MTP joint in flexion and extension (unlike gout)
4. Painless resisted flexion and extension of the MTP joint, isometrically performed

(1) Acute inflammation is present over the medial aspect of the first MTP joint. Swelling, redness, and warmth are present over a quarter-sized area. Tenderness is maximal over the medial aspect of the joint (as opposed to the diffuse tenderness over the entire MTP joint with gout). The inflammatory signs and local tenderness rarely extend beyond the confines of the bursal sac unless a concurrent cellulitis is present (rare). (2) The typical bunion deformity, hallux valgus, is present. (3) The range of motion of the joint is limited due to arthritis of the underlying joint. Mild to moderate pain is present at the extremes of motion. This is in distinct contrast to the severe pain and severe limitation of joint movement seen with acute podagra. (4) Isometrically resisted toe flexion and extension are painless. The extensor and flexor tendons of the foot are not involved.

X-RAYS. X-rays of the foot are recommended. The underlying arthritic change at the MTP joint predominates. Joint-space narrowing, bony spurs, and the valgus angulation are obvious changes and are usually advanced in degree. Soft-tissue swelling may be apparent on the anteroposterior projection. Calcification does not occur.

SPECIAL TESTING. None.

DIAGNOSIS. The diagnosis is made by physical exam. The acute inflammatory change located medially, the presence of the typical valgus deformity, and the absence of signs of gouty arthritis strongly suggest the diagnosis. Local anesthetic block placed in the superficial tissue layers above the joint will differentiate involvement of the bursa and acute gout or acute osteoarthritic flare of the MTP joint. When inflammatory change is extensive, the diagnosis must be confirmed by aspiration. Bursal fluid analysis (negative Gram stain, culture, and crystal analysis) is mandatory if infection is suspected.

TREATMENT. The goals of treatment are to reduce the acute swelling and inflammation and to prevent recurrent bursitis by avoiding pressure and friction. Local corticosteroid injection combined with antifriction measures are the treatments of choice.

Step 1: Obtain x-rays of the foot, aspirate the bursa if sufficient swelling is present, and inspect the aspirate or send the aspirate for lab analysis (Gram stain, culture, crystals).

Perform a local injection of K40 if infection is unlikely (no penetrating trauma, no diabetes, no vascular insufficiency, etc.).

Recommend wide–toe-box shoes.

Recommend a felt ring be placed over the medial aspect of the MTP joint (p. 305).

Suggest a bunion shield for advanced valgus deformity (p. 304).

The NSAIDs (e.g., ibuprofen [Advil, Motrin]) are ineffective.

Step 2 (4 to 6 weeks for persistent cases): Repeat the injection in 4 to 6 weeks if the pain and swelling have not decreased by 50%.

Reemphasize the importance of padding and proper shoes.

Step 3 (8 to 10 weeks in the recovery phase): Reinforce the need to wear well-fitting shoes and use a felt ring for prevention.

Consider surgical referral if the bunion deformity is severe and especially if bursitis has been difficult to treat.

PHYSICAL THERAPY. Physical therapy does not play a significant role in the treatment of this local musculoskeletal condition. Ice and elevation are always recommended for the acute inflammatory flare. Stretching exercises to preserve range of motion are indicated for the underlying arthritis of the MTP joint.

INJECTION. Local anesthetic block is used to differentiate this periarticular condition from gout. Corticosteroid injection is used to control the symptoms of the acute inflammatory flare.

Positioning: The patient is in the supine position with the leg extended and the foot externally rotated.

Surface Anatomy and the Point of Entry: The bursa lies directly over the medial prominence of the MTP joint. The point of entry is directly over the center of the bursa.

Angle of Entry and Depth: The needle is inserted perpendicular to the skin. The depth is no greater than 1/4 to 3/8".

Anesthesia: Ethyl chloride is sprayed on the skin. Local anesthesia is placed in the subcutaneous tissue (1/4 ml).

Technique: A *medial approach* is preferred. After anesthesia is placed, the needle is advanced down to the hard resistance of the bone and then withdrawn 1/4" (the bursa is located just outside the capsule of the joint!). Attempts to aspirate fluid are usually unsuccessful. With the needle held carefully in place, 1/2 ml of K40 is injected.

INJECTION AFTERCARE

1) *Rest* for 3 days, avoiding all unnecessary weightbearing.

2) Recommend loose-fitting, wide–toe-box shoes with extra padding (double socks, felt ring, molefoam) combined with a padded insole.

3) Use a toe spacer to improve alignment.

4) *Ice* (15 minutes every 4 to 6 hours) and *Tylenol ES* (1000 mg twice a day) for soreness.

5) *Protect* the great toe for 3 to 4 weeks by avoiding all unnecessary walking and standing.

6) Recommend shortening the stride: "Take extra time when walking to and from work!"

7) Begin *passive stretching* of the great toe in flexion and extension at 3 to 4 weeks.

8) Repeat *injection* of corticosteroid at 6 weeks if pain recurs or persists.

9) Request *plain x-rays* of the foot and a *consultation* with a surgical orthopedist or podiatrist if two consecutive injections fail to control pain and swelling.

SURGICAL PROCEDURE. Bursectomy is almost always combined with bunionectomy.

PROGNOSIS. Medical therapy with local injection is usually very effective. Recurrent bursitis occurs in the setting of bunions with severe angulation deformity. Surgery is usually directed to the underlying bunion. Bursectomy without surgical correction of the underlying bunion deformity is usually ineffective.

DESCRIPTION. Gout is an acute monoarticular arthritis of the MTP joint of the great toe. Acute swelling, redness, and heat develop as an inflammatory response to precipitation of monosodium urate crystals in the synovial fluid. The synovial fluid

Gout

Enter medially on the metatarsal side of the joint line.

Needle: ⅝", 25 gauge for anesthesia or 1", 21 gauge for aspiration

Depth: ⅜ to ½", depending on swelling

Volume: 1 to 2 ml of anesthetic plus ¼ to ½ ml of K40

Note: Multiple attempts to enter the joint may be damaging. With the needle flush against the periosteum—under the synovial membrane—the injection is intra-articular; manual pressure may yield sufficient fluid for analysis.

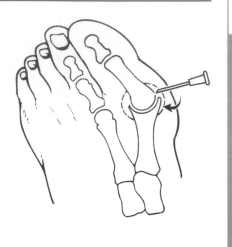

Figure 11–3. Injection for podagra

becomes supersaturated with uric acid crystals as a result of overproduction of uric acid (hemolytic anemias, leukemia, psoriasis, tumors with rapid cell turnover, and so forth cause 10% of cases) or undersecretion of uric acid (renal disease, aspirin, niacin, diuretics, and so forth cause 90% of cases). Patients with recurrent gouty attacks should undergo laboratory evaluation to determine the cause of their altered metabolism. Gout can also affect the olecranon and prepatellar bursa, the tenosynovial sheaths of the dorsum of the foot and instep, and the other small joints of the foot.

SYMPTOMS. The patient complains of severe toe pain, swelling, redness, and an inability to walk because of the pain.

"I woke up in the night with severe, sharp pain in my big toe."
"The pain in my toe was so bad that I couldn't stand having the sheet on my foot."
"My big toe is very red and swollen."
"Doc, I've got the gout in my big toe again."
"I can't put any weight down on my foot because of the severe pain in my big toe."
"There's no way I can walk. I can't bend my big toe."
"My arthritis has hurt in the past, but never like this."

EXAM. Each patient is examined for the degree and extent of the inflammation affecting the first MTP joint.

EXAM SUMMARY ● ● ● ● ● ● ● ● ● ● ● ● ● ●

1. Acute swelling, redness, and heat arising from the MTP joint
2. Severe tenderness at the MTP joint
3. Pain aggravated by even the slightest movement of the joint

(1) The toe is swollen, red, and hot. The inflammation envelops the joint and may extend 1" proximally and distally, involving the soft tissues. The greatest degree

of swelling is along the medial border of the joint. (2) Severe tenderness is present around the entire joint, with the greatest sensitivity medially (by contrast, the tenderness of adventitial bursitis is located only on the medial aspect of the joint). (3) Movement of the toe in any direction is extremely painful. The patient often exhibits great anxiety at the thought of moving the toe.

X-RAYS. X-rays of the foot are optional in patients presenting with their first attack and recommended in patients with recurrent and chronic gout. Patients presenting with a first attack do not demonstrate bony or joint abnormalities. Patients with recurrent or chronic tophaceous gout may show periarticular or intra-articular erosions, round or oval erosions typically surrounded by a thin sclerotic margin.

SPECIAL TESTING. The demonstration of monosodium urate crystals is the diagnostic test of choice. Light microscopy reveals the characteristic needle-shaped monosodium urate crystals that appear bright yellow under polarized light, also referred to as negative birefringence.

[handwritten margin note: needle-shaped bright yellow neg birefring.]

DIAGNOSIS. The diagnosis of an acute inflammatory monoarticular arthritis of the first MTP joint is not difficult. However, there is difficulty in differentiating the acute attack of gout from the much less common infective arthritis, two conditions with identical physical examination findings. A presumptive diagnosis of gout is much more likely if there has been a history of gouty attacks, if the serum uric acid is elevated, and if risk factors for infection (diabetes, vascular insufficiency, an absence of penetrating trauma, etc.) are absent. In addition, statistically, gout is at least 100 times more likely than infection.

Absolute confirmation of the diagnosis requires demonstrating the presence of urate crystals when analyzing the joint fluid. In patients with risk factors for infection, aspiration is mandatory to exclude infection.

TREATMENT. The goal of treatment is to rapidly reduce the acute inflammation within the first MTP joint.

Step 1: Assess the patient's risk factors for infection (diabetes, vascular insufficiency, immunocompromise, etc.), aspirate the joint for synovial fluid analysis (crystals, cell count, Gram stain, and culture), obtain a serum uric acid level, and either proceed to local injection of corticosteroids or wait for the results of lab analysis.

Recommend application of ice and elevation of the foot.

Eliminate low-dose aspirin, alcohol, diuretics (if possible), and any other drug that interferes with the secretion of uric acid.

Recommend avoiding pressure from shoes.

A prescription of any NSAID (e.g., ibuprofen [Advil, Motrin]) or colchicine or an injection of any of the cortiocosteroid derivatives will effectively treat the severe inflammation.

Step 2 (2 to 4 days acute follow-up): Measure the 24-hour urinary uric acid excretion to determine whether the patient is an overproducer or undersecretor.

If the patient is an overproducer of urates, perform an evaluation of the causes of urate overproduction. *[handwritten: hemolysis, leukemia, psoriasis, rapid turn...]*

Prescribe probenecid (for the undersecretors) or allopurinol (for the overproducers) for the long-term prevention of gout.

Prescribe an NSAID or colchicine to protect against precipitating gout when initiating probenecid or allopurinol (1 month for recurrent acute gout and 6 months for chronic tophaceous gout).

Step 3 (4 to 8 weeks for long-term follow-up): Recheck the uric acid to assess whether long-term preventive therapy has reduced uric acid production to the normal range.

Adjust the dosages of probenecid or allopurinol to keep the uric acid in the normal range.

PHYSICAL THERAPY. Physical therapy does not play a significant role in the treatment of gout. Ice and elevation are always recommended, but definitive treatment requires medication.

INJECTION. Corticosteroid injection is indicated when the NSAIDs cannot be used because of peptic ulcer disease, concurrent use of warfarin (Coumadin), renal failure, and so forth. The general treatment of gout is very similar to the treatment of bunions (see p. 194). Injection with local anesthetic is also used to aspirate the joint for crystal analysis (see below).

Special Technique: A *medial approach* to aspirating the joint is the safest and easiest to perform. After placing the anesthetic just outside the synovial membrane, the needle is advanced to the periosteum of the metatarsal and 1/4 ml of anesthetic is placed under the synovial membrane. With the needle held carefully in place, gentle manual pressure is exerted over the lateral and medial aspects of the joint to express one or two drops of synovial fluid for crystal analysis. Leaving the needle in place, 1/2 ml of K40 is injected into the joint. *Caution:* Do *not* advance the needle into the center of the joint!

PROGNOSIS. The NSAIDs and colchicine are very effective in reducing the acute joint inflammation, usually within 1 to 2 days. Intra-articular corticosteroid injection is also very effective and often reduces the pain, swelling, and erythema in a matter of hours. Either treatment will effectively control all symptoms and signs within 3 to 4 days.

Long-term control of gout rests on prevention. Low-dose aspirin, alcohol, foods high in purine, and certain medications (most notably the diuretics and niacin) must be avoided. For patients with recurrent episodes of acute gout and patients with chronic gout, allopurinol or probenecid should be prescribed. Allopurinol—a xanthine oxidase competitive inhibitor—is the drug of choice for patients who are overproducers of uric acid. Probenecid is the drug of choice for prevention of gout in patients who are undersecretors of uric acid. Because 90% of patients with gout are undersecretors, probenecid is the logical choice for most patients. Note that patients who are found to be overproducers should be thoroughly examined for the specific cause of excess production of urates!

DESCRIPTION. Hammer toes is the term used to describe the toe deformity caused by contracted extensor tendons of the foot. As the tendons slowly lose their flexibility, the MTP joints gradually extend and the proximal interphalangeal (PIP) joints gradually flex. The hammer-like deformity results. Pressure over these joints leads to plantar surface calluses and to dorsal surface corns, both of which consist of hypertrophic skin over the bony prominences.

Note the hammer toe deformity is the end result of years of tight, inflexible extensor tendons. The first sign of the condition is metatarsal pain (metatarsalgia) with a physical examination showing tight dorsal tendons.

SYMPTOMS. The patient complains of pain over the ball of the foot, calluses, or abnormal-looking toes.

"My toes are crooked."
"I can't bend my toes any more."
"It's like walking on marbles. I have these thick calluses on the bottom of my feet."
"The skin over the top of my toes is starting to thicken."
"My toes are rubbing on my shoes."
"At the end of the day my toes ache. The whole ball of my foot hurts."

Hammer Toes

Enter from above, midway between the MTP joints.

Needle: ⅝″, 25 gauge

Depth: ⅜ to ½″ to the periosteum of the MT head

Volume: 1 ml of anesthetic plus ¼ ml of K40

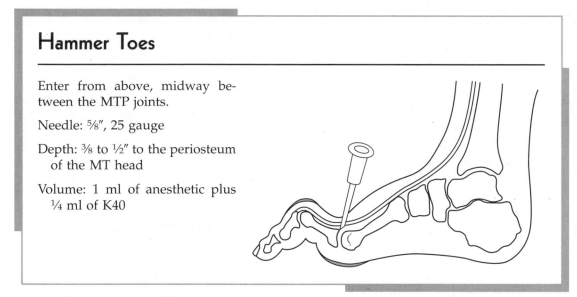

Figure 11–4.   MTP injection for hammer toes

EXAM.   The extensor tendons of the toes are assessed for flexibility, the MTP joints are assessed for irritation and thickening, and the corns and calluses are documented.

EXAM SUMMARY   • • • • • • • • • • • • • • •

1. Tight extensor tendons, especially when the ankle is placed in plantarflexion
2. Tenderness directly over the MTP joint
3. A positive MTP squeeze sign
4. Corns and calluses
5. Hammer toe deformity

(1) The hammer toe deformity is characteristic of the endstage of this condition. All patients present with tight or contracted extensor tendons over the dorsum of the foot. This is best appreciated when placing the ankle in extreme plantarflexion. In this position, the patient experiences tightness, pain, or both. This tightness may be experienced just over the dorsum of the foot or up the anterior surface of the leg. (2) Individual MTP joints may be tender. Tenderness is best elicited by compressing the joint from above and below and rolling the MTP head between the fingers. (3) If the joints are particularly inflamed, the MTP squeeze sign will be painful. In this maneuver, all the joints are compressed simultaneously by side pressure (medial to lateral) while holding the second, third, and fourth MTP joints in line with the opposite hand. (4) Corns over the top of the PIP joints and calluses below the MTP joint are seen as the deformity progresses. Both of these abnormalities consist of hypertrophic skin, a result of the constant pressure over the bony prominences. (5) The typical hammer toe deformity is seen in well-established cases.

X-RAYS.   X-rays of the foot are not recommended routinely. Although the lateral view will demonstrate the typical hammer toe deformity in the advanced case, x-rays rarely provide additional information that could not be assessed on the basis of the physical examination. However, x-rays should be obtained in the atypical case (severe swelling, unusual coloration, unequal involvement of the toes, and so forth). Dramatic tenderness and swelling in a symmetric pattern suggest rheumatoid arthritis. Excessive bony enlargement suggests degenerative changes at the MTP joints. Extensive swelling and discoloration suggest reflex sympathetic dystrophy or infection.

SPECIAL TESTING.   Bone scanning is rarely indicated. Joint aspiration is not possible.

DIAGNOSIS.   The diagnosis is based on a history of pain over the balls of the feet, an exam showing localized metatarsal tenderness and, in the advanced case, the typical hammer toe deformity. The diagnosis is less evident when the typical deformity is not present. These early presentations are often labeled simply as metatarsalgia. These patients need to be examined closely for the painful tight extensor tendons.

TREATMENT.   The goals of treatment are to stretch the dorsal extensor tendons and to reestablish normal toe alignment. Passive stretching of the extensor tendons is the treatment of choice.

Step 1: The stage of the condition is determined (early metatarsalgia vs. advanced hammer toe deformity), x-rays are obtained in the advanced case, and the number of MTP joints involved is documented.
Prescribe passive stretching exercises of the extensor tendons.
Prescribe padded insoles to reduce the pressure over the metatarsal heads (p. 303).
Recommend wide–toe-box shoes.
Prescribe a hammer toe crest for the advanced case with established deformity. Pare the large corns and calluses with sharp dissection in the office and recommend maintenance care at home with a pumice stone or hand-held file. Suggest cotton ball, foam, or rubber spacers for padding between the toes.

Step 2 (4 to 6 weeks for persistent cases): Perform a local injection of K40 at the most painful MTP head (limit injection to one to two toes).
Reemphasize the importance of the stretching exercises.

Step 3 (3 to 4 months for chronic cases): Consider surgical referral for flexor tenotomy or arthroplasty if symptoms and deformity are persistent.

PHYSICAL THERAPY.   Physical therapy plays an important role in the active treatment and prevention of hammer toes. The focus of therapy is passive and active stretching of the extensor tendons. After soaking the feet in warm to hot water for 15 minutes (a vibrating water massage appliance is ideal), the toes are held firmly at the MTP joints and the toes are passively flexed downward in the direction of plantarflexion. Sets of 20 to 25 stretches are performed once or twice a day. Initially, these are performed with the ankle and foot in the neutral position. As flexibility improves, the ankle is plantarflexed more and more to accentuate the stretching. A pulling sensation should be felt in the anterior portion of the lower leg!

Following the passive stretching program, active stretching exercises are begun to increase the flexibility and prevent future problems. These active exercises include curling the toes up and down, grasping plush carpet with the toes, picking up marbles one by one, or picking up a small rolled-up towel.

INJECTION.   Treatment focuses on stretching exercises, padding, treatment of the secondary corns and callouses, and wide–toe-box shoes. Local corticosteroid injection is most often indicated for the acute inflammatory flare localized to one or two joints.

Positioning: The patient is to be in the supine position with the leg extended and the foot plantarflexed.

Surface Anatomy and the Point of Entry: The heads of the MTP joints are palpated from above and below and marked. The point of entry is centered between the two MTP joint heads, approximately 1/2″ back from the web space.

Angle of Entry and Depth: The needle is inserted into the skin at a 45-degree angle directed toward the most severely affected joint. The depth to the synovial membrane is 3/8 to 1/2".

Anesthesia: Ethyl chloride is sprayed on the skin. Local anesthesia is placed in the subcutaneous tissue (1/4 ml) and just outside the synovial membrane at 3/8" (1/4 ml). All anesthesia should be kept outside of the joint, for it will hold only a small volume!

Technique: A *dorsal approach* is taken to the MTP joint. The 25-gauge needle is introduced midway between the MTP joints and advanced at a 45-degree angle down to the bone of the metatarsal head (typically 1/2" down). Anesthesia is placed just outside the synovial membrane. The first syringe is removed and is replaced with the syringe containing the corticosteroid. The needle is advanced to the periosteum, and with the needle held flush against the bone, 1/4 ml of K40 is injected. Note that an injection placed underneath the synovial membrane is an intra-articular injection.

INJECTION AFTERCARE

1) *Rest* for 3 days, avoiding all unnecessary weightbearing.

2) Recommend loose-fitting, wide–toe-box shoes with extra padding (double socks, padded insoles, padded arch supports when indicated, or a hammer toe crest).

3) Use a toe spacer to improve alignment and minimize pressure.

4) *Ice* (15 minutes every 4 to 6 hours) and *Tylenol ES* (1000 mg twice a day) for soreness.

5) *Protect* the toes for 3 to 4 weeks by avoiding all unnecessary walking and standing.

6) Recommend shortening the stride: "Take extra time when walking to and from work!"

7) Begin *passive stretching* of the toes in flexion at 3 to 4 weeks (manual stretching, picking up marbles, grasping a towel, grabbing plush carpet, etc.).

8) Repeat *injection* at 6 weeks with corticosteroid if pain recurs or persists.

9) Request *plain x-rays* of the foot and a *consultation* with a surgical orthopedist or podiatrist if two consecutive injections fail to control pain and swelling, the PIP joints have fixed contractures, and the patient is willing to undergo possible fusion.

SURGICAL PROCEDURE.   Arthroplasty with or without fusion with K wires.

PROGNOSIS.   Medical treatment for the early stage of this condition (the painful metatarsalgia stage, before the toes have become irreversibly deformed) is very successful. Stretching exercises performed regularly over a period of months should reduce the deformity, aid in reducing the reactive hypertrophic corns and calluses, and obviate the need for surgery.

If the MTP and PIP joints have become rigid as a result of progressive extensor tendon contracture, surgery can be considered. The flexor tendons can be cut (flexor tenotomy) or combined with removal of the head of the proximal phalanx (arthroplasty).

DESCRIPTION.   Morton neuroma is a chronic irritation/inflammation of the digital nerve as it courses between the metatarsalphalangeal heads. Pressure from below (walking or standing on hard surfaces with poorly padded shoes) and pressure from the sides (tight shoes) cause the nerve to enlarge gradually; the pathologic changes consist of perineural thickening and fibrosis. The digital nerve between the third and fourth toes is affected most commonly.

SYMPTOMS.   The patient complains of pain between the toes or numbness along the sides of two adjacent toes.

Morton Neuroma

Enter from above, ½″ distal to the MTP joint.

Needle: ⅝″, 25 gauge

Depth: ⅝ to ¾″ (below the transverse metatarsal ligament)

Volume: ½ ml of K40

Note: This is identical to a digital block.

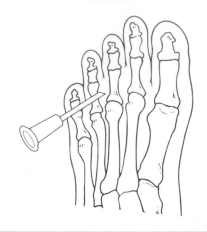

Figure 11–5.   Morton neuroma injection

"My two toes have gone numb."
"I have sharp pain between my toes."
"Certain tight shoes cause my toes to tingle."
"If I put all my weight on my right foot, I get a shooting pain through my toes."
"Sandals are the only shoes that feel comfortable."
"My third and fourth toes feel dead."

EXAM.   The space between the metatarsal heads is assessed for local tenderness, and the skin of the adjacent two toes is tested for loss of sensation.

EXAM SUMMARY   • • • • • • • • • • • • • • • •

1.   Maximum tenderness in the web space
2.   Pain aggravated by the MTP squeeze sign
3.   Passive range of motion of the MTP joints that is painless
4.   Loss of sensation along the inner aspects of the adjacent two toes (advanced case)
5.   Digital nerve block to confirm the diagnosis

(1) Local tenderness is greatest in the web space between the MTP heads. This is in contrast to the tenderness at the MTP heads in metatarsalgia. Firm pressure must be applied to elicit pain in the web space! (2) Pain can be reproduced by squeezing the MTP heads from either side (medial to lateral). This compression may cause an electricity-like pain to shoot to the ends of the adjacent two toes. (3) Passive range of motion of the MTP joints should be painless in an uncomplicated case. (4) Advanced cases may show a loss of sensation along the inner aspects of the adjacent two toes. Light touch or pain sensation may be decreased. (5) Finally, a digital nerve block should eliminate the local tenderness and pain with MTP squeeze.

X-RAYS. X-rays of the foot are normal. No characteristic changes are seen on plain films.

SPECIAL TESTING. Local anesthetic block is used to confirm the diagnosis.

DIAGNOSIS. A presumptive diagnosis is based on the pain and local tenderness in the web space between two adjacent MTP joints. Confirmation of the diagnosis requires relief with local digital nerve block placed just below the transverse tarsal ligament. If the diagnosis is still in question and the patient's symptoms are unrelieved with conservative care, surgical exploration may be indicated for definitive diagnosis.

TREATMENT. The goals of treatment are to reduce the pressure over the nerve and to eliminate the associated inflammation. The treatments of choice combine a padded toe spacer with soft insoles placed in wide–toe-box shoes.

Step 1: Recommend wide–toe-box shoes.
Suggest soft, padded insoles (p. 303).
Demonstrate the use of a cotton or rubber spacer taped or placed between the affected toes (p. 306).
The NSAIDs are ineffective because of poor penetration into these tissues.

Step 2 (4 to 6 weeks for persistent cases): Perform a local injection of K40.
Reemphasize the importance of proper shoes.
Repeat the injection in 4 to 6 weeks if symptoms have not decreased by 50%.

Step 3 (3 months for chronic cases): Consider a referral to a podiatrist or an orthopedist for a definitive neurectomy.
Educate the patient: "Surgery may cause permanent toe numbness!"

PHYSICAL THERAPY. Physical therapy does not play an important role in the treatment of Morton neuroma.

INJECTION. Local anesthetic injection is often used to confirm the diagnosis. Local corticosteroid injection is indicated when padding, protection, and change in shoes fail to control symptoms.

Positioning: The patient is to be in the supine position with the leg extended and the foot plantarflexed to 30 degrees.

Surface Anatomy and the Point of Entry: The heads of the MTP joints are palpated from above and below and marked. The point of entry is centered between the two MTP joint heads, approximately 1/2" back from the web space.

Angle of Entry and Depth: The needle is inserted perpendicular to the skin and advanced down and through the transverse tarsal ligament (between the metatarsal heads). The depth is 3/8 to 1/2" to the transverse tarsal ligament and 5/8 to 3/4" to the nerve.

Anesthesia: Ethyl chloride is sprayed on the skin. Local anesthesia is placed in the subcutaneous tissue (1/4 ml), the transverse tarsal ligament (1/4 ml), and just below the ligament (1/4 to 1/2 ml). If the injection is placed accurately under the transverse tarsal ligament, the inner aspects of the adjacent toes should be numb!

Technique: A *dorsal approach* is taken. The proximal phalangeal heads are palpated. The 25-gauge needle is inserted halfway between the MTP heads and advanced to the firm resistance of the transverse tarsal ligament (subtle!). Following anesthesia at this level, the needle is advanced through the ligament. Often a giving-way or popping sensation is felt. The patient is reexamined after 1/4 to 1/2 ml of anesthetic is injected. If the local tenderness and the MTP squeeze sign are relieved, K40 is injected.

INJECTION AFTERCARE

1) *Rest* for 3 days, avoiding all unnecessary weightbearing.

2) Recommend loose-fitting, wide–toe-box shoes with extra padding (double socks, padded insoles, and padded arch supports when indicated).

3) Use a toe spacer to improve alignment and minimize pressure.

4) *Ice* (15 minutes every 4 to 6 hours) and *Tylenol ES* (1000 mg twice a day) for soreness.

5) *Protect* the toes for 3 to 4 weeks by avoiding all unnecessary walking and standing.

6) Recommend shortening the stride: "Take extra time when walking to and from work!"

7) Repeat *injection* at 6 weeks with corticosteroid if pain recurs or persists.

8) Request *plain x-rays* of the foot and a *consultation* with a surgical orthopedist or podiatrist if two consecutive injections fail to control pain and the patient is willing to undergo an operation that may result in permanent numbness.

SURGICAL PROCEDURE.   Neurectomy.

PROGNOSIS.   Two consecutive injections with K40, 6 weeks apart, are effective in reducing the perineural inflammation and fibrosis around the digital nerve. The condition should be observed for at least 2 months prior to proceeding to surgery. Nerve injuries take months to improve once the inflammation has been reduced and the offending irritation has been eliminated. A neurectomy can be considered for persistent symptoms. The patient should be informed that surgery can leave the adjacent two toes permanently numb.

Fractures

chapter 12

Fractures Frequently Encountered in Primary Care

INTRODUCTION TO FRACTURES

Although most fractures associated with major skeletal trauma (hip fracture, spiral fracture of the tibia, and so forth) are evaluated in the emergency room and are referred directly to a fracture specialist, fractures associated with lesser degrees of trauma or with cumulative trauma are often evaluated in urgency care centers and medical offices. It is frequently the responsibility of the primary care practitioner (1) to order the initial x-rays, (2) to diagnose the type and severity of the fracture, (3) to identify complicated fractures that require referral to a fracture specialist, and (4) to provide the initial treatment. The primary care provider plays a critical role in the initial evaluation, in the triage process, and in the development of the treatment plan. Lack of knowledge of the management of bony fractures can lead to delays in diagnosis, neurovascular complications, poor healing (malunion or nonunion), or medicolegal entanglements.

Nearly half the population will experience a bony fracture at some time, which makes it one of the most common conditions presenting to the medical office. The 10 most common fracture locations are listed in Table 12–1. Fractures of the ankle (distal fibula) and wrist (radius) predominate (approximately 40%). The 10 most common fractures account for 90% of all fractures. Because only 10 to 15% of all fractures require open reduction and internal fixation (ORIF) or specialized reduction and cast management, the primary care provider should be familiar with and feel confident about managing the most common bony fractures.

The enhancement of fracture management skills requires that the primary care provider understand (1) the classification of fractures, (2) which fractures can be managed nonoperatively, (3) which fractures require the expertise of a fracture specialist, and (4) which braces, splints, and casts are used for immobilization.

Fractures are classified according to location, involvement of the adjacent joint, displacement of the fracture fragments, number of fragments, stability of the fragments, and involvement of the soft tissues. Fractures that do not involve the adjacent joint are called *extra-articular fractures*. Nearly all extra-articular fractures that are not displaced can be managed nonoperatively. On the other hand, *intra-articular fractures*, especially those that disrupt the normal integrity of the articular surfaces or the stability of the supporting structures of the joint, commonly require open reduction and internal fixation and hence should be referred to an orthopedic surgeon. Similarly, fractures that demonstrate multiple fragments *(comminution)*, dramatic displacement *(angulation)*, or penetration of the skin *(compound)* are nearly always unstable or at risk for infectious complication and should be referred to an orthopedic surgeon as well.

Certain unique types of fractures, particularly those that do not involve an obvious traumatic event, nearly always present to the primary care provider, placing

TABLE 12–1. FRACTURE DISTRIBUTION

Fracture Location	Frequency (%)
Ankle	23
Wrist	17
Fingers (Tuft/Phalanges)	14
Toes	7
Ribs	7
Knee (Tibia/Patella)	7
Clavicle	6
Elbow	6
Tarsus	3
Hip	2
Other	9

the practitioner in the critical role of identifier, evaluator, and initiator of treatment. Such fractures include (1) most of the *avulsion fractures* and nondisplaced fractures associated with severe sprains, (2) the *stress fractures* in athletes, dancers, and military recruits, (3) the *vertebral compression fractures* associated with advanced osteoporosis, (4) the *rib fractures* in elderly or emphysematous patients, (5) the *segmental collapse fractures* in avascular necrosis of the femoral head, (6) the *occult fractures* of the femoral head, and (7) the *pathologic fractures* of metastatic involvement of the spine, femur, tibia, and humerus. All of these fractures require a high index of suspicion for early diagnosis and often require confirmation by specialized radiographic testing.

The following section describes the fractures that affect the peripheral skeleton—the classification, the criteria for referral to a surgical orthopedist, the general treatment plan for those that are managed surgically, and the details of treatment for those that are managed nonoperatively. The list is extensive but not comprehensive. If there is any question about the stability of the fracture, its intra-articular extension, or the optimal type or length of immobilization, referral to a surgical orthopedist is recommended. More detailed descriptions of the management of any given fracture can be found in the standard texts of orthopedics.

Lastly, associated soft-tissue injury must be assessed in all patients with bony fractures. The neurovascular status must be assessed distal to the site of the fracture. Pulse pressure and capillary fill times as well as light touch, two-point discrimination, and pain sensation must be assessed distal to the fracture site and compared side to side. In addition, the integrity of the muscular compartments of the forearm, thigh, and lower leg must be assessed and followed closely for signs of compromise with the fractures of the long bones in these areas.

FRACTURES THAT ARE MANAGED OPERATIVELY

Fracture/Dislocation	Reason for Orthopedic Referral
Fractures that Require Referral to Orthopedic Surgery	
Multifragment intra-articular	Risk of arthritis and malunion
Fracture dislocations	Difficulty of reduction, risk of arthritis
Metastatic lesion of bone	Risk of pathologic fracture
Comminuted fractures	Risk of nonunion and angulation
Compound fractures	Risk of infectious complication
Fractures associated with neurovascular compromise	Soft-tissue injury

See Appendix 1–1 for individual fracture management.

FRACTURES THAT ARE MANAGED NONOPERATIVELY

Fracture/Dislocation	Nonoperative Immobilization or Treatment
General Categories of Fractures Managed Nonoperatively	
All stress fractures	Reduced running, standing, repetitious use
All nondisplaced extra-articular fractures	Casting for 3 to 6 weeks
Most small (flecks) avulsion fractures	Casting for 2 to 4 weeks
Some nondisplaced, single-fragment intra-articular fractures	Casting for 4 to 6 weeks

Humerus

Fragment displacement < 1 cm or angulation < 45 degrees	Hanging cast plus pendulum stretching exercises

Clavicle

Nonarticular proximal third	Figure-of-eight splint or simple sling
Middle third	Figure-of-eight splint or simple sling
Nondisplaced distal third	Figure-of-eight splint or simple sling

Elbow

Dislocation without fracture	Closed reduction with distal distraction
Nondisplaced radial head fracture	Simple sling and range-of-motion (ROM) exercises
Nondisplaced fracture of the radius or ulna	Long-arm cast with collar and cuff

Wrist

Most distal radius fractures without foreshortening of the radius or with less than 20 degrees of angulation	Chinese finger-trap traction plus sugar-tong splint plus short-arm cast

Hand

Boxer fracture of the fifth metacarpal with less than 40 degrees of angulation	Removable volar splint
Volar dislocation of the MTP with avulsion fracture < 2 to 3 mm	Radial or ulnar gutter splinting
Extra-articular metacarpal fracture of the thumb without displacement in any plane	Thumb spica cast plus ROM exercises of the thumb
Dorsal dislocation of the MP joint of the thumb if a single reduction succeeds	Dorsal hood splint
Gamekeeper's thumb, incompletely ruptured	Dorsal hood splint
Extra-articular fractures of the proximal and middle phalanges (nondisplaced and without rotation or angulation)	Buddy-tape plus ROM exercises
The acute boutonnière injury without avulsion fracture	Splinting of the PIP joint in extension plus ROM exercises of the finger joints
Dislocation of the PIP joint without volar lip fracture	Radial or ulnar gutter splinting for 2 weeks, then buddy-taping
All distal phalanx fractures	Stack splint
Most mallet fingers	Stack splint or dorsal aluminum splint in full extension
Mallet fractures, displacement < 2 to 3 mm	Stack splint

Chest

Rib fracture, without pulmonary injury	Wide bra, Ace wrap, or chest binder

Pelvis

Nondisplaced, nonarticular, with minimal pain	Touch-down–weightbearing crutches

Hip

Hip fracture in a debilitated patient	Prolonged bedrest
Impacted fractures that are weeks old	Non-weightbearing crutches followed by touch-down–weightbearing crutches
Stress fractures	Bedrest vs. crutches vs. reduced running
Avascular necrosis	Crutches

Knee

Patellar, nondisplaced and intact quads	Long-leg cast, well molded at the patella
Avulsion fracture at the joint line	Velcro straight-leg brace
Osteochondritis dissecans without mechanical locking or effusion	Straight-leg raises and observation
Tibial plateau rim, if < 10 degrees	Long-leg cast

Tibia

All tibial stress fractures	No running vs. decreased running schedule
Most minimally displaced tibial fractures, if < 1 cm leg shortening or < 5 to 10 degrees of angulation	Long-leg casting with suprapatellar and medial tibial molding; neutral ankle position; knee flexed to 5 degrees
Fibula, all fractures	Short-leg walking cast for pain control vs. reduced standing and walking
Gastrocnemius tear	No running, reduced standing and walking, tape

Ankle

Isolated small avulsion fractures	Short-leg walking cast for 2 to 4 weeks
Nondisplaced single malleolar fractures	Jones dressing followed by a short-leg walking cast for 4 to 6 weeks
Stable bimalleolar fractures	Jones dressing followed by a short-leg walking cast for 4 to 6 weeks
Posterior process of the talus	Short-leg walking cast for 4 to 6 weeks
Lateral process of the talus, nondisplaced	Short-leg walking cast for 4 to 6 weeks

Calcaneus

Most extra-articular fractures (except the displaced posterior process fracture)	Bedrest for 5 days, Jones dressing, short-leg walking cast with crutches and non-weightbearing, then gradual weightbearing

Talus

Chips, avulsions, nondisplaced neck fractures	Short-leg walking cast for 8 to 12 weeks

Navicular

All avulsion, stress, and tuberosity fractures (except with large fragments)	Short-leg walking cast for 4 to 6 weeks

Foot

Heel-pad syndrome	Heel cups or padded insoles
All fifth MTP avulsion fractures	Short-leg walking cast for 2 to 4 weeks
Jones fracture of the fifth metatarsal, nondisplaced	Jones dressing followed by a short-leg walking cast for 3 to 4 weeks
Nondisplaced metatarsal fractures	Short-leg walking cast with crutches and non-weightbearing for 2 to 3 weeks plus casting and weightbearing for an additional 2 weeks
All stress fractures of the metatarsals	Well-supported shoe plus limited standing and walking
Nearly all great toe fractures without comminution or soft-tissue injury	Taping plus a well-supported shoe vs. short-leg walking cast for 2 weeks
Nearly all sesamoid fractures without comminution or soft-tissue injury	Short-leg walking cast for 3 to 4 weeks, then a well-supported shoe
Lesser toe fractures	Cotton ball between the toes plus taping

FRACTURES OF THE HUMERUS: SHAFT AND PROXIMAL NECK

SUMMARY ▌

Fractures of the humerus constitute approximately 2% of all fractures. The incidence increases with age and with osteoporosis (especially in the humeral neck). Humeral fractures are classified according to location: proximal neck, humeral shaft, and supracondylar. The proximal neck and humeral shaft fractures are grouped together, separate from the supracondylar fractures, because they are usually treated by nonoperative means. Supracondylar fractures are more complex, can involve the elbow joint, and may require open fixation *(Sx)*.

SEQUENCE OF TREATMENTS

1) Order *x-rays,* classify the type of fracture, determine the degree of displacement or dislocation of the adjacent joints, and assess the integrity of the radial nerve by testing wrist strength.

2) Obtain *surgical orthopedic referral* (see below).

3) Immobilize in a *hanging cast* (p. 286) with collar and cuff appliance.

4) *Adjust* the length of the sling and its position at the wrist to correct for anterior or posterior bowing or valgus or volar angulation.

5) Begin daily finger stretches (p. 263) and Codman pendulum stretching exercise (p. 256) after the acute pain subsides.

■ FRACTURES OF THE HUMERUS

Fractures of the humerus are classified according to location: proximal neck, shaft, and supracondylar.

Proximal neck fractures are classified into two-part, three-part, and four-part fractures with or without dislocation of the shoulder joint (Neer classification).

Humeral shaft fractures are classified by fracture line (spiral, transverse, longitudinal, comminuted) and by location relative to the pectoralis and deltoid insertions.

Supracondylar fractures are grouped with fractures of the elbow; nearly all are referred to surgery *(Sx)*.

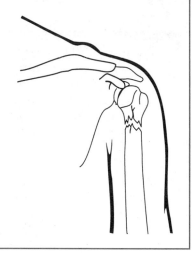

Figure 12–1. Fractures of the humerus

6) Obtain weekly *x-rays* to assess for angulation, bowing, and callus formation.

7) Refer to *physical therapy* if frozen shoulder intervenes.

8) Begin *isometric toning exercises* at 6 to 8 weeks to restore full function of the shoulder (p. 254).

9) Limit *overhead reaching and positioning* if impingement signs are present and limit *lifting, pushing, and pulling* until full strength has been restored.

SURGICAL CONSULTATION. Internal fixation is necessary for (1) shaft fractures that are open, severely comminuted, or transverse (where there is a higher degree of nonunion) and (2) for neck fractures showing dislocation of the shoulder, fragment displacement greater than 1 cm, or fragment angulation greater than 45 degrees.

COMPLICATIONS. Frozen shoulder (proximal neck fractures); chronic impingement (angulation of the greater tubercle); osteoarthritis of the shoulder (fracture/dislocation); radial nerve injury (lower-third shaft fractures); brachial artery injury (shaft fractures); nonunion (transverse and comminuted shaft fractures).

FRACTURES OF THE CLAVICLE

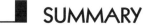 ## ■ SUMMARY

Fracture of the clavicle is the most common fracture of childhood and is a very common fracture in shoulder-girdle trauma in adults. These fractures are classified according to location (proximal-, middle-, and distal-third fractures), involvement of the adjacent articular cartilage of the SC joint or the AC joint, and position of distal fractures relative to the coracoclavicular ligaments. Fracture of the middle third is the most common (80%). The second most common fracture is the interligamentous, nondisplaced fracture of the distal third (10%).

Displacement of the fracture fragments is dependent on the pull of the sternoclei-

FRACTURES OF THE CLAVICLE

Fractures of the clavicle are classified according to location: proximal, middle, and distal third.

Fractures of the proximal third are classified as nondisplaced, displaced, or intra-articular.

All middle-third fractures are grouped together.

Fractures of the distal third are classified according to displacement, location relative to the coracoclavicular ligaments, and whether the fracture line enters the AC joint.

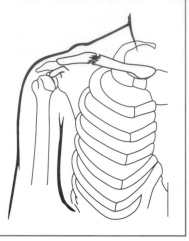

Figure 12–2.   Proximal, middle, and distal third fractures of the clavicle

domastoid muscles (the proximal fragments are pulled superiorly) and the pectoralis major muscles (the distal fragments drop forward).

SEQUENCE OF TREATMENTS

1) Order *x-rays,* classify the type of fracture, and determine the degree of displacement or dislocation of the adjacent joints.

2) Refer to a *surgical orthopedist* (see below).

3) Immobilize in a *simple sling* or *figure-of-eight splint* (pp. 285–286).

4) Adjust the figure-of-eight to maintain close approximation of the fragments.

5) Note that Codman exercises are not necessary if the glenohumeral joint is not directly involved.

6) Begin *isometric toning exercises* in abduction and external rotation (rotator cuff tendons) at 4 to 6 weeks (p. 254).

7) Limit *overhead reaching and positioning* for the first 3 months and limit *lifting, pushing, and pulling* until full strength has been restored to the rotator cuff tendons.

8) Gradually increase active general shoulder conditioning exercises at 3 months.

SURGICAL CONSULTATION.   Surgery must be considered in the case of any fracture associated with first-rib, pneumothorax, or neurovascular injury (less than 3%); in distal-third fractures with displacement (because of the greater risk of nonunion); and in nonunion that includes shoulder dysfunction or chronic pain.

COMPLICATIONS.   Complications include dislocation of the AC or SC joint; head and neck injuries (displaced fractures); first-rib fracture; pneumothorax (3%); brachial plexus injury (caused by severe and forceful blows in a downward direction); subclavian vessel or internal jugular vein injuries (caused by rare, severe blows); nonunion, which is rare; and malunion with cosmetic deformity, which is common.

DISTAL HUMERAL FRACTURES: SUPRACONDYLAR FRACTURE

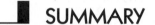 SUMMARY

Supracondylar fractures of the distal humerus are categorized as elbow fractures or dislocations and can be further classified as extension or flexion types, depending on the force of the injury. The most common injury is a fall to the outstretched hand. Because the fracture can extend into the elbow joint and involve either the brachial artery or the median nerve, referral to a surgical orthopedist is strongly advised *(Sx)*. Nondisplaced or minimal fractures that do not enter the elbow joint can be treated with a *posterior splint* for 1 to 2 weeks, followed by early ROM exercises of the elbow.

DISTAL HUMERAL FRACTURES: INTERCONDYLAR FRACTURE

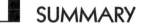 SUMMARY

Intercondylar fractures should be referred immediately to an orthopedic surgeon *(Sx)*. The T- or Y-configuration fractures of the distal humerus are the most difficult to manage of fractures of the upper extremity. Open reduction with rigid internal fixation is the preferred treatment in order to optimize the alignment and continuity of the articular surfaces of the elbow.

ELBOW DISLOCATION WITHOUT CONCOMITANT FRACTURE

 SUMMARY

Elbow dislocation occurs mostly in the young (10 to 20 years) and in the elderly. The elbow usually dislocates posteriorly. Neurovascular evaluation of the brachial artery, median nerve, and ulnar nerve is mandatory before proceeding to reduction. Closed reduction involves distraction with or without hyperextension to unlock the olecranon, followed by anterior translation. Open reduction is rare.

REDUCTION

1) The patient is to be in a *prone position*.

2) The *arm is hung* over the side of the examination table with *weight* applied to the wrist or with *traction* applied by the examiner.

3) With constant traction, and as the olecranon is felt to slip distally, the elbow is gently flexed.

4) The *range of motion* of the elbow in flexion to 30 degrees and in supination/ pronation is performed to ensure the stability of the reduction.

5) A *posterior splint* is applied for 2 to 3 weeks.

6) Gentle, *passive range-of-motion* exercises are performed within 1 to 2 weeks to prevent contracture.

7) With improving motion, *isometric toning exercises* of elbow flexion and extension are begun.

NONDISPLACED RADIAL-HEAD FRACTURE

SUMMARY

The preferred management with a *sling* (p. 285) and range-of-motion exercises is a classic example of the application of early physical therapy. It can be combined with aspiration of the hemarthrosis and intra-articular injection of local anesthetic (p. 60) to assist in early exercising. Note that associated injuries to the medial collateral ligament, interosseus membrane, and wrist should be excluded.

Displaced radial head fractures should be referred to an orthopedic surgeon for radial head excision *(Sx)*.

NONDISPLACED FRACTURES OF THE SHAFTS OF THE RADIUS AND ULNA

SUMMARY

Fixed immobilization in a *long-arm cast*—axilla to metacarpals—with a collar and cuff suspension at the proximal forearm is the treatment of choice for a nondisplaced fracture.

Displaced fractures must be evaluated by an orthopedic surgeon *(Sx)*. Open reduction and fixation is the preferred method of counteracting the opposing muscular forces, restoring the proper length of the bones, and achieving axial and rotational alignment. Similarly, open reduction and internal fixation is the preferred treatment for a Monteggia fracture in an adult (displaced fracture of the ulna with radial head dislocation).

FRACTURES OF THE DISTAL RADIUS

SUMMARY

Of the variety of fractures that affect the wrist, the Colles fracture is the most common. Nondisplaced fractures and displaced fractures that are readily reduced and stable can be managed with casting for 3 to 6 weeks. Colles fractures that are reducible but unstable, comminuted, or intra-articular and Smith fractures and Barton fractures may require open reduction and internal fixation *(Sx)*. These fractures should be managed by an orthopedic surgeon.

SEQUENCE OF TREATMENT FOR COLLES FRACTURES

1) Order *x-rays*, classify the type of fracture, determine the degree of displacement or dislocation of the adjacent joints, and assess the integrity of the median nerve.

2) Refer to a *surgical orthopedist* (see below).

3) Perform hematoma, axillary, or Bier block anesthesia.

4) Perform closed reduction using *finger-trap traction* (p. 292) with proximal brachial countertraction.

5) Repeat the *x-rays* to ensure a slightly volar tilt and restoration of the length of the radius.

6) Use a *sugar-tong splint* (p. 291) for the first 48 hours to allow room for swelling.

7) After 48 hours, replace the splint with a *short-arm cast* (p. 288) for undisplaced

FRACTURES OF THE DISTAL RADIUS

Fractures of the distal radius are classified according to the direction of angulation of the radius and whether the radiocarpal joint, radioulnar joint, or both are involved.

The Colles fracture involves the distal 2 cm of the radius, is angled dorsally, and may or may not involve the joints.

The Smith fracture is identical to the Colles fracture except for the volar angulation.

The Barton fracture is a fracture/dislocation with the predominant finding of wrist dislocation by both clinical criteria and x-ray findings.

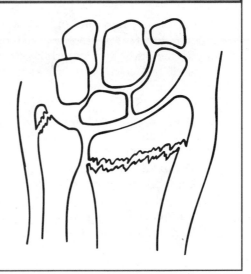

Figure 12–3.   Fractures of the distal radius: Colles, Smith, and Barton

fractures or a *long-arm cast* (p. 290) with slight flexion and ulnar deviation for displaced fractures (if unstable, refer to surgery).

8) Repeat *x-rays* at 4 to 6 weeks to assess for healing.

9) Use a *Velcro wrist splint with a metal stay* (p. 288) for 3 to 4 weeks after immobilization.

10) Start passive range-of-motion exercises of the wrist in dorsiflexion and volarflexion after fixed immobilization.

SURGICAL PROCEDURE.   Pin fixation or open reduction is necessary for a fracture that remains unstable despite closed reduction, for a Barton fracture/dislocation, for a comminuted fracture, and for a displaced fracture (especially an intra-articular fracture).

COMPLICATIONS.   Intra-articular and extra-articular fractures that result in a foreshortened or angled radius (> 5 mm or 20 degrees, respectively) have a greater incidence of poor range of motion of the wrist, osteoarthritis of the wrist, and median nerve damage.

NAVICULAR FRACTURE/SEVERE WRIST SPRAIN

SUMMARY

A patient presenting with mild to moderate symptoms and signs of a sprained wrist can be treated by recommending ice, limited use for 7 to 10 days, and immobilization with a simple wrist band (p. 288) or Velcro wrist brace (p. 288) and will have uniform good results. However, it is imperative to evaluate for and aggressively treat navicular fracture, lunate dislocation, carpal avascular necrosis, and so forth if wrist pain is severe, if tenderness over the first carpal row and in the snuffbox is severe, and if the range of motion of the wrist is limited to 50%. Failure to identify and treat

FRACTURES OF THE NAVICULAR

Patients who fall onto an outstretched hand or suffer a direct blow to the wrist may suffer a simple, self-limited injury to the supporting ligaments of the wrist, but are at risk for several serious injuries.

Patients with substantial injury, severe pain, or dramatic degree of dorsal swelling should be carefully evaluated for:

1. Navicular fracture
2. Perilunate dislocation
3. Chondral fracture of the radius
4. Carpal instability
5. Radiocarpal dissociation
6. Carpal bone fractures.

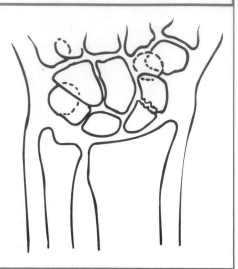

Figure 12—4.   Navicular fracture and other injuries associated with severe wrist sprain

these advanced wrist conditions can result in the medicolegal predicament of delay in diagnosis.

SEQUENCE OF TREATMENTS FOR SEVERE WRIST SPRAINS

1) Order six views of the wrist (including PA and lateral views, flexion and extension lateral views, and radial and ulnar deviation PA views), apply *ice* immediately, and *immobilize* the wrist with a posterior splint (especially if there is a dramatic degree of swelling) or a short-arm cast (p. 288).

2) Refer to a *surgical orthopedist* (see below).

3) Order *special testing* to assess for navicular fracture or other carpal bone fracture (which are rare): oblique views of the wrist, carpal tunnel views, wrist tomography, or an MRI of the wrist.

4) *Measure* the scapholunate gap (abnormal: more than 4 mm), the scapholunate angle (abnormal: more than 80 degrees), and capitolunate angle (abnormal: more than 30 degrees) for perilunate dislocation.

5) Prescribe a *long-arm thumb-spica* (p. 290) cast that uses three-point pressure at the volar scaphoid, dorsal radius, and dorsal capitate (displacement < 1 mm and a scapulolunate angle < 60 degrees).

6) With improvement, begin *passive stretching exercises* in flexion and extension.

7) As motion returns, begin gradual *grip strengthening* exercises and *isometric toning exercises* in flexion and extension, and follow the progress with sequential dynometric measurements.

8) Gradually return to greater degrees of active motion.

9) *Restrict* heavy gripping and grasping, exposure to vibration, and repetitive impact in cases that have had poor or incomplete healing.

SURGICAL PROCEDURE.   Primary ligament repair of the wrist can be considered for severe ligamentous injuries associated with joint instability. Displaced scaphoid fractures should be stabilized with internal fixation. Severe perilunate instability may have to be surgically fused (arthrodesis).

COMPLICATIONS.   Wrist instability, chronic wrist pain, osteoarthritis of the radiocarpal joint, and nonunion or malunion of the fracture fragments are the most common sequelae of severe wrist sprains.

METACARPAL FRACTURES

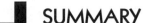 **SUMMARY**

Fractures of the metacarpals are classified according to location—head, neck, shaft, and base. These fractures are difficult to manage because of fracture angulation, fragment rotation (especially the oblique fractures of the shaft), inherent instability after reduction, and postfracture stiffness that can occur as a result of improper immobilization. For these reasons, open reduction and pin fixation are suggested *(Sx)*.

However, the Boxer fracture of the fifth metacarpal neck can be treated nonoperatively. If the fracture is not comminuted, angulation is less than 40 degrees, and the patient is willing to accept a deformity on the back of the hand, good function will result from 4 weeks of wearing a removable *volar splint* (p. 288).

VOLAR DISLOCATION OF THE METACARPOPHALANGEAL JOINTS

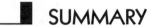 **SUMMARY**

Dislocation of the MP joints involves injury to the lateral collateral ligaments and is an uncommon condition. Immobilization with a *radial or ulnar gutter splint* (p. 289) is the preferred treatment unless an avulsion fracture greater than 2 to 3 mm is present. In the case of a large avulsion fracture, pin fixation is the preferred surgical procedure.

Often, a patient presents with similar symptoms weeks to months after an injury to the MP joint. Intra-articular corticosteroid injection combined with 3 weeks of immobilization using a *radial or ulnar gutter splint* (p. 289) is effective, although symptoms may persist for 9 to 12 months.

EXTRA-ARTICULAR METACARPAL FRACTURES OF THE THUMB

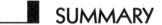 **SUMMARY**

Transverse or oblique fractures of the shafts of the metacarpal (totally extraarticular in all views) can be treated with closed reduction with good results. The fracture is immobilized for 4 weeks in a well-molded *thumb-spica cast* (p. 292) and followed by passive range-of-motion exercises of the thumb. Metacarpal fractures that involve the carpometacarpal joint are inherently unstable and must be managed surgically (see below).

INTRA-ARTICULAR METACARPAL FRACTURES OF THE THUMB

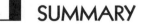 **SUMMARY**

Comminuted metacarpal fractures or fractures that involve the carpometacarpal joint are inherently unstable and must be managed surgically *(Sx)*. A Bennett fracture is a fracture/dislocation of the base of the metacarpal and is unstable because of the dorsal and radial pull of the abductor pollicis longus. A Rolando fracture is a comminuted fracture of the base of the thumb and is even more unstable than the Bennett fracture. Both fractures should be managed by an orthopedic surgeon because of the difficulty in maintaining anatomic reduction without internal pin fixation.

DORSAL DISLOCATION OF THE MP JOINT OF THE THUMB
SUMMARY

If a single attempt at closed reduction is unsuccessful, an orthopedic surgeon should be consulted. Closed reduction is impossible with a trapped volar plate.

GAMEKEEPER'S THUMB, COMPLETE RUPTURE
SUMMARY

The gamekeeper of the royal court injured the ulnar collateral ligament and volar plate of the MP joint when twisting the necks of the fowl and rabbits hunted for the king. Today, ski pole injuries are the most common cause of this condition. A minority of cases have an associated avulsion fracture at the base of the proximal phalanx.

The physical examination is used to distinguish a partial tear from a complete disruption of the ligament. Gross radial deviation instability provoked by abduction stress applied across the joint suggests complete disruption of the ligament. A partial tear is suggested by abduction-stress–produced pain and minor opening of the joint. Local anesthesia may be necessary to distinguish the two conditions.

Gamekeeper's Thumb, Complete Rupture

Enter ¼" distal to the prominence of the distal metacarpal head on the ulnar side of the joint. Local anesthesia is used to differentiate this soft-tissue injury from involvement of the joint.

Needle: ⅝", 25 gauge

Depth: ⅛ to ¼", just under the skin and above the ligament

Volume: ¼ ml of anesthetic (Corticosteroid is not used for this condition.)

Note: To locate the proper depth of injection, advance the needle to the hard resistance of the bone and then withdraw ⅛".

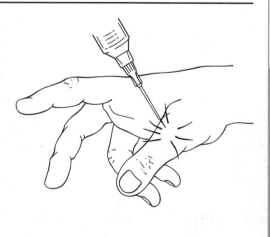

Figure 12–5.   Ulnar collateral ligament injury to the metacarpal joint

SEQUENCE OF TREATMENTS

1) Apply *ice* to the ulnar side of the MP joint.

2) Refer to *orthopedic surgery* if the ligament is completely ruptured (see below).

3) Perform a *local anesthetic block* placed subcutaneously in order to assist in staging the ligament injury or to determine involvement of the joint.

4) Prescribe a *dorsal hood splint* (p. 289) or a well-molded *thumb-spica cast* (p. 292) for 4 to 6 weeks.

5) Begin gentle, *passive range-of-motion* exercises in flexion and extension after immobilization (p. 263).

6) Begin gradual *isometric toning exercises* of gripping (p. 262).

7) *Restrict* pinching, gripping, and grasping until motion and strength are restored.

8) Refer to *orthopedic surgery* if several weeks of immobilization and physical therapy fail to improve the patient's function or resolve the pain.

SURGERY. Primary repair of a completely torn ligament is more successful when performed in the acute stage. Tendon graft repair or arthrodesis are performed if the thumb remains unstable or if the joint is complicated by late-onset osteoarthritis.

COMPLICATIONS. Whether by injury or repetitive use, the disrupted ligament can cause instability of the joint, poor pinching and opposition function, or late-onset degenerative change.

FRACTURES OF THE PROXIMAL AND MIDDLE PHALANGES

▌ SUMMARY

Fractures of the phalanges are classified by location, configuration (transverse or oblique), and the effects of the fracture on the rotation and foreshortening of the digit. The majority of these fractures can be managed nonsurgically. Extra-articular fractures that do not exhibit displacement, rotation, or angulation can be treated with *buddy-taping* (p. 293) and active range-of-motion exercises. Nearly all transverse fractures can be managed in this fashion.

In addition, small chip fractures of the collateral ligaments, dorsal chip fractures of the central slip of the extensor tendon at the base of the middle phalanx, and nondisplaced marginal fractures of the base of the proximal phalanx, can be managed with *buddy-taping* (p. 293).

However, transverse fractures at the base or neck of the proximal phalanx, nearly all spiral oblique fractures, and all comminuted and condylar (intra-articular) fractures must be evaluated by an orthopedic surgeon for possible open reduction and internal fixation *(Sx)*.

All phalangeal fractures must be assessed for late complications, including malrotation, lateral deviation, recurvatum angulation, shortening, intra-articular malunion, nonunion, tendon adherence, joint stiffness, and nailbed interposition.

ACUTE BOUTONNIÈRE INJURY

▌ SUMMARY

Finger injuries leading to an acute boutonnière deformity—tissue disruption of the central slip of the extensor tendon combined with tearing of the triangular ligament on the dorsum of the middle phalanx—can be treated by closed reduction as long as no bony chip fracture is present. The PIP joint is immobilized in full extension with a *PIP splint*, and active and passive range-of-motion exercises are performed daily. As with all finger and thumb injuries, postimmobilization stiffness must be guarded against.

DISLOCATIONS OF THE PIP JOINT

SUMMARY

There are three types of dislocation of the PIP joint: dorsal, volar (rare), and rotatory (uncommon). The dorsal or volar plate injury (with or without a small volar avulsion fracture) is the most common type of dislocation and is the result of hyperextension of the joint. Reduction is accomplished by closed means. The PIP joint is immobilized with a *PIP splint* (p. 294) for 2 weeks (no more than 15 degrees of flexion) or with *buddy-taping* (p. 293) for 3 to 6 weeks. Buddy-taping has the advantage of allowing early active motion (guarding against residual joint stiffness) while preventing hyperextension. Range-of-motion exercises are continued for several weeks after immobilization.

Surgical consultation is strongly recommended for dorsal dislocations associated with volar lip fractures involving more than 20% of the articular surface and for nonreducible dislocations *(Sx)*.

FRACTURE OF THE DISTAL PHALANX

SUMMARY

Fractures of the distal phalanx are classified as longitudinal, transverse, or crushed-eggshell types. These account for 50% of all hand fractures. Simple protective splinting for 3 to 4 weeks using a *fingertip guard or Stack splint* (p. 293) is combined with specific treatment of the soft-tissue injuries (laceration, subungual hematoma, etc.). The splint should not be placed close to the PIP joint so as to avoid joint stiffness.

MALLET FRACTURES

SUMMARY

The extensor tendon has avulsed a large fragment of bone (greater than one third of the articular surface) from the dorsal articular surface of the DIP joint. Management is controversial. Open reduction and fixation are advocated by some surgeons if the avulsed fragment is large, volar subluxation is present, and the fragment has been displaced more than 2 to 3 mm *(Sx)*.

RUPTURE OF THE EXTENSOR TENDON: MALLET FINGER

SUMMARY

The mallet finger deformity can result from stretching or partially tearing the extensor tendon or from complete rupture or rupture with avulsion fracture of the distal phalanx. Treatment consists of splinting the DIP joint in full extension or slight hyperextension for 1 to 2 months, using a *dorsal aluminum splint* and tape (p. 294) or a *Stack splint* (p. 293). The patient should be advised that function may be impaired in up to 30% of cases, especially in patients over age 60 and in patients with RA or peripheral vascular disease, if treatment is delayed over 4 weeks, and if immobilization lasts less than 4 weeks.

Patients with large avulsion fractures should be evaluated by an orthopedic surgeon *(Sx)*.

RUPTURE OF THE EXTENSOR TENDON OF THE THUMB: MALLET THUMB

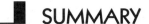

■ SUMMARY

Mallet thumb results from a rupture of the extensor pollicis longus insertion. Treatment with IP joint splinting and operative repair provide similar results *(Sx)*.

RUPTURE OF THE FLEXOR DIGITORUM PROFUNDUS TENDON

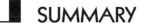

■ SUMMARY

This is an uncommon injury caused by forced hyperextension of the DIP joint. Early operative treatment is the treatment of choice *(Sx)*.

COMPRESSION FRACTURE OF THE VERTEBRAL BODY

■ SUMMARY

Compression fracture of the vertebral body is the most common fracture of the spine. The leading causes are structural weakness due to osteoporosis, trauma, and

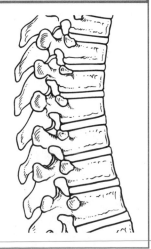

■ COMPRESSION FRACTURE OF THE VERTEBRAL BODY

Osteoporosis and trauma are the most common causes of vertebral body compression fracture; metastatic cancer and osteomyelitis are much less common causes.

Trauma and osteoporosis most often affect the lower thoracic spine and lumbar vertebrae.

As a general rule, if a compression fracture occurs above thoracic vertebra number 7, metastatic disease or infection must be excluded.

Figure 12–6. Wedge-shaped compression fracture of the vertebral body

metastatic disease. The lower thoracic vertebrae and the lumbar vertebrae are the sites most often affected. Metastatic disease should always be suspected if the fracture occurs above thoracic vertebra number seven (T7).

SEQUENCE OF TREATMENTS

1) Order x-rays of the spine, obtain baseline laboratory values (CBC, calcium, alkaline phosphatase, and ESR), and evaluate the neurologic status of the patient.

2) Obtain a *neurosurgical consultation* if angulation exceeds 35 degrees, if the fracture is unstable, or if neurologic compromise is present.

3) Prescribe adequate *analgesia* for this painful condition.

4) Recommend *bedrest* for 3 to 5 days for the patient with acute and severe pain.

5) Educate the patient: "The fracture may take several months to heal!"

6) Prescribe a *lumbosacral corset* (p. 295) or a three-point brace (p. 296) if pain control has been difficult to achieve.

7) Follow the alkaline phosphatase, calcium, and CBC to assess healing.

8) Perform a *bone densitometry* to assess the degree of bone loss.

9) Prescribe *calcium, vitamin D, and/or hormonal replacement* with estrogen and progesterone.

10) Gradually increase the level of activities after the acute pain has subsided and strongly encourage an aerobic exercise program.

SURGICAL PROCEDURE. Fracture stabilization is performed for severely angulated or unstable fractures.

COMPLICATIONS. Depending on the underlying cause, the number of fractures, their locations, and their effects on the underlying neurologic structures, vertebral body compression fractures can be complicated by chronic pain (in the case of multiple fractures), neurologic impairment (epidural metastasis, epidural abscess, or severe collapse), pulmonary insufficiency (multiple fractures), chronic osteomyelitis, and overlying skin ulceration (multiple fractures leading to an exaggerated kyphosis).

RIB FRACTURE

SUMMARY ▌

Rib fractures are classified as nondisplaced ("cracked") or displaced. They result from blunt trauma to the chest or from severe paroxysms of coughing. Nondisplaced fractures should be suspected if the patient has localized chest wall pain that is aggravated by direct palpation over the rib, deep breathing, coughing or sneezing, or chest wall compression. If the fracture is not a result of blunt trauma and the patient does not have generalized osteoporosis, a pathologic fracture should be suspected.

SEQUENCE OF TREATMENTS

1) The lungs should be carefully auscultated for diminished lung sounds and the soft tissues palpated for crepitance.

2) Order *x-rays* of the chest and rib in selected patients.

3) Apply *ice* directly over the rib.

4) Prescribe an *antitussive* if appropriate or use Tylenol with codeine compound to control both pain and cough.

▉ RIB FRACTURE

Rib fractures are commonly encountered in primary care.

Nondisplaced fractures can be managed with chest wall splinting, analgesics, and antitussives as indicated.

Greater attention must be paid to patients with displaced rib fractures. The entire bony thorax, the great vessels, and the pulmonary tree and parenchyma must be assessed for additional injury.

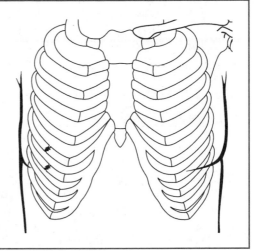

Figure 12–7.   Nondisplaced and displaced rib fractures

5) Educate the patient: "A fractured rib may take several weeks to heal."

6) Perform an *intercostal nerve block* with local anesthesia for severe localized pain.

7) Suggest a well-fitted bra, a snug jogging bra, an Ace wrap, or a *rib binder* to provide chest wall support.

8) Advise the patient that overmedication or excessive chest-wall binding can lead to local areas of lung collapse or pneumonia.

SURGICAL PROCEDURE.   None.

COMPLICATIONS.   Blunt trauma of a sufficient degree to the chest can cause damage to the internal organs, great vessels, or other structures of the thorax (the sternoclavicular joint, sternum, and vertebral bodies). The patient must be observed closely for progressive respiratory distress (pneumothorax or hemothorax). A patient with significantly compromised lung function due to emphysema, asthma, or other illness may require temporary hospitalization.

PELVIC FRACTURES

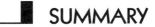

▉ SUMMARY

The successful management of a fractured pelvis requires the combined clinical skills of the primary care provider, the orthopedic surgeon *(Sx)*, and the urologist. Blunt trauma severe enough to fracture the sacrum, ilium, ishium, or pubic bones often leads to injury of the underlying organ system. Life-threatening hemorrhage, urologic injury to the bladder, urethra, or ureters, or gastrointestinal injury to the colon must be quickly assessed for possible emergent treatment.

After the patient has been stabilized medically, specific x-rays should be obtained to determine the severity and classification of the injury. The x-rays should include cervical spine, chest, PA pelvis, and inlet and outlet views of the pelvic ring. If the acetabulum is involved, special iliac and obturator views or a CT scan of the entire pelvis must be obtained. With these x-rays the fractures can be classified according to the degree of pelvic ring disruption, the involvement of the acetabulum, and the degree of displacement and instability of the bony fragments in the vertical and rotational directions.

Hospitalization, sling traction, and close observation for the first 24 to 48 hours, including hemodynamic monitoring, is combined with early pin placement for external fixation or open reduction and internal fixation *(Sx)*. Unstable patients with ongoing retroperitoneal hemorrhage should be evaluated by pelvic angiography and treated with embolization.

HIP FRACTURES AND FRACTURES OF THE FEMUR

SUMMARY

Fractures of the femur are divided into fractures involving the hip joint and fractures of the femur. Hip fractures are further subdivided into impacted, occult, avascular necrosis, stress, and the nondisplaced and displaced neck fractures. Fractures of the femur are further subdivided into intertrochanteric, trochanteric process, subtrochanteric, shaft, and supracondylar fractures (although the latter is traditionally grouped with fractures of the knee). All of these fractures are treated surgically (internal fixation, hemiarthroplasty, or total hip replacement) with the exception of certain impacted and occult fractures, stress fractures of the femoral neck, and avascular necrosis. The primary care physician must be able to diagnose and initiate the early treatment of these four fractures (see below).

EMERGENCY DEPARTMENT TREATMENT FOR HIP FRACTURE. The patient presents with a displaced femoral neck fracture with a foreshortened leg that is externally rotated. Transfers should be made with great attention to support of the extremity. The patient must be evaluated for a cardiovascular event that could have caused the fall. Appropriate analgesia by the intravenous route should be provided. Traction should be applied at 5 to 10 pounds, depending on the size of the patient and the bulk of the quadriceps. Consultation with an orthopedic surgeon should be made emergently.

METASTATIC INVOLVEMENT OF THE FEMUR AND TIBIA

SUMMARY

Metastatic involvement of the weightbearing bones of the lower extremity poses a special management problem. Secondary fracture through these bones has a disastrous effect on a patient's quality of life and can create a potential medicolegal dilemma for the provider. Protected weightbearing, radiation therapy, and prophylactic intrameduallary rod placement are used to prevent secondary fracture.

If metastatic disease is identified by bone scanning, the patient should be placed on limited weightbearing immediately. Plain x-rays of the pelvis, femur, and tibia are obtained to determine the compromise of the cortical structural bone, and urgent referral is made to an orthopedic surgeon *(Sx)* and radiation oncologist. These patients must be followed regularly and closely.

AVASCULAR NECROSIS OF THE HIP

SUMMARY

Avascular necrosis of the hip results from an interruption of the normal blood supply to the proximal portion of the femoral head. Common causes include trauma,

■ AVASCULAR NECROSIS OF THE HIP

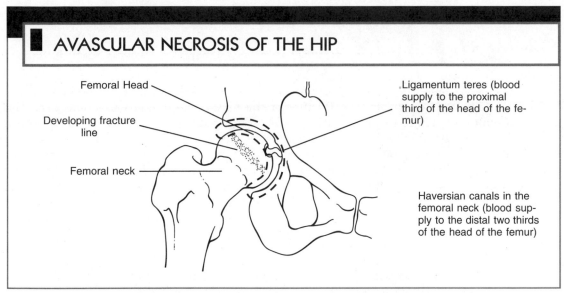

Femoral Head

Developing fracture line

Femoral neck

Ligamentum teres (blood supply to the proximal third of the head of the femur)

Haversian canals in the femoral neck (blood supply to the distal two thirds of the head of the femur)

Figure 12–8. Avascular necrosis of the femoral head

diabetes, alcoholism, high viscosity hematologic states, and oral corticosteroids (especially in the young asthmatic). The diagnosis is difficult to make early because of the nonspecific presenting complaints and physical signs. The diagnosis should be suspected if (1) the patient is at risk, (2) anterior groin pain is progressive, (3) weightbearing causes severe pain, and (4) rotation of the hip causes severe pain. Note that x-rays obtained in the first few weeks of the process are almost always unremarkable. If the diagnosis is suspected, a radionuclide bone scan or an MRI should be obtained.

SEQUENCE OF TREATMENTS

1) Advise the patient to immediately begin *non-weightbearing ambulation with crutches.*

2) Order an *MRI* to evaluate for a fracture line at the proximal third of the femoral head.

3) Perform baseline lab testing: CBC, ESR, glucose, LFTs, SPEP, calcium, and alkaline phosphatase.

4) Order urgent *orthopedic surgical consultation* to assist in the management.

5) Repeat *plain x-rays* in 2 to 3 weeks to assess for segmental collapse.

6) Begin *range-of-motion exercises* (p. 272) and progressive ambulation after the patient stabilizes.

Initiate weightbearing when rotation of the hip is no longer painful and healing has been demonstrated on plain x-rays.

SURGICAL PROCEDURE. Core decompression can be considered in the acute stage of the condition. Total hip replacement is appropriate for the patient who has lost significant range of motion, has segmental collapse, or is in persistent pain.

COMPLICATIONS. The principal goal of treatment is to prevent the segmental collapse of the proximal femoral fragment leading to the classic "step-off" of the articular surface, the flattening of the superomedial portion of the head (coxa plana), and loss of the true fit of the femoral head into the acetabulum. This dreaded complication causes chronic pain, loss of function, and accelerated osteoarthritis.

OCCULT FRACTURE OF THE HIP

SUMMARY ▮

The diagnosis of hip fracture is straightforward in most cases. However, a nondisplaced or incomplete fracture of the femur may elude early detection. This occult fracture occurs as a result of a fall. Elderly patients with advanced osteoporosis are at particular risk. The diagnosis must be suspected when examination of the hip discloses severe pain and extreme guarding with hip rotation. Plain x-rays do not show an obvious fracture line when advanced osteopenia is present. Weightbearing must be restricted until the diagnosis is confirmed or excluded by studies. In order to avoid the medicolegal issues of delay in diagnosis or inappropriate management, weightbearing must be restricted to avoid completing the fracture.

SEQUENCE OF TREATMENTS

1) *Examine* the patient's tolerance of weightbearing and the severity of pain with passive internal and external rotation.

2) Order an AP pelvis *x-ray.*

3) If the diagnosis is suspected, weightbearing must be *restricted acutely* by using crutches or by strict bedrest.

4) Order an MRI to evaluate for a subtle occult fracture.

5) Obtain an urgent *consultation* with an orthopedic surgeon.

6) Repeat the *plain x-rays* in 2 to 3 weeks.

7) Resume weightbearing when rotation of the hip is free of pain and significant healing has been demonstrated on plain x-rays.

SURGICAL PROCEDURE.   Although debilitated patients can be treated with prolonged bedrest, physical therapy range-of-motion exercises, and gradual weightbearing, there is a substantial risk of medical complications such as pneumonia, deep

▮ OCCULT FRACTURE OF THE HIP

Occult fracture of the hip must be suspected if:
1. A fall has occurred and the patient is elderly and is known to have osteoporotic bones,
2. Weightbearing is impossible due to moderate to severe hip pain, and
3. Internal and external rotation of the hip causes moderate to severe hip pain on examination.
Note: Plain x-rays of the hip do not demonstrate true fracture lines because the bones are too osteoporotic.

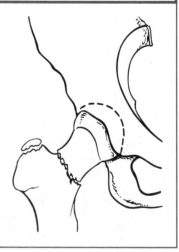

Figure 12–9.   Occult fracture of the hip

venous thrombosis, stasis ulceration, and so forth. For this reason, early percutaneous fixation of the hip or total hip replacement are the treatments of choice. The patient and the patient's family should be advised of the morbidity associated with prolonged confinement to bed.

COMPLICATIONS.   The risk of full weightbearing (conversion of an occult fracture into a displaced fracture) is so great that percutaneous pinning is performed in all but severely debilitated patients. Patients treated with combined bedrest and limited weightbearing are at risk for deep venous thrombosis and infectious complications.

FRACTURES OF THE KNEE: TIBIAL PLATEAU AND DISTAL FEMUR

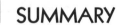 **SUMMARY**

Owing to the diversity of fractures that occur at the knee (tibial plateau) and the distal femur (supracondylar), the intra-articular extension of a sizable proportion of these fractures, the associated injuries to the supporting ligaments, and the need for specialized traction and cast-bracing, most patients with these fractures should be referred to an orthopedic surgeon for management *(Sx)*.

Fractures that can be treated nonoperatively include avulsion fractures at the joint line (medial collateral and lateral collateral ligament injuries), nondisplaced osteochondritis dissecans fractures that do not cause mechanical locking, minimally depressed tibial plateau rim fractures (depression less than 10 degrees), and certain patellar fractures (see below).

FRACTURES OF THE PATELLA

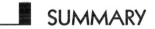 **SUMMARY**

Patellar fractures are classified as transverse, stellate, longitudinal, marginal or, rarely, osteochondral. Over half the fractures are transverse, and the majority of these are the result of a direct blow to the patella that is magnified by the tremendous pull of the quadriceps mechanism. Most show little or no separation of the fragments due to the intact medial and lateral quadriceps muscle "expansions." Nonoperative treatment with *long-leg casting* (p. 299) and gradual restoration of weightbearing is the treatment of choice for nondisplaced fractures.

Surgery involves cerclage wiring or lag-screw internal fixation for displaced fragments or total patellectomy for the severely comminuted fracture *(Sx)*.

SEQUENCE OF TREATMENTS

1) *Aspirate* the hemarthrosis.

2) *Assess the quadriceps mechanism* by asking the patient to lift the leg against gravity. This can be more accurately determined after aspiration of the hemarthrosis and intra-articular anesthesia.

3) Refer to a *surgical orthopedist* if the quadriceps mechanism is ruptured or the fragments are separated by more than 2 to 3 mm.

4) Immobilize with a *long-leg cast* (p. 299) for 4 to 6 weeks.

5) Allow partial weightbearing until the pain is significantly decreased, then full weightbearing.

6) Perform *straight-leg–raising exercises* (p. 276) as soon as the pain has lessened.

7) *Restrict* squatting and kneeling and avoid repetitious bending for 3 to 6 months.

8) Obtain bilateral *sunrise x-rays* at 1 year to assess for early osteoarthritic changes.

OSTEOCHONDRITIS DISSECANS OF THE MEDIAL FEMORAL CONDYLE

SUMMARY

Osteochondritis dissecans is an osteochondral fracture (bone and cartilage) at the site of attachment of the posterior cruciate ligament on the lateral aspect of the medial condyle. As to its exact cause, direct trauma, ischemia, and true avulsion are theorized. Patients present with nonspecific knee complaints or with mechanical locking due to an associated loose body. Patients with large fragments, persistent knee effusion, and mechanical locking should be referred to orthopedic surgery to consider posterior cruciate ligament repair, drilling of the fragment (to stimulate revascularization), or repair of any other associated injuries to ligaments or meniscal cartilage *(Sx)*.

TIBIAL SHAFT FRACTURES

SUMMARY

Most tibial shaft fractures should be managed by an orthopedic surgeon *(Sx)*. Fractures with no less than 1 cm of shortening, 5 degrees of varus or valgus angulation, or 10 degrees of anteroposterior or rotational angulation can be managed nonoperatively. After closed reduction using intravenous sedation, a *long-leg cast* with suprapatellar and medial tibial molding is applied. The foot and ankle are kept in the neutral position and the knee is flexed to 5 degrees. Healing time averages 5 months. Cast wedging is used to correct any postreduction angulation. When adequate callus formation is noted on x-rays, the cast can be replaced with a patellar tendonbearing cast or brace to complete the healing process. During the recovery period, the patient must be carefully monitored for deep venous thrombosis, anterior compartment syndrome, and distal ischemia.

TIBIAL STRESS FRACTURE

SUMMARY

Stress fractures of the tibia result from repeated microtrauma to the proximal third of the bone, often occurring in the section of the tibia with the smallest cross-sectional area. The condition is seen almost exclusively in runners, professional ballet dancers, and military recruits, although patients with severe osteoporotic bones are also susceptible. Radiographically, the periosteum of the proximal third (runners) and the middle third (ballet dancers) of the tibia is thickened. A true fracture line is seen infrequently. Stress fracture must be distinguished from the more common "shin splints," anterior compartment syndrome, and lumbosacral radiculopathy localized to the outer lower leg.

SEQUENCE OF TREATMENTS

1) Obtain *x-rays* of the tibia and compare them with old films, if available.

2) Repeat the plain x-rays in 2 to 3 weeks or obtain a *bone scan* to confirm the diagnosis.

▌ TIBIAL STRESS FRACTURE

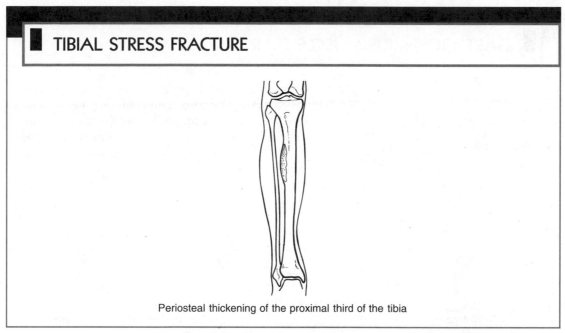

Periosteal thickening of the proximal third of the tibia

Figure 12–10.   Tibial stress fracture

3) Running and other high-impact sports are *restricted acutely* for at least several weeks, and crutches are recommended for severe pain.

4) Most cases respond to reduced activities. Persistent cases may require fixed *immobilization* with an air cast or short-leg walking cast (p. 301).

5) Nonimpact muscle-toning exercises are the *exercises of choice,* and they can be continued throughout the treatment period.

6) Padded arch supports are to be worn continuously in well-fitted shoes for prevention.

SURGICAL PROCEDURE.   None.

COMPLICATIONS.   Recurrence can be seen at 2 to 3 months if running and dancing are resumed prior to complete healing. Completion of the fracture is unusual.

COMBINED TIBIAL AND FIBULAR SHAFT FRACTURES

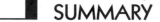

▌ SUMMARY

This combined fracture should be referred to an orthopedic surgeon because of the presence of instability, angulation, greater degrees of soft-tissue injury, and so forth *(Sx).*

ISOLATED FIBULAR SHAFT FRACTURE

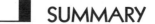

▌ SUMMARY

This fracture is much less common than the tibial/fibular fracture. It usually occurs as a result of a direct blow. Immobilization is used for pain control only. The fracture can be treated with a shortened stride, decreased weightbearing activities, or

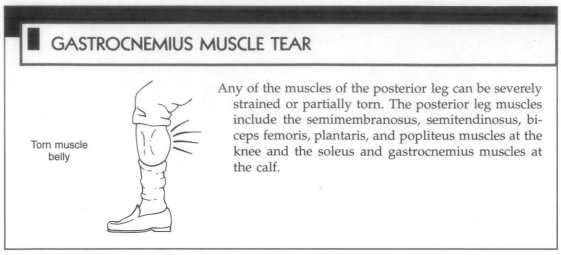

> ### GASTROCNEMIUS MUSCLE TEAR
>
> Torn muscle belly
>
> Any of the muscles of the posterior leg can be severely strained or partially torn. The posterior leg muscles include the semimembranosus, semitendinosus, biceps femoris, plantaris, and popliteus muscles at the knee and the soleus and gastrocnemius muscles at the calf.

Figure 12–11.   Gastrocnemius muscle tear

immobilization with a *short-leg walking cast* (p. 301). Fixed immobilization with casting is recommended when weightbearing pain is troublesome.

GASTROCNEMIUS MUSCLE TEAR
SUMMARY ▌

Gastrocnemius muscle tears occur in the proximal third of the muscle and are nearly always a result of trauma. This soft-tissue injury must be distinguished from a ruptured Baker cyst and lower extremity deep venous thrombosis.

SEQUENCE OF TREATMENTS

1) Exclude *deep venous thrombosis* in patients with significant risk factors for thrombosis.

2) *Restrict* running, walking, prolonged standing, and other weightbearing activities for 1 to 3 weeks.

3) Advise limited weightbearing with *crutches* for the first week.

4) Prescribe an Ace wrap (p. 297) or athletic taping (the *most common immobilizer*) and combine this with ice applications in the first few days.

5) Begin passive stretching of the ankle in dorsiflexion (p. 279) followed by the gradual return to regular activities.

SURGICAL PROCEDURE.   None.

FRACTURES OF THE ANKLE
SUMMARY ▌

Fractures of the ankle are probably the most difficult of all fractures to manage, in part because of the complexity of the ankle joint but also because of the diversity of fractures that can occur. Various combinations of injuries to ligaments and interosseous membranes and bony fractures are possible. Classification is based on the injury

■ FRACTURES OF THE ANKLE

Using the mortise view, ankle alignment and stability are assessed by the following measurements:

Talar tilt lines	Talocrural angle	Tibiofibular line
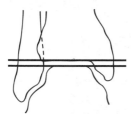	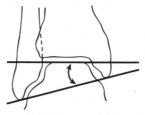	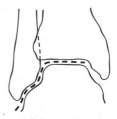
Should be parallel in the static position or up to 5 degrees with inversion stress	Normal angle of 8 to 12 degrees or no greater than 2 to 3 degrees from the opposite side	Should be a continuous line unless the fibula is shortened, rotated, or displaced

Figure 12–12.   Ankle fracture alignment measurements

pattern, the particular bones and ligaments that have been injured, the degree of fragment displacement, and the degree of incongruity of the articular surface. The Henderson system identifies malleolar, bimalleolar, and trimalleolar fractures. Lauge-Hansen classifies according to injury forces, that is, the supination-adduction injury pattern corresponds to the classic turned-in ankle sprain. Danis-Weber classifies the fractures according to the location of the fibular fracture relative to the syndesmosis, which correlates well with fracture instability.

The goal of the primary care physician is to diagnose the extent of the injury accurately by assessing the severity of the injury, the radiographic abnormalities, and the stability of the fracture and joint. The PA, lateral, and mortise x-rays are used to define the number and locations of the fractures. Measurements of the tibiofibular line, talocrural angle, talar tilt, and medial clear space from these views are used to determine fracture stability and displacement. Angle measurements on stress views of the ankle are used to determine ligamentous injuries. CT scans are used to define complex fracture patterns.

Small-fragment avulsion fractures, nondisplaced single malleolar fractures, and stable bimalleolar fractures can be treated nonoperatively. Initially, a *Jones compression dressing* with plaster splint reinforcement (p. 302) is used until swelling begins to resolve. Subsequently, a *short-leg walking cast* (p. 301), fracture brace, or walking boot (p. 301) is prescribed. Weightbearing is limited until pain has decreased and fracture healing is documented.

Most fractures at the syndesmosis, all fractures above the syndesmosis, and fractures with significant displacement (radiographically, by line measurement or stress views) should be placed in a Jones dressing. The patient should be given crutches and referred to an orthopedic surgeon *(Sx)*.

FRACTURES ACCOMPANYING SEVERE ANKLE SPRAIN

■ SUMMARY

Inversion injury with extreme equinus positioning can cause a *fracture of the posterior process of the talus,* which must be distinguished from the os trigonum, an accessory bone that is located posterior to the talus. This stable fracture can be treated with a compressive dressing or a *short-leg walking cast* (p. 301) for 4 to 6 weeks.

Inversion injury with the ankle dorsiflexed can cause a *fracture of the lateral process of the talus*. A mortis view or PA tomograms are necessary to demonstrate the fracture line. Small and minimally displaced fragments can be treated with a *short-leg walking cast* (p. 301) for 4 to 6 weeks. If the fragment is large, surgical referral for internal fixation is required *(Sx)*.

Inversion injury with rotation can cause excessive pressure on the peroneus brevis tendon and result in an *avulsion fracture of the base of the fifth metatarsal*. Small and minimally displaced fragments can be treated with a *short-leg walking cast* (p. 301) for 4 to 6 weeks.

Malleolar fractures are also very common with severe ankle sprains.

FRACTURES OF THE CALCANEUS
SUMMARY

The calcaneus is the tarsal bone that is most commonly fractured. Most fractures result from vertical falls and twisting injuries. Fractures are classified as extra-articular or intra-articular. Extra-articular fractures are further subdivided into anterior, tuberosity, medial process, sustentacular, and body fractures. Radiographically, PA, lateral, axial-calcaneal, and oblique views are combined with CT scans to define the location and intra-articular extension of the fragments.

Most extra-articular fractures can be treated nonoperatively. After 5 to 6 days of strict bedrest with leg elevation to control swelling (including hospitalization in selected cases) and a *Jones compression dressing* (p. 302) for 2 to 3 days, a *short-leg walking cast* (p. 301) is applied. Ambulation is restricted to non-weightbearing crutches until union is definitely seen on repeat x-rays (typically, several weeks). Subsequently, weightbearing is graduated through partial to full weightbearing, as tolerated.

Surgical referral is indicated for nonunion of the anterior process fracture, for displaced posterior process fractures (to restore the integrity of the Achilles tendon), and for all intra-articular fractures *(Sx)*.

Intra-articular fractures heal unpredictably. The clinician must apprise the patient of the potential of long-term complications, including subtalar joint pain, subtalar posttraumatic arthritis, peroneus tendinitis, bone spur formation, calcaneocuboid osteoarthritis, or entrapment of the medial and lateral plantar nerves.

FRACTURES OF THE TALUS
SUMMARY

The incidence of talus fractures is second only to that of calcaneal fractures. Classically, these are the result of hyperdorsiflexion injuries, as in hitting the brakes. Fractures are classified as chips, avulsions, or nondisplaced or displaced neck fractures. Surgical referral is advisable for the displaced neck fracture which is often accompanied by subtalar joint dislocation, as a favorable outcome demands a perfect reduction of the articular cartilage *(Sx)*.

The remaining fractures respond to 8 to 12 weeks of immobilization with a *short-leg walking cast* (p. 301) in a slightly equinus position for the first month, followed by 1 to 2 months in the neutral position. As soon as union is documented on repeat x-rays, range-of-motion exercises can be started.

Unfortunately, despite perfect reduction, healing can be complicated by avascular necrosis of the body in as many as 50% of cases.

FRACTURES OF THE NAVICULAR

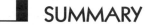

SUMMARY

The *cortical avulsion fracture of the dorsal navicular* occurs adjacent to the talus and is the result of a twisting injury. Unless the fragment is large, these fractures should be treated with 4 to 6 weeks of a *short-leg walking cast* (p. 301).

The *tuberosity fracture* occurs medially and is often confused with the accessory navicular bone. If the tuberosity is not displaced, a *short-leg walking cast* (p. 301) in neutral position for 4 to 6 weeks is the preferred treatment.

The *navicular stress fracture* occurs in young athletes. Plain x-rays are difficult to interpret. If the long-distance runner has persistent local tenderness and difficulties with arch pain, a bone scan can be ordered to identify this uncommon stress fracture.

HEEL PAD SYNDROME

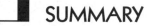

SUMMARY

Traumatic irritation of the specialized fat tissues of the heel is referred to as "heel pad syndrome." It is characterized by local tenderness of the fat pad reproduced by direct pressure and by squeezing the fat from both sides. Radiographic studies are normal. The goal of treatment is to protect the fat pad from pressure, allowing the tissues to return to normal.

SEQUENCE OF TREATMENTS

1) Examine the Achilles tendon, the pre-Achilles bursa, the plantar fascia, and the configuration of the arch to determine if the heel pad syndrome alone is responsible for the symptoms.

2) *X-rays* of the ankle and heel are necessary if associated conditions are present.

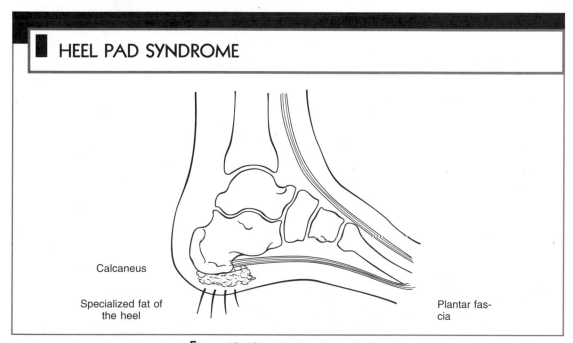

Figure 12–13. Heel pad syndrome

3) The most commonly prescribed *immobilizers* are rubber heel cups or padded arch supports (p. 303) worn continuously for 1 to 2 weeks in well-fitted shoes.

4) *Restrictions* during the acute phase involve limited weightbearing ranging from using crutches for the first few days to limited walking and standing and avoidance of hard surfaces.

5) Standing on a *fatigue mat* is recommended at the work station.

6) Ice applications over the heel will control the acute symptoms during the first few days.

7) In the *recovery phase,* passively performed range-of-motion exercises of the ankle are performed daily and are followed by Achilles tendon stretches.

SURGICAL PROCEDURE.   None.

COMPLICATIONS.   None.

FRACTURES OF THE MIDTARSALS

SUMMARY ▌

Midtarsal fractures are rare because of the rigidity of the midfoot.

CHARCOT, OR NEUROPATHIC, FRACTURES

SUMMARY ▌

Patients with impaired sensation due to peripheral neuropathy are at risk for fracture and for impaired fracture healing. Often such patients present with localized swelling and erythema that is disproportionate to the average amount of reactive soft-tissue change for that particular fracture. The midfoot is often the site of these fractures. Nonunion and malunion of the fracture is common because of the delay in diagnosis.

ACCESSORY BONES OF THE FEET (See Figure 12–14, page 241.)

SUMMARY ▌

The accessory bones occur in a variety of locations. Radiographically, they are sharply defined, well-circumscribed, oval or round ossifications adjacent to the tarsal or metatarsal bones. They are significant only from the standpoint of their being frequently misinterpreted as fractures. Their specific locations and distinctive anatomic features should differentiate them from avulsions and small-fragment fractures of the bones of the feet.

FRACTURES OF METATARSALS 1 THROUGH 4

SUMMARY ▌

A metatarsal fracture is most often caused by a direct blow to the top of the foot. Such fractures are classified according to the mechanism of injury (stress fractures),

■ ACCESSORY BONES OF THE FEET

The accessory bones of the feet are significant because they can mimic fractures.

1. Os trigonum
2. Os sustentaculum
3. Talus accessories
4. Os subcalcis
5. Os tibiotibiale
6. Calcaneus secundarium
7. Os supranaviculare
8. Os supratalare
9. Os tibiale externum
10. Os intercuneiforme
11. Os peroneum
12. Os vesalianum
13. Os intermetatarseum

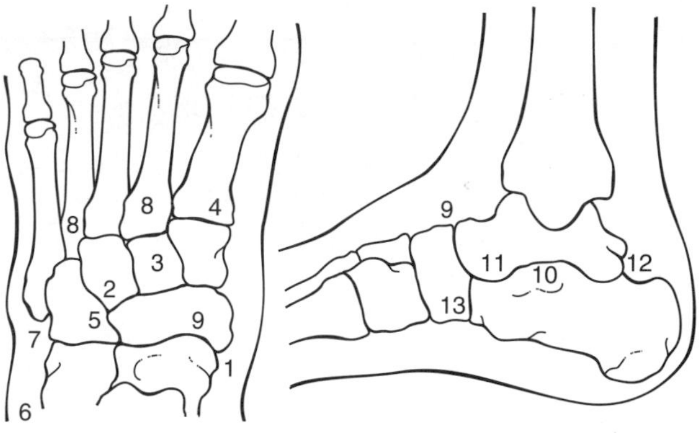

Figure 12–14.   The accessory bones of the feet in the differential diagnosis of foot fractures

the location (base, neck, or shaft), the direction of the fracture line (transverse or spiral), and the displacement. Nondisplaced fractures of the neck or shaft of metatarsals 2 through 4 can be treated with ice, elevation, analgesia, and a *short-leg walking cast* (p. 301). Nondisplaced fractures of the first metatarsal are treated similarly, but with the addition of a 2- to 3-week period of non-weightbearing casting followed by a short-leg walking cast to complete the 5-week immobilization. Displaced metatarsal fractures should be referred to an orthopedic surgeon for reduction *(Sx)*.

STRESS FRACTURES OF THE METATARSALS: MARCH FRACTURE

■ SUMMARY

Athletes, military recruits, and patients with osteoporosis who walk and stand for prolonged periods of time are at risk for the microfracturing of the metatarsal bones. The diagnosis should be suspected if the examination of the foot demonstrates dramatic swelling over the dorsum of the foot, local tenderness of the metatarsal, and pain when the metatarsals are squeezed from either side. Plain x-rays may show periosteal thickening, but that is a late finding. Nuclear-medicine bone scanning will demonstrate the abnormality in the early stages.

SEQUENCE OF TREATMENTS

1) *Wide–toe-box shoes* will lessen the side-to-side pressure.

2) *Padded insoles* (p. 303) worn continuously will lessen the effects of impact.

3) *Weightbearing,* both walking and standing, must be restricted until the pain has dramatically lessened.

4) Walking with a *shortened stride* will lessen the impact on the bones.

5) Persistent symptoms can be treated with a *short-leg walking cast* (p. 301).

METATARSAL STRESS FRACTURES (MARCH FRACTURE)

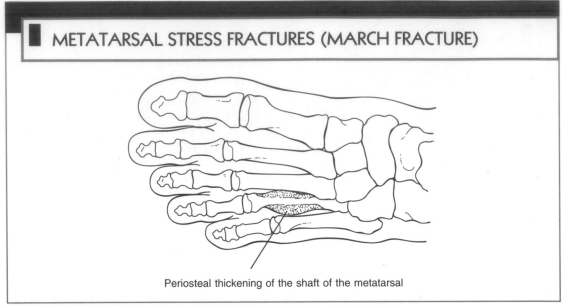

Periosteal thickening of the shaft of the metatarsal

Figure 12–15.   Stress fracture of the metatarsals

6) *Surgical consultation* is indicated if the bone fails to heal with restrictions and protection or if a completed fracture occurs with angulation.

SURGICAL PROCEDURE.   Open reduction and internal fixation are necessary for the rare case of complete fracture with displacement or angulation.

FRACTURES OF THE FIFTH METATARSAL BONE

SUMMARY

Fractures of the fifth metatarsal are unique. Severe inversion injuries of the ankle can cause the avulsion of a fleck of bone from the most proximal portion of the metatarsal. The peroneus brevis tendon detaches a small portion of cortex when the ankle is turned in. A *short-leg walking cast* (p. 301) is the treatment of choice. Immobilization should be continued for 3 to 4 weeks to allow the tendon to reattach securely to the metatarsal.

The Jones fracture involves the tuberosity of the base of the metatarsal. It should not be confused with a transverse fracture of the base, which has a much different prognosis. The Jones fracture is commonly located within 3/4" of the most proximal portion of the metatarsal. It is usually treated with a *bulky Jones dressing* (p. 303) for the first 24 to 36 hours and non-weightbearing followed by a *short-leg walking cast* (p. 301) for 3 to 4 weeks.

A transverse fracture of the shaft of the fifth metatarsal is treated with a *short-leg walking cast*. Unfortunately, there is a high incidence of delayed union and of nonunion of this fracture despite proper immobilization.

TURF TOE: STRAIN OF THE GREAT TOE

SUMMARY

Hyperextension of the first MTP joint causes stretching of and strain on the capsule of the joint and the plantar plate of the great toe. Occasionally a capsular avulsion fracture occurs. Treatment includes *buddy-taping* of the joint (p. 306), stiff shoes, and a stiff orthotic for 2 to 3 weeks.

FRACTURES OF THE GREAT TOE

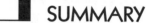 SUMMARY

Fracture of the proximal phalanx of the great toe occurs as a result of direct trauma (dropped objects) or a stubbing injury. Most fractures show minimal displacement. Treatment includes *buddy-taping* (p. 306), stiff shoes, or a *short-leg walking cast* (p. 301) with a toe plate for 2 weeks. Displaced intra-articular fractures can be reduced with *finger traps* (p. 292) and then treated in the same fashion as the nondisplaced fractures.

FRACTURES OF THE SESAMOID BONE

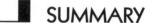 SUMMARY

Fractures of the sesamoid bone (medial-aspect fractures occur much more frequently than lateral-aspect fractures) must be distinguished from the congenital bipartate sesamoid. True fractures have rough edges, are transverse in direction, and eventually show callus formation. Bipartate sesamoid fractures occur bilaterally and have smooth, sharply bordered edges. Most fractures occur as a result of direct trauma, avulsion forces, or repetitive stress. Treatment with a *short-leg walking cast* (p. 301) for 3 to 4 weeks is followed by a stiff shoe and a metatarsal bar or pad.

FRACTURES OF THE TOES

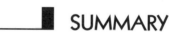 SUMMARY

Fractures of the lesser toes are easily reduced with manual pressure or with finger traps. *Buddy-taping* (p. 306) to the adjacent larger toe with cotton placed in the toe web is the treatment of choice. The patient should wear wide–toe-box shoes until the toe has healed.

Exercise Instruction Sheets

chapter 13

Exercise Instructions for Home Physical Therapy

INTRODUCTION

Physical therapy treatments—passive stretching exercises, isometric toning exercises, ultrasound, local massage, phonophoresis, and thermal applications—play an essential role in the complete management of the soft-tissue injuries and bony fractures that affect the skeleton. This is especially true for those conditions that have a strong element of *mechanical dysfunction* when compared to the degree of inflammation and those conditions that are associated with *disuse atrophy*. For example, the Codman pendulum stretching exercise is the treatment of choice for the subacromial impingement that accompanies rotator cuff tendinitis. The gluteus medius stretching exercise is fundamental to reducing the direct pressure of the tendons that accompanies trochanteric bursitis. Passive stretching exercises in abduction and external rotation are essential to restoring full range of motion to the glenohumeral joint in cases of frozen shoulder. Each condition demands a unique set of treatments.

Physical therapy treatments must be recommended at the appropriate *time* and at the appropriate *stage* of recovery. For example, stretching exercises to restore full range of motion after severe ankle sprain are started after 2 to 4 weeks of immobilization. The acute inflammation and pain must be arrested and the ligament securely reattached to the bone before range-of-motion exercises are begun. Similarly, isometric toning exercises to restore the strength of the rotator cuff tendons cannot be started until the inflammation of the rotator cuff tendon has been nearly resolved. Ideally, the optimal timing and extent of these treatments should be determined individually. The decision to initiate any physical therapy treatment must be assessed by the primary care provider and should be based on (1) the phase of recovery, (2) the patient's ability and willingness to carry out a home exercise program, and, most important, (3) the patient's tolerance of the specific exercise, as determined by the health care provider in the office. Performing the exercise in the office engenders greater confidence in the provider's treatment plan, provides hands-on explanation of the exercise, and allows the provider to assess the patient's understanding and tolerance of the exercise.

The recommendations in this book should serve as guidelines for prescribing physical therapy. The timing of these treatments, the frequency of performance, and the number of repetitions represent averages. Any specific physical therapy treatment must be adjusted according to the individual patient's understanding, cooperation, and tolerance. The information that follows represents general recommendations for physical therapy.

GENERAL CARE OF THE NECK

ANATOMY. The neck is made up of *seven neck bones* (vertebrae) connected together by a network of ligaments and muscles, all of which serve to protect the spinal cord and the spinal nerves. Seven pairs of spinal nerves exit the spinal column and travel down the neck through the shoulder and into the lower arm. Each nerve must pass by one of the disks and through an opening (foramen) formed by two adjacent neck bones.

CONDITIONS. Everyone will develop a problem in the neck at some time. Arthritis is a universal problem that develops with age. Gradual stiffness, especially when turning from side to side, and the forward positioning of the head are its common manifestations. Neck strain—muscular irritation in the neck and upper back—is an exceedingly common condition caused by tension, emotional strain, and poor posture. Many patients suffer recurrent neck stiffness, headaches, and pain from another very common cause, whiplash. A rapid-deceleration injury as a result of a motor vehicle accident or a heavy blow to the head can cause permanent damage to the neck's supporting ligaments and muscles. Some patients develop symptoms down the arm

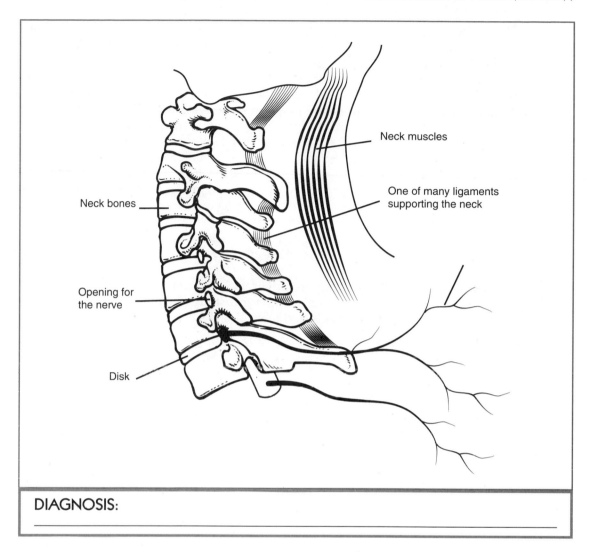

Neck muscles

One of many ligaments
supporting the neck

Neck bones

Opening for
the nerve

Disk

DIAGNOSIS:

that result from a pinched nerve due to large bony spurs, caused by arthritis (90%) or a herniated disk (10%), that impair spinal nerve function.

PHYSICAL THERAPY.   Physical therapy is fundamental to the treatment and prevention of conditions affecting the neck.

Ice should be applied directly to the affected muscles of the neck. An iced towel wrapped around the neck, blue ice packs, or a simple ice bag will effectively control the acute muscle spasms that accompany neck strain. The ice must be left in place for 15 to 20 minutes so it can penetrate to the deeper tissues.

PHYSICAL THERAPY SUMMARY

1. Ice applied directly to an acute muscle spasm
2. Heat and massage for chronic muscle spasms
3. Neck muscle stretching exercises, passively performed
4. Stress reduction
5. Posture improvement
6. Ultrasound
7. Vertical cervical traction

Heat should be applied to the muscles of the neck prior to performing the passive stretching exercises. A shower, a hot bath, and a moist towel warmed in a microwave and applied for 10 to 15 minutes are all effective.

Massage is applied to both sides of the neck and the upper back muscles using hand pressure or an electric, hand-held vibrator. The neck muscles should be relaxed during massage either by supporting the head or by lying down.

Reduction in *stress* and improvement in *posture* help reduce the tension and pressure in the neck. Upper back massage, gentle vibration with heat, relaxation techniques, or meditation can be very helpful in selected cases.

Passively performed *stretching exercises* are used to increase flexibility and preserve motion. Each exercise is performed in sets of 20, gradually increasing the stretch through the muscles. Mild discomfort is to be expected. Sharp pain or electricity-like pain is a sign of excessive stretching or spinal nerve irritation.

Ultrasound of the neck and upper back muscles can be combined with deep massage and stretching exercises. Neck strain and whiplash respond well to this combination.

Vertical cervical traction is reserved for chronic whiplash, chronic neck strain, and arthritis associated with a pinched nerve. Vertical stretching of the neck muscles and ligaments must be started gradually and increased slowly.

Good Body Mechanics.   The following recommendations emphasize correct posture, neutral neck positions, and preventive measures.

Sitting with the shoulders back

Sleeping with the head aligned with the torso: on the back with a small pillow or on the side with enough pillows to keep the head straight

Using seat belts and an air bag

Using arm rests to keep the shoulders slightly shrugged

Taking periodic breaks from desktop work

Avoiding continuous sitting or standing

Choosing a chair with good lumbar support

Activity Limitations.   The preferred activities and body positions emphasize neutral neck position and a minimum of tension across the supporting muscles and ligaments of the neck. The extremes of range of motion, activities, and body positioning that cause constant tension across the upper back and at the base of the neck must be minimized or avoided. The limitations include:

Not doing overhead work for long periods of time, especially if looking up is necessary

Not sleeping on the stomach with the neck turned or rotated

Avoiding stressful situations

Relying upon the hip belt rather than the over-the-shoulder straps when backpacking

Carrying heavy objects close to the body rather than with outstretched arms

Not carrying a heavy purse over the shoulder

Avoiding continuous sitting

Avoiding slumping over the workstation; adjusting the level of the work so that good posture can be maintained.

Avoiding looking down at a computer monitor; adjusting it to eye level

Precautions. Stretching exercises are not always tolerated by patients with advanced arthritis (large bone spurs), with limited mobility, or with the symptoms of a pinched nerve. Extremes of neck turning and neck extension can be painful (the bones are forced together) or harmful (the pressure over the nerve is increased).

Likewise, the deep heating and resultant swelling caused by ultrasound treatments may aggravate the symptoms associated with a pinched nerve.

Vertical cervical traction has to be used cautiously in patients with severe muscle irritation. Overly aggressive traction (too much weight or too long a period of traction) may aggravate the underlying muscular irritability. Note that a neck x-ray must be obtained before any vertical traction stretching program is begun.

NECK MASSAGE

Heat your upper back and the neck for 15 minutes. Lie down on your stomach with your head aligned with your body. (Place a pillow under your chest and neck). Ask your partner to press firmly with circular motions along the side of your neck and over the upper back muscles.

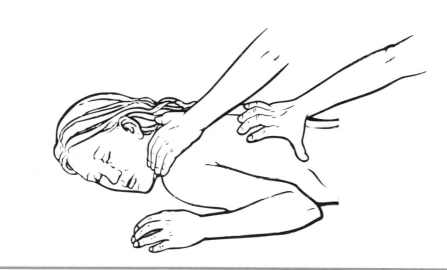

STRETCHING EXERCISES FOR THE NECK

Heat your neck and upper back in a bathtub, in a shower with a water massage, or with moist towels heated in a microwave. Gently stretch the muscles in sets of 10 to 15, with each held for 5 seconds. Expect mild, achy muscle pain but not sharp or electric pain. Relax the muscles in your neck during the exercises. Perform these exercises in the morning to relieve stiffness and just before sleeping.

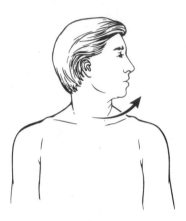

Neck Rotation
Slowly turn your head to the right. Place tension on your chin with your fingertips. Hold for a few seconds and return to the center. Repeat to the left.

Neck Tilting
Tilt your head to the right, trying to touch your ear to the tip of your shoulder. Place tension on the temple with your fingertips. Hold for a few seconds and return to the center. Repeat to the left.

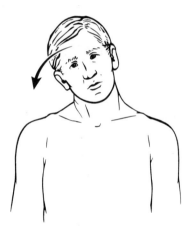

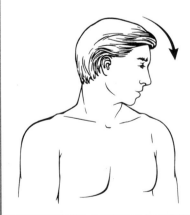

Neck Bending
Try to touch your chin to your chest. Hold for a few seconds and return to the neutral position. Breathe in gradually, and exhale slowly with each exercise. Relax the neck and back muscles with each neck bend.

HOME CERVICAL TRACTION

Home traction using a cervical water bag traction unit can be started after an evaluation by a physical therapist. Traction is begun using 4 to 5 pounds of water weight for 5 minutes and is slowly increased to 12 to 15 pounds for 10 minutes. Each week, the weight and/or time is increased by 1 to 2 pounds and/or 1 to 2 minutes. The neck muscles should be relaxed. Heat application prior to treatment is advised.

Note:

Traction can aggravate some conditions, particularly some disk herniations. If symptoms worsen, stop the traction and reevaluate. Arthritis of the neck may have to be treated three times a week for an indefinite period.

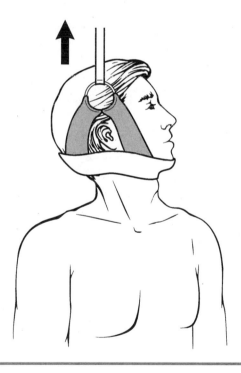

GENERAL CARE OF THE SHOULDER

ANATOMY.   The shoulder is a ball-and-socket joint formed by the upper arm bone (the humerus), the cap of the shoulder (the acromion process), and the bony socket (the glenoid of the scapula). It has many moving parts, including the following:

One major joint	The ball-and-socket joint
Three auxillary joints	The end of the collar bone (the AC joint); the joint of the collar bone and the breast plate (the SC); and the wing over the ribs (the scapulothoracic)
Eight major tendons	The rotator cuff tendons (four), biceps, triceps, deltoid, and pectoralis
One major lubricating bursal sac	The subacromial bursa
Four major ligaments	Three over the end of the collar bone and one encircling the ball-and-socket joint

CONDITIONS.   There are many causes of shoulder pain, including tense neck and upper back muscles, a pinched nerve in the neck, shoulder strain or separation, tendinitis, bursitis, and arthritis. However, tendinitis of the rotator tendons and frozen shoulder resulting from disuse account for two thirds of all problems. Shoulder separation occurs at the end of the clavicle. Arthritis at the end of the clavicle occurs to some degree or another in everyone, but only a small percentage of patients develop symptoms from it. Arthritis of the ball-and-socket joint is infrequent.

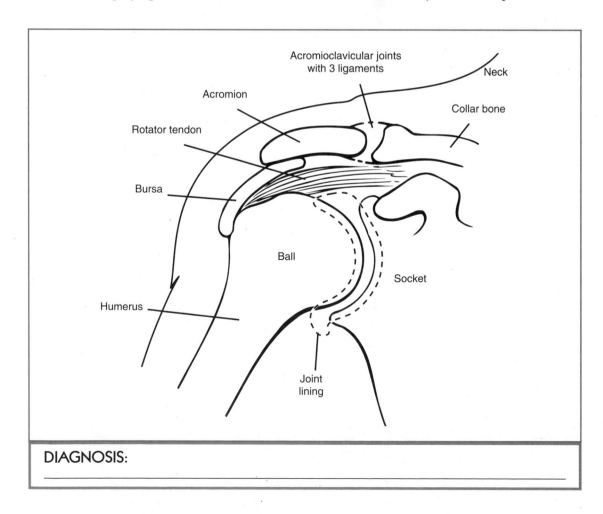

DIAGNOSIS:

PHYSICAL THERAPY.   Physical therapy plays a major role in the active treatment and rehabilitation of conditions involving the shoulder.

Ice applications can be used as the initial anti-inflammatory treatment for any of the shoulder conditions. However, the response is unpredictable. The shoulder joint and its supporting structures (the rotator tendons) are located deep in the tissues, 1 to 1 1/2″ below the skin.

Deep *heat* and *massage* are used to increase the blood flow to these tissues and prepare the shoulder for stretching. The shoulder is heated in a shower or warm bath for 10 to 15 minutes. Total body heating is preferable to local heat (a moist heating pad or a towel warmed in a microwave), again because of the depth of the tissues.

The *weighted pendulum stretching exercise* has a dual function in the active treatment of the shoulder. Its primary role is to gently stretch the tendon space between the ball-and-socket joint and the cap (see below). Its secondary role is to prevent frozen shoulder by providing passive movement of the shoulder joint. The muscles of the shoulder are relaxed, allowing the weight to open the shoulder and provide room for the shoulder bursa and the rotator tendons. A weight of 5 to 10 pounds is held in the hand; a filled gallon milk jug weighs 8 pounds, but any weight that can be easily hand-held will do. The arm is kept vertical and close to the body, thus avoiding further tendon impingement. The exercise is begun as a pure stretch, dangling the arm. With improvement, the arm is allowed to swing freely but no farther than 1 foot in any direction. The exercise is performed after heating for 5 minutes once or twice a day.

Muscle toning exercises for the supporting tendons are used to strengthen and tighten the joint. These should always follow the weighted pendulum stretching exercises. Rotation and lifting exercises are performed in sets of 20, each held 5 seconds with moderate tension. Flexible rubber tubing, bungee cords, or large rubber bands provide the necessary resistance. These exercises are gradually increased to restore the strength of the weakened tendons and muscles and put them in balance with their shoulder counterparts. Mild soreness should be expected. Sharp or severe pain may indicate a flare of the underlying condition.

Good Body Mechanics.   Safe activities and positions involve keeping the arm down and in front of and close to the body. A good rule of thumb is to perform all activities with the elbow held at the sides:

Lifting objects close to the body

Weight training with light weights below shoulder level

Sidestroke or breaststroke when swimming

Side-arm or underhand ball throwing

Volleying rather than serving in tennis

Desktop writing, assembly, and so forth with good posture

PHYSICAL THERAPY SUMMARY   • • • • • • • • • • • • • •

1. Heat and massage
2. Weighted pendulum stretching exercises, performed with relaxed shoulder muscles
3. Muscle toning exercises in lifting and turning out
4. Activity limitations
5. Stress reduction

PENDULUM STRETCH EXERCISES FOR THE SHOULDER

Prior to exercise or heavy work, shoulders should be stretched in a downward direction. This exercise provides greater space for the rotator cuff and the bicep tendons, allowing them to work more effectively and efficiently. Regular use of pendulum exercises can increase the space under the cap of the shoulder by ¼".

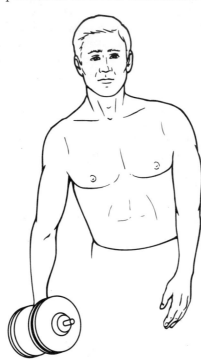

Weighted Pendulum Stretch
Heat the shoulder with moist towels or in a hot bath or hot shower. A weight of 5 to 10 pounds is held lightly in the hand (a filled gallon container weighs 8 pounds). The muscles of the shoulder are to be relaxed! The arm is kept vertical and close to the body (bending over too far may cause pinching of the rotator cuff tendons). The arm is allowed to swing back and forth or in a small-diameter circle (no greater than 1' in any direction). A properly performed stretching exercise may cause a deep achy pain, either in the armpit or down the inner aspect of the arm. This exercise can be performed just as effectively while sitting.

This exercise is very helpful for shoulder tendinitis (rotator cuff and biceps tendinitis), shoulder bursitis, frozen shoulder, and rotator cuff tendon tears. It is not appropriate for shoulder separation/strain or upper back/neck muscle strain.

STRENGTHENING EXERCISES FOR THE ROTATOR CUFF TENDONS

The rotator cuff tendons are the weakest and most susceptible to injury of the eight major tendons in the shoulder. Isometric exercises are necessary to improve the strength of these tendons. These exercises will balance the strength of the shoulder muscles. Flexible rubber tubing, bungee cords, or large rubber bands are used to develop muscle tone and strength. First, the shoulder is heated and then it is prepared by stretching, using the weighted pendulum swing exercise. Following a 2- to 3-minute rest, sets of 15 to 20 exercises, each held 5 seconds, should be performed daily.

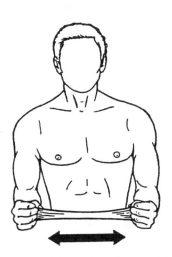

Outward Rotation Isometric
The elbows are held at 90°, close to the sides. The rubber bands are grasped with the hands. The forearms are rotated outward only 2 to 3″ and held 5 seconds. The forearms swing out like a door.

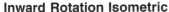

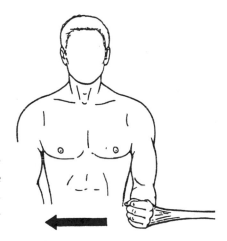

Inward Rotation Isometric
The elbow is held at 90°, close to the side. The rubber bands are hooked onto a door handle and grasped with the hand. The forearm is rotated inward only 2 to 3″ and held 5 seconds. The forearm swings in like a door.

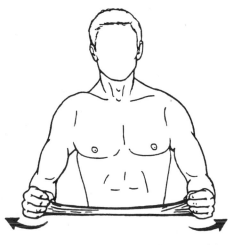

Lifting Isometric
The elbows are bent to 90°. The rubber bands are placed near the elbows. The arms are lifted up only 4 to 5″ away from the body and held 5 seconds.

These exercises are used for shoulder tendinitis, shoulder bursitis, and rotator cuff tendon tears and are begun 3 to 4 weeks after the acute inflammation has resolved. Ideally, the outward and inward rotation strength should be restored before moving on to the lifting exercise. Note: If begun too soon, these exercises may result in a flare-up of the underlying condition! During the healing process, heavy work must be restricted!

STRETCHING EXERCISES FOR A FROZEN SHOULDER

These exercises, performed once or twice a day for several months, should loosen the tightened shoulder lining and restore normal range of motion. First, heat the shoulder for 15 to 20 minutes and perform a 5-minute pendulum swing. Then perform sets of 10 to 20 of the following three exercises. A mild muscle-type pain along the front or side of the shoulder is to be expected. Severe discomfort is unusual and suggests overstretching.

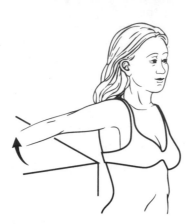

Armpit Stretch

Use your good arm to lift the arm onto a shelf, a dresser, or any object about breast high. Gently bend at the knees, opening up the arm pit. Try to push the arm up just a little bit farther with each stretch.

Finger-Walk Up the Wall

Face a wall about three quarters of an arm s length away from it. Using only your ngers (*not* your shoulder muscles) raise your arm up to shoulder level. Repeat this exercise.

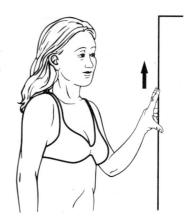

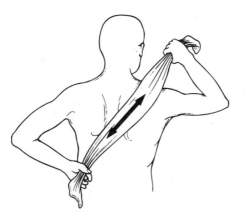

Towel-Stretch Behind the Back

Take a 3'-long towel, grasp it with both hands, and hold it at a 45-degree angle. Use the upper, good arm to pull the arm toward the lower back. This can be repeated with the towel in the horizontal position.

Activity Limitations.   Activities and positions that require repetitive reaching out, up, or back are to be minimized or avoided altogether:

Overhead reaching	Serving and the overhead smash in tennis
Throwing	Overhead military press
Sleeping with the arm over the head	Incline bench press
Sleeping directly on the shoulder	Chin-ups and push-ups
Leaning on the elbows, jamming the shoulder	The crawl and backstroke when swimming
Lifting heavy objects with the arms extended	Archery, pulling a 90-pound bow
Heavy pushing and pulling	

Associative Conditions.   Reductions in stress and improvements in posture help reduce the pressure over the ball-and-socket joint, the shoulder tendons, and the bursa. Upper back and neck massage, gentle vibration with heat, relaxation techniques, and meditation may be very helpful in selected cases.

Precautions.   Weighted pendulum stretching exercises should be avoided if there is any history or suggestion of dislocation or partial dislocation of the ball-and-socket joint. Likewise, these exercises should be used with caution by patients with a history of shoulder separation at the clavicular joint. Either condition can be aggravated by downward traction! Isometric toning exercises must be properly prescribed to be beneficial. Chronic shoulder tendinitis or shoulder tendinitis complicated by a torn tendon can be aggravated by overly aggressive toning. It is always safest to start out with low tension and gradually increase as tolerated!

GENERAL CARE OF THE ELBOW

ANATOMY. The elbow works like a simple door hinge. It is formed by the two forearm bones (the **radius** and **ulna**) and the upper arm bone (the **humerus**). It is capable of moving in only two directions, bending and straightening (**flexing and extending**). Forcing the arm backwards (**hyperextension**) causes the ulna to break or the elbow joint to dislocate. Movement at the elbow always affects the wrist joint. Conditions affecting the elbow often cause problems at the wrist and vice versa. Elbow anatomy includes:

One major joint	The hinge joint
One companion joint	The wrist
Four major tendon groups	The biceps (in front), the triceps (in back), the muscles that extend the wrist and fingers up (on the outside), and the muscles that flex the wrist and fingers down (on the inside)
One major lubricating bursal sac	The olecranon bursa over the back of the elbow
Two major ligaments	The hinge ligaments on the outside and inside of the elbow

CONDITIONS. Tendinitis is the most common condition to affect the elbow. Tennis elbow is an inflammation of the outer tendon; it is ten times more common than golfer's elbow, an inflammation of the inner tendon. Both result from heavy use of the wrist and forearm muscles. Bursitis occurs over the back of the elbow and is caused by direct pressure in most cases (draftman's elbow). Arthritis of the elbow is uncommon and is almost always the result of a previous injury.

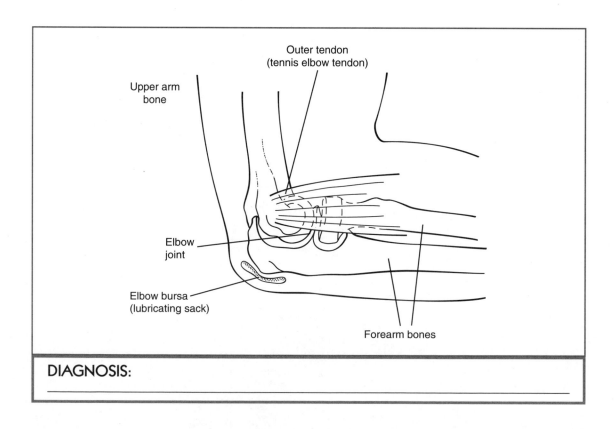

DIAGNOSIS:

PHYSICAL THERAPY.   Physical therapy plays a major role in the rehabilitation of elbow tendinitis and conditions that interfere with the normal range of motion of the elbow joint (arthritis, fractures, chips of the joint cartilage).

The elbow joint and its supporting tendons (the wrist extensors on the outside and the wrist flexors on the inside) are located just under the surface. Local applications of *ice* for 10 to 15 minutes 3 to 4 times a day are very effective in controlling pain and inflammation.

Phonophoresis with a hydrocortisone gel applied directly over the inner and outer tendons of the elbow is effective in reducing the mild to moderate inflammation that accompanies elbow tendinitis. Once again, the superficial location of the tendons allows good penetration of the medication, leading to a reduction in the degree of local swelling and heat.

Muscle toning exercises involving gripping and wrist motion are fundamental to restoring full support to the elbow and wrist. A graduated program of exercises is necessary. It should begin at the lowest tolerated level of gripping and be followed by a stepwise increase in the toning of the forearm muscles responsible for the maintenance of forearm tone, wrist strength, and elbow support. The importance of performing these exercises in sequence cannot be overemphasized. They should be taken just to the edge of discomfort over several weeks to gradually improve the strength of the elbow and wrist without inciting recurrent tendon inflammation.

Good Body Mechanics.   A healthy elbow joint requires a healthy wrist joint, well-toned and strong biceps and triceps muscles that move the joint, and well-toned and strong forearm muscles that support the elbow as well as the wrist. The use of good body mechanics includes:

Lifting objects close to the body with the elbow in a partially flexed position

Keeping the wrist in a neutral position when performing repetitive forearm work or weight training

Using wrist supports when weightlifting

Using leverage to reduce the effects of torque (a cheater bar when using a torque wrench, keeping the elbow close to the body, and so forth)

Avoiding tight gripping; increasing the gripping surface of tools with gloves or padding

Using a hammer with extra padding to reduce tension and impact

Holding heavy tools with two hands

Using the double backhand in tennis

Applying grip tape or oversized grips to golf clubs

PHYSICAL THERAPY SUMMARY   • • • • • • • • • • • • • • •

1. Local applications of ice over the tendons or the joint
2. Phonophoresis with a hydrocortisone gel
3. Gripping exercises, performed initially with half grips and gradually increasing
4. Toning exercises of wrist extension (tennis elbow) or wrist flexion (golfer's elbow)

Activity Limitations.   Activities that cause impact and tension at the wrist and forearm cause the greatest aggravation of the elbow. They include:

Lifting with the elbow fully extended

Doing heavy work, unless gripping strength is good and the forearm muscles are well toned

Leaning on the elbows

Allowing unprotected repetitive impact and tension

Associative Conditions.   Poorly toned forearm muscles and a poorly supported, weak wrist contribute substantially to injuries of the elbow. Similarly, the single most important means of protecting the elbow is to maintain the strength of the gripping muscles and the muscles that support the wrist.

TENNIS ELBOW STRENGTHENING EXERCISES

These exercises are begun 2 to 3 weeks after the acute pain and local tenderness have subsided. They strengthen the muscle and the tendon, reducing the risk of recurrent tendinitis. Muscle soreness in the forearm (2 to 3″ down from the elbow) is common. If sharp or intense pain is felt in the outer elbow, the exercises should be discontinued (recurrence?).

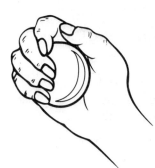

Grip Strengthening
Gripping exercises should always precede wrist isometrics. Begin with a small, compressible rubber ball (e.g., an old tennis ball or silicone ball). Grip firmly but not hard. Perform 20 to 25 mild squeezes, holding each for 5 seconds. With increasing strength, advance to a spring-loaded metal gripper.

Wrist Isometrics
After 2 to 3 weeks of gripping exercises, isometric strengthening of wrist bending can be started. Perform 15 to 20 sets per day. Keep the wrist in a neutral position while pulling on a large rubber band, bungee cord, or flexible rubber tubing. Achy pain should be felt in the forearm, but sharp pain over the elbow may indicate recurrent tendinitis.

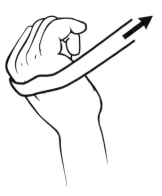

These exercises are preventive measures. In addition to these exercises, switch to a two-handed backhand, use power tools, wear a tennis-elbow band, try to lift objects with two hands, and emphasize lifting with the palms up.

GENERAL CARE OF THE WRIST AND HAND

PHYSICAL THERAPY. Physical therapy plays a major role in the prevention of carpal tunnel syndrome, trigger finger, and the scarring that occurs in the palms of the hands (Dupuytren contracture).

STRETCHING OF THE WRIST AND HAND TENDONS

These stretching exercises help to rehabilitate and prevent trigger finger, thickened palms (Dupuytren contracture), and carpal tunnel syndrome. They are begun 3 to 4 weeks after the acute pain and inflammation have resolved. The hand and wrist are heated for 15 to 20 minutes. The wrist and fingers are bent back using very light finger pressure.

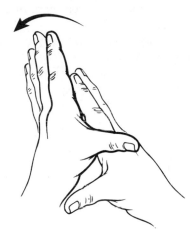

Wrist Stretching
Bend the wrist back as far as is comfortable. Enhance the stretch with gentle, constant tension against the fingers. A pulling sensation should be felt in the forearm. Perform sets of 15 to 20 per day.

Finger Stretching
Massage the palm and base of the fingers with lanolin cream for 5 minutes. Stretch the affected fingers back with gentle finger pressure. Perform sets of 15 to 20 per day.

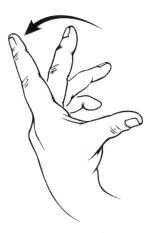

Gradual stretching exercises should be performed over several months to prevent a reucrrence or to slow down the progression of the problem. In addition, avoid vibrating tools, heavy gripping and grasping of tools, and any tools that place pressure over the wrist or the palm tendons.

GENERAL CARE OF THE BACK

ANATOMY. The lower back (the lumbosacral spine) consists of *five back bones* (verte-brae) connected together by a network of ligaments and muscles all of which protect the spinal cord and spinal nerves. Five pairs of spinal nerves exit the spinal column and travel down the back through the pelvis and buttocks and into the lower legs. Each nerve passes by one of the spinal disks and through a bony passage formed by the two adjacent back bones.

CONDITIONS. Back problems are exceedingly common. Everyone will develop some degree of arthritis and at least one episode of low back strain. Poor posture, excessive weight, lack of exercise, and improper lifting all contribute to acute lumbar strain. Some patients develop symptoms down into the leg because of a pinched nerve. The most common cause of a pinched nerve in the lower back is a herniated disk.

PHYSICAL THERAPY. Physical therapy is essential to all phases of treatment of the low back.

In the *first few days and weeks* of an acute back condition, *cold, heat, massage, and gentle stretching exercises* are used to treat muscle irritation and spasm.

Cold, heat, or cold alternating with heat are effective in reducing pain and muscle spasm. Some patients respond to one better than another. A bag of frozen corn, an iced towel from the freezer, or an ice pack should be left in place for 15 to 20 minutes 3 to 4 times a day. Moist heat is preferable and is used similarly.

Massage of the lower back muscles is effective in reducing muscle spasm. It should always be performed on a comfortable surface while the patient is lying on

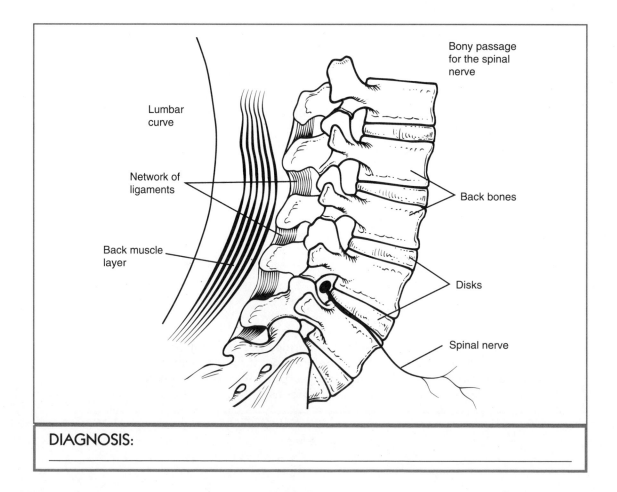

DIAGNOSIS:

PHYSICAL THERAPY SUMMARY

1. Cold applications for acute muscular spasm
2. Heating prior to stretching exercises
3. Stretching exercises of the back and side muscles
4. Aerobic exercises (e.g., walking, swimming, cross-country ski machine, etc.)
5. Strengthening exercises of the muscles of the back
6. Vertical stretching of the ligaments of the back
7. Ultrasound
8. Lumbar traction
9. Chiropractic manipulation

the stomach. Hand pressure or pressure from an electric vibrator is applied from the lower rib cage to the top of the pelvis. Up-and-down and circular motions are performed on both sides. Massage is especially effective just before going to bed.

Low back muscle *stretching exercises* are performed to restore lost flexibility. These exercises are especially important for patients suffering from scoliosis, fractured vertebrae, or other structural back disorders. Side bends, knee-chest pulls, and pelvic rocks are designed to stretch the low back muscles, the buttocks muscles, and the sacroiliac joints. These are begun after the most intense muscle spasms have resolved (usually days). Initially, they should be performed while lying down in bed. As the pain and muscle spasms diminish, stretching can be performed in the standing position. Sets of 20 of each exercise are performed to the point of mild muscular aching. Any sharp pain or any electricity-like or shooting pain down the leg may be a sign of nerve irritation or overstretching!

Ultrasound treatments are used in selected cases. A physical therapist or chiropracter must administer them. The device causes a vibration-like feeling but is actually heating the deep tissues. *Diathermy* is another special machine that provides deep heating. Both are used for difficult-to-treat muscle spasms. A patient with a herniated disk should avoid these treatments.

Chiropractic manipulation is an effective alternative to home physical therapy. Realignment by adjustment of the spinal elements has been shown to provide temporary benefit for lumbar strain. It is not appropriate to consider chiropractic treatments if there has been or if there is a serious possibility of a compression fracture, a disk herniation, or disease directly involving the bones of the back!

Patients with severe symptoms unresponsive to the treatments above may require in-hospital *lumbar traction*. This type of treatment is rarely used today. Several days of pelvic traction at 20 to 25 pounds are combined with intense use of a strong muscle relaxer and narcotic medications.

In the *recovery and rehabilitation phase,* greater emphasis is placed on progressive stretching exercises, muscle toning exercises, aerobic exercises, and vertical traction. These treatments are important for prevention, as well. They are typically begun around 3 to 4 weeks after the acute symptoms have resolved.

Toning exercises of the abdominal and low back muscles consist of modified sit-ups, weighted side-bends, and gentle extension exercises. These are always performed after heating and stretching (see above).

Aerobic exercise is one of the best ways to prevent recurrent back strain. General toning of the body improves posture, muscular support, and flexibility. Swimming and cross-country ski machine workouts are probably the best overall exercises that will not aggravate the back. Swimming, in particular, is an excellent way to recover lost muscular tone and function after a herniated disk, compression fracture, or spinal surgery. Fast walking and light jogging are acceptable forms of exercise also. Exercise apparatus that places excessive bend or torque on the back are to be avoided.

BACK-STRETCHING EXERCISES

Back-stretching exercises play a vital role in the treatment of lumbosacral muscle spasms. The lower back is heated for 15 to 20 minutes. Sets of 10 to 20 stretches, each held for 5 seconds, are performed on each side. The muscles are kept relaxed. Rest for 1 to 2 minutes between exercises. Mild muscle soreness is to be expected. Severe pain, electric-like sharp pain, or severe muscle spasms suggest overstretching.

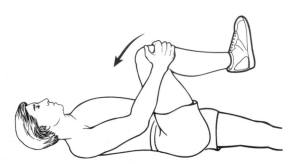

Knee-Chest Pulls
Bring your knee slowly up to your chest, holding it in place with your hands. Relax the buttock and back muscles. Do the left side, then the right side, and then both simultaneously (curling up in the fetal position).

Pelvic Rocks
With knees bent, rotate your pelvis forward and then backwards. The abdominal muscles do the work, as the back muscles are relaxed.

    Caution: Do not overextend when arching the back!

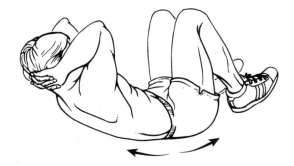

Side Bending
While lying down, crawl your fingers down the side of your thigh. Hold in this tilted position for 5 seconds. Return to a neutral position. Repeat on the other side.

Initially, these should be performed while lying down or while floating in the bath or hot tub. With improvement, these exercises can be performed standing or sitting. Follow these movements with exercises to strengthen the back.

ADVANCED BACK-STRETCHING EXERCISES

This exercise is not appropriate for everyone. A strong upper body is a prerequisite as well as a 2- to 4-week period of basic back exercises. The vertical stretch elongates the support ligaments, lengthens the back muscles, and allows the back bones to pull apart and realign. (I refer to this exercise as "the poor man's chiropractic adjustment.") Suspension between parallel bars is ideal, but any method to allow the weight of the legs to pull down on the back will work (e.g., leaning on a countertop, using crutches, or supporting your weight between two bar stools).

Vertical Stretching Exercise

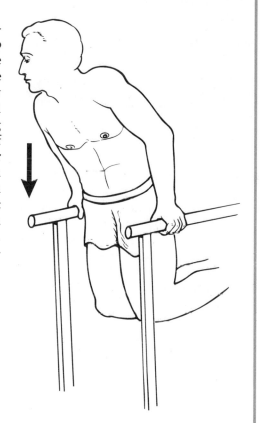

Starting in a standing position, gradually shift the weight of your body to your outstretched arms. The toes are kept on the ground for balance. The back muscles should be relaxed. Allow the weight of your legs to draw out and pull out the lower back bones. Popping sensations or a gentle sensation of stretching should be felt in the lower back. Additional pulling occurs if you lean forward slowly. Hold this position for 30 to 60 seconds. Gradually shift your weight back to the legs and then stand up straight. Repeat once or twice. This exercise is especially helpful before going to bed.

This is a great way to keep the back limber and the back muscles supple. This exercise can be performed daily to prevent recurrent back strain.

Vertical traction can be used at home as a part of a comprehensive back treatment program. The weight of the lower body and legs is used to pull the lumbar segments apart. Leaning on a countertop, suspending the body between two bar stools, or using inversion equipment for 1 to 3 minutes at a time will allow the back's bones, ligaments, and muscles to gradually stretch apart and lengthen. Several vertical stretches are performed each day. It is extremely important to relax the whole lower body when performing these exercises and to slowly return to full weightbearing by lowering down onto the legs very gradually.

For chronic cases that do not respond to traditional physical therapy, a transcutaneous electric nerve stimulator (TENS) can be prescribed to block or attenuate the persistent pain. This type of treatment should be combined with a thorough evaluation by a pain clinic.

BACK-STRENGTHENING EXERCISES

Before starting a strengthening program for the back, flexibility must be restored with 3 to 6 weeks of daily back stretching. Strengthening exercises should be performed when the body is well-rested. First, the back muscles are stretched out for 5 to 10 minutes. Then sets of 15 to 20 of the following are performed daily for 6 weeks. As the strength of the back increases, the frequency can be reduced to three times a week.

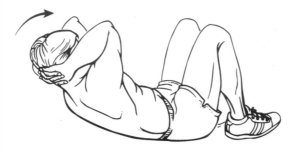

Modified Sit-ups

The knees are kept bent. The lower back is kept flush with the ground. The hands can be kept either behind the neck or held over the chest. The head and neck are raised 3 to 4″ and held for 5 seconds. The abdominal muscles will gradually strengthen.

Weighted Side-bends

In a standing position, a 5- to 15-pound weight is held in the hand. The back is tilted to the weighted side and is immediately brought back to center. The back should be tilted only a few inches! The farther away from the body the weight is held, the greater is the amount of muscle work! After a set of 15 to 20, the weight is switched to the opposite side.

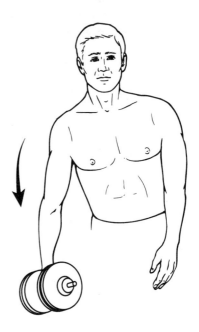

These specific exercises are complementary to a regular aerobic exercise program. No single exercise is better than another. If you are having problems doing any specific exercise, discuss it with your health care provider.

Good Body Mechanics.   The positions and activities that follow are safest to perform, and over time they reduce the possibility of reinjury of the muscles and ligaments:

Sitting and standing up straight

Lifting by using the legs and knees

Lifting and carrying weight close to the body

Lifting using an external lumbar support

Sleeping on a firm mattress, placing a pillow under the knees

Keeping one's weight down

Wearing seat belts and purchasing a car with an airbag

Low-weight, high-repetition weightlifting

Swimming, a cross-country ski machine (with low-tension arm setting to avoid back twisting or torque), a soft-platform treadmill, or fast walking

Activity Limitations.   These positions and activities place excessive load or torque on the muscles, ligaments, and bones of the back:

Lifting heavy objects

Lifting objects away from the body (with the arms held out)

Lifting in a twisted position

Working in a stooped position

Bending at the waist with excessive frequency

Full sit-ups

Bending over to touch the toes (at least in the recovery period)

A rowing machine, heavy weightlifting, or any apparatus that puts too much bend, torque, or pressure onto the lower back

Precautions.   Stretching and toning exercises should always be increased gradually. If sharp pain, electricity-like pain, or shooting pain down the leg develop, the exercises must be interrupted. These symptoms suggest nerve irritation!

Ultrasound treatments should be avoided in patients with herniated disks. Deep heating may cause the disk to swell further!

Chiropractic manipulation must be avoided with bony compression fractures, disk herniations, and disease of the back bones!

Vertical traction must be used with caution. A patient must possess strong upper body strength and be free of cardiovascular disease (blood can pool in the legs and lead to fainting). The health care provider should be contacted before this type of aggressive stretching is begun.

GENERAL CARE OF THE HIP

ANATOMY.   The hip is a *ball-and-socket joint* formed by the bony pelvis (the socket) and the end of the femur bone (the ball). Both bones are covered with a smooth layer of protective cartilage (articular cartilage). Loss of this cartilage from wear and tear, inflammation, or injury is called arthritis. The anatomy of the hip includes:

One main joint	The ball-and-socket joint
Five large lubricating bursal sacs	Two at the outer hip, three surrounding the major muscles attached to the pelvis
Four major muscle groups	Three buttock muscles and tendons, the top of the quadriceps muscle of the thigh, the tops of the hamstring muscles, and the large hip flexor muscle
One ligament	One thick capsule surrounding the joint to hold the hip in place and contain the lubricating fluid

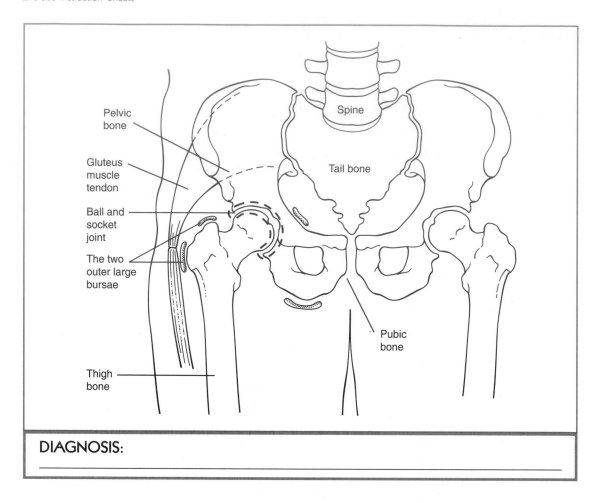

Pelvic bone

Gluteus muscle tendon

Ball and socket joint

The two outer large bursae

Thigh bone

Spine

Tail bone

Pubic bone

DIAGNOSIS:

CONDITIONS.   Bursitis is the most common cause of hip pain. It is an inflammation of one of the five lubricating sacs that surround the hip and ensure smooth motion. The two large outer bursal sacs become inflamed when the walking gait has been disturbed by any cause. Arthritis is the second most common problem affecting the hip. Damage to the normal protective layer of cartilage that covers the ball-and-socket joint can occur because of age, wear-and-tear, injury, or rheumatism. Tendinitis is a very uncommon problem at the hip. Some patients experience pain at the hip that has been referred from the back (sciatic nerve pain) or from impaired circulation in the abdominal and pelvic arteries.

PHYSICAL THERAPY.   Physical therapy is essential to the treatment, rehabilitation, and prevention of the conditions that affect the hip and its surrounding supporting structures.

Heating the hip is necessary to stimulate blood flow deep in the tissues and to loosen those tissues prior to stretching. The hip is heated in a shower or warm bath

PHYSICAL THERAPY SUMMARY   ● ● ● ● ● ● ● ● ● ● ● ● ● ●

1.   Heat applications to the front and side of the joint
2.   Stretching exercises of the supporting tendons and joint lining
3.   Toning exercises of the buttock and flexor muscles
4.   Activity limitations

for 10 to 15 minutes. Total body heating is preferable to local heat, which should come from a moist heating pad or a moist towel warmed in a microwave.

Stretching the supporting tendons (the outer and groin tendons) and the joint lining is the single most important exercise for the conditions affecting the hip. Patients with arthritis need to stretch the hip capsule (the lining of the joint) and the groin muscles that have tightened from disuse. Knee-chest pulls, figure-of-four, and Indian sitting stretches are performed in sets of 15 to 20 after heating.

Similarly, patients with bursitis should perform sets of 15 to 20 cross-leg pulls and side stretches to reduce the pressure of the large buttock tendons over the two large outer bursal sacs. Once again, deep heating is performed prior to performing these stretching exercises.

Last, some patients should combine the primary hip stretching exercises with the flexion exercises of the lower back. The hip and lower back are so intertwined that stiffness in either area contributes to problems in the other.

Ultrasound treatments are prescribed for patients who suffer recurrent or chronic bursitis. A physical therapist or chiropractor must administer such treatments. The ultrasound waves cause a vibration-like feeling but are actually heating the deep tissues. *Diathermy* is another specialized treatment that provides deep heating.

Muscle toning exercises of the hip are rarely indicated. However, if deconditioning has occurred as a result of prolonged bedrest, cast immobilization, or lengthy inactivity, straight-leg–raising and leg-extension exercises can be performed.

Good Body Mechanics.   These positions and activities are safest and reduce the possibility of reinjury to the hip joint and the bursal sacs that surround the hip:

Sitting in a partially reclined position

Sitting up straight with the leg turned out

Standing with the weight equally distributed between the right and left legs

Lifting and carrying weight close to the body

Sleeping on the back with the legs spread apart

Sleeping on the unaffected side with a large pillow between the knees

Keeping weight down

Low-weight, high-repetition weightlifting

Swimming with the crawl kick (legs kept straight)

Using a cross-country ski machine with low tension

Activity Limitations.   To reduce the chance of an arthritic flare of the hip joint, the extremes of motion should be avoided, and jarring and impact must be minimized. The limitations include:

Avoiding running and jumping

Limiting stop-and-go sports to reduce direct impact and jarring

Not using a trampoline

Avoiding any positions that cause a wide spreading of the legs

Activity Limitations.   Patients with bursitis must reduce direct pressure over the outer hip and minimize repetitive bending. Limitations include:

Avoiding direct pressure

Avoiding prolonged sitting with the hip in a bent position

Minimizing stair climbing

Minimizing working in a stooped position

STRETCHING EXERCISES FOR ARTHRITIS

Home physical therapy for hip arthritis consists of stretching and strengthening exercises. First, the hip is heated in a hot tub or bath or with moist heat for 20 minutes. Then 15 to 20 knee-chest, figure-of-four, and Indian-style exercises are performed to stretch the muscles and ligaments around the hip. After relaxing for 5 minutes, weighted straight-leg raises and leg extensions are performed to strengthen the hip (see knee exercises).

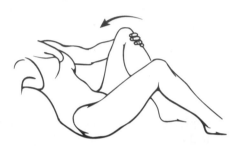

Knee-Chest Pulls
Bend the hip and knee to 90 degrees. Grasp the upper shin, and pull the knee onto the chest. Hold this position for 5 seconds, and then relax back to 90 degrees. These exercises should be performed lying down.

Figure-of-Four Stretch
The foot is placed over the knee. The leg is gently rocked outward. The higher the foot is raised on the leg, the greater is the stretch. Perform this exercise while lying down.

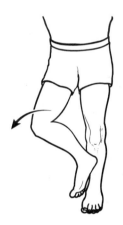

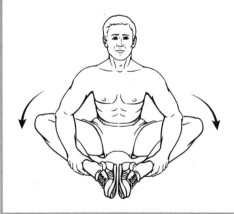

Indian Sitting Stretch
In a seated position, pull the feet up toward the buttocks. Lean forward gradually to increase the stretch.

Limiting repetitive bending at the hip

Replacing full sit-ups with partial sit-ups

Not bending over to touch the toes (at least in the recovery period)

Avoiding the repetitive bending involved in the use of the rowing machine, stationary bicycle, stair-stepper, and glider

STRETCH EXERCISES FOR HIP BURSITIS

The large buttock tendon over the outer hip has to be stretched to reduce the pressure over the bursal sac. First, the area is heated either in a tub or with moist heat. Sets of 15 to 20 stretches are performed daily. Begin these 2 to 4 weeks after the outer-hip pressure and pain have resolved.

Cross-leg Pulls

In a sitting position, either in a chair or on the floor, cross the affected leg over the other. Grasp the knee and pull the leg to the opposite side. Keep the buttocks flat and avoid twisting the back. A gentle pulling sensation should be felt in the outer buttocks or hip areas. Sharp pain suggests irritation of the bursa.

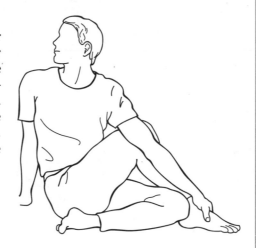

Outer-thigh Stretches

Stand an arm's length away from a wall, with the affected leg toward the wall. Cross the leg behind the outer leg. Carry all the weight on the good side. Lean into the wall, stretching the entire leg and lower side muscles. Perform sets of 15 to 20. The farther away from the wall you stand, the greater the stretch will be.

GENERAL CARE OF THE KNEE

ANATOMY.   The knee is a **hinge joint** that connects the thigh bone (the femur) and the lower leg bone (the tibia). The knee cap (the patella) sits in front of the joint, embedded in the large quadriceps tendon, providing protection and additional leverage to the quadriceps muscle. The hardest bone in the body (the femur), the body's thickest and strongest tendon (the quadriceps), and the body's largest and strongest muscle (the quadriceps) require the greatest amount of lubrication. Surrounding the quadriceps mechanism are five large lubricating sacs.

The knee joint is supported by the hinge ligaments (the collateral ligaments), the crossing ligaments in the center of the joint (the cruciates), and the large thigh muscles (the quadriceps and hamstrings).

The bones are covered with a thick layer of cartilage (articular cartilage) and are protected from the ravages of repetitive impact by the "shock-absorber cartilages" (the meniscal, or football, cartilages). In summary, the knee is composed of the following parts:

Three joint compartments	The inner (medial), outer (lateral), and knee cap
Two major muscle groups	The quadriceps (front of the thigh) and hamstrings
Two hinge ligaments	The inner (medial collateral) and outer (lateral collateral)
Five lubricating bursal sacs	The prepatellar, infrapatellar, suprapatellar, anserine, and baker cyst
Two shock-absorber cartilages	The inner (medial) and outer (lateral) meniscus

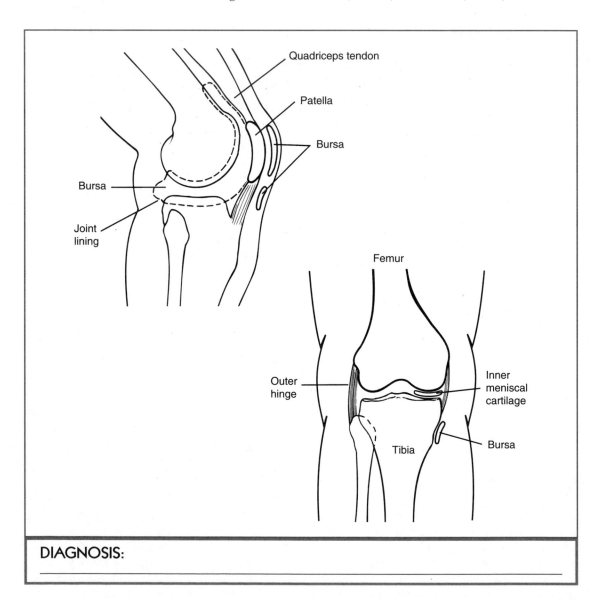

DIAGNOSIS:

CONDITIONS.   Any part of the knee can wear out, suffer injury, or become inflamed by overuse. However, injury and irritation of the undersurface of the knee cap (painful knee caps) and wear-and-tear arthritis (degenerative arthritis) are the most common problems, accounting for nearly two-thirds of all complaints. Twisting injuries most often injure the inner hinge ligament and, less commonly, the inner meniscal cartilage.

Any of the conditions that affect the joint can cause "water on the knee," the knee's response to injury.

PHYSICAL THERAPY.   Physical therapy plays a vital role in the treatment of the variety of conditions that affect the knee and its supporting structures and it is especially important in the rehabilitation of an injured knee. Specific exercises are fundamental to improving knee support and stability.

Ice is useful for the control of pain and swelling. Cold is applied for 15 to 20 minutes as often as every 2 to 4 hours. A bag of ice, a bag of frozen corn, or an iced towel cooled in the freezer work well.

Ice and elevation are indicated for the acutely swollen knee. The knee should be kept above the level of the heart.

Rehabilitation of the knee begins with gentle toning exercises. *Straight-leg–raising* and *leg-extension* exercises are used to strengthen the quadriceps and hamstring muscles, to provide support to the joint, and to counteract the giving-out sensation caused by disuse or weakened ligaments. Begin with sets of 10 leg lifts and gradually work up to 20 to 25 lifts, each held 5 seconds. At first these are performed without weight, but with improvement, weight is added to the ankle. Start with a 2-pound weight (a heavy shoe, fishing weights or coins in a sock, a purse with a large book in it, etc.) and gradually increase to a weight of 5 to 10 pounds. Twisting and rotating the leg must be avoided. To secure the leg in the straight position cock the ankle up!

If the straight-leg–raising exercises do not cause any aggravation of the underlying condition, weighted leg lifts with bended knee can be started. Initially, these should be performed at 30 degrees, using the same amount of weight and number of repetitions used with the straight-leg exercises. The amount of bending is gradually increased as tolerated, in increments of 30 to 45 to 60 to 90 degrees of bending.

Activity limitations, proper exercises, and proper exercise equipment involve limiting exposure to repetitive impact, jarring, and bending (depending on the severity of the knee condition). Ideally, activities and exercises should maximize the toning of the thigh muscles, provide smooth motion to the knee, minimize impact, and emphasize the least amount of bending to accomplish the muscle toning.

Activity Limitations.   These positions and activities place excessive pressure on the knee joint and must be limited until the pain and swelling resolve:

Squatting

Kneeling

Twisting and pivoting

Repetitive bending (stairs, getting out of a seated position, clutch and pedal pushing, etc.)

Jogging

Jazzercize

Playing stop-and-go sports (basketball and sports that require the use of rackets)

Swimming using the frog or whip kick

Bicycling

KNEE-STRENGTHENING EXERCISES

Nearly all conditions that affect the knee cause loss of tone in the thigh muscles (quadriceps and hamstrings). The strength of these muscles must be restored to restore knee stability.

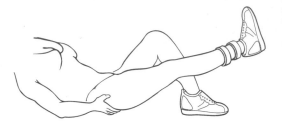

Straight-leg Raises

While sitting on the edge of a chair or while lying down with the opposite leg bent, the leg is raised 3 to 4″ off the ground. Sets of 15 to 20 leg raises (each held for 5 seconds) are performed daily. Bending the knee should be avoided. After 2 to 4 weeks, the exercises are performed with a 5- to 10-pound weight placed at the ankle (e.g., a sock with fishing weights, an old purse with a large book in it, Velcro ankle weights).

Leg Extensions

While lying on the stomach or while up on all fours, the leg is raised, perfectly straight, 3 to 4″ off the ground. Sets of 15 to 20 extensions (each held 5 seconds) are performed daily. After 2 to 4 weeks, the exercise is performed with a 5- to 10-pound weight added to the ankle.

   Note: This exercise must be performed while lying flat if the knee cap is the source of knee irritation!

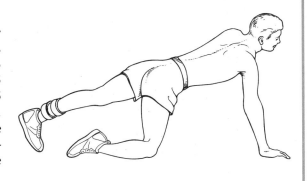

PHYSICAL THERAPY SUMMARY • • • • • • • • • • • • • • •

1. Direct applications of ice to the front and sides of the joint
2. Elevation to assist in the reabsorption of knee fluid
3. Toning exercises of the quadriceps and hamstring muscles to provide muscular support
4. Activity limitations
5. Exercises and exercise equipment that minimize repetitive impact and bending

Equipment Limitations.   These types of exercise equipment place excessive pressure on the knee joint and must be limited until the pain and swelling resolve:

Stair-stepper

Stationary bicycle

Rowing machine

Universal gym utilizing leg extensions

Acceptable Activities.   These activities place much less tension on the knee by limiting impact and repetitive bending:

Fast walking

Water aerobics

Swimming, using the crawl stroke

Cross-country ski glide machines

Soft-platform treadmill

Trampoline

Weight loss is always an important issue in retarding and preventing future problems of the knee!

GENERAL CARE OF THE ANKLE

ANATOMY.   The ankle is a **hinge joint** that allows flexing up and down, but also allows the foot to turn in and out. It is held together by a network of ligaments along the sides of the joint (the "hinges") and is supported by four major tendons. To function normally, the ankle must be properly aligned with the lower leg, must have intact and strong ligaments, and must have flexible and well-toned tendons. The ankle is made up of the following elements:

Two joint compartments	The main hinge joint (tibial-talar) and the swivel joint (subtalar)
Four major tendons	The Achilles (back), tibialis (inner), peroneus (outer), extensors (front)
Two hinge ligaments	The medial (inner) and lateral (outer)
Two lubricating bursal sacs	The heel bursa (pre-Achilles) and the ankle bursa (retrocalcaneal)
One thick arch ligament	The plantar fascia

CONDITIONS.   The most common condition to affect the ankle is the common ankle sprain, which causes pain along the outer ankle joint. Twisting injuries and a violent turning of the ankle inward cause the supporting ligaments to split, partially separate, or completely tear. Pain below the ankle (heel pain) is often an inflammation of the origin of the arch ligament (plantar fasciitis). This is often associated with weak ankles (pronation) or loss of the strength of the arch (flat feet). Tendinitis at the ankle most commonly affects the Achilles tendon located behind the ankle. Arthritis is almost always caused by a previous injury (fracture, severe ankle sprain, and so on). Bursitis at the ankle is not common.

Physical Therapy.   Physical therapy does not play an active role in the treatment of acute ankle conditions. However, stretching and toning exercises are vitally important in the recovery, rehabilitation, and prevention of ankle conditions.

Ice is useful for the temporary control of pain and swelling of acute sprains,

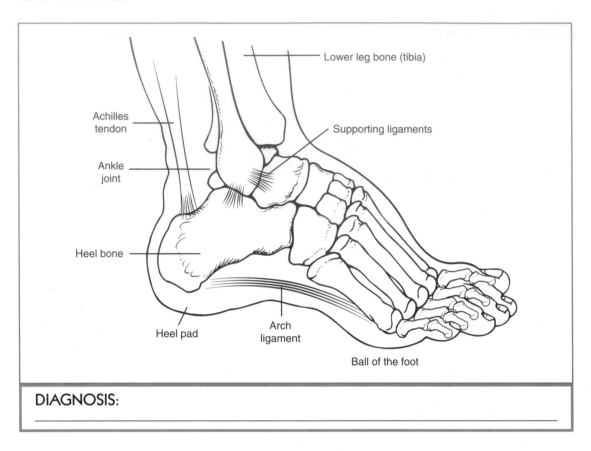

Lower leg bone (tibia)

Supporting ligaments

Achilles tendon

Ankle joint

Heel bone

Heel pad

Arch ligament

Ball of the foot

DIAGNOSIS:

tendinitis, and the occasional case of ankle arthritis. Ice is applied for 15 to 20 minutes as often as every 2 to 4 hours. A bag of ice, a bag of frozen corn, or an iced towel cooled in the freezer work well.

Heat is commonly recommended for recurrent or chronic ankle conditions that require stretching and toning exercises. Heating provides additional blood flow and facilitates stretching.

Stretching exercises are commonly used to treat and rehabilitate Achilles tendinitis and the inflammation of the arch ligament. They should always be preceded by heating for 10 to 15 minutes. Stretching exercises should be carried out over many weeks to avoid aggravating the underlying condition. Successful stretching should gradually improve over weeks.

Isometric toning exercises are the most important means of improving ankle stability that has been weakened by disuse or injury. Large rubber tubing, a TheraBand, or large rubber bands are used to gradually build up the tone and tension in the lower leg muscles. Each direction of ankle motion (bending up and down and turning in

PHYSICAL THERAPY SUMMARY ● ● ● ● ● ● ● ● ● ● ● ● ● ● ●

1. Direct applications of ice to the front and sides of the joint
2. Heating prior to the stretching exercises
3. Stretching exercises of the ankle joint and the Achilles tendon
4. Toning exercises of the outer ankle tendons
5. Activity limitations
6. Exercises and exercise equipment that minimize repetitive impact and bending

ACHILLES TENDON STRETCHING EXERCISES

Rehabilitation for Achilles tendinitis involves a long period of protection and gradual stretching exercises. Four weeks after the swelling and inflammation have resolved, the tendon is gradually stretched. The ankles are heated in water for 15 to 20 minutes. For the first 5 to 7 days, the ankle is pulled up by hand in sets of 20. With progress, the following two active exercises are performed.

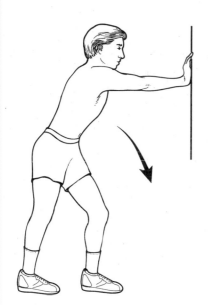

Wall Stretch
Face the wall and place your outstretched arms on the surface. Keep the affected leg in back. Partially flex the unaffected leg. While keeping the affected foot flat on the ground, gently lean forward. A pulling sensation should be felt in the calf, below the knee. Keep all of your body weight on the front leg!

Toe-ups
The balls of the feet are placed on a 3" block or on the edge of the stairs. The muscle is tightened by tiptoeing. Then the muscle is relaxed and allowed to stretch when the heel drops below the level of the block. Do sets of 20 exercises.

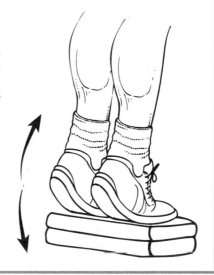

ANKLE ISOMETRIC TONING EXERCISES

Isometric toning exercises of the ankle tendons are indicated for strengthening and stabilizing the ankle after disuse, injury, or immobilization. Large rubber tubing, a bungee cord, or larger rubber bands are used to tone the lower leg muscles. Heating and stretching are performed prior to toning.

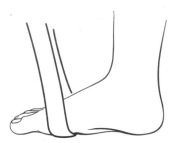

Achilles Tendon Toning
The rubber tubing is placed under the ball of the foot. The ankle is held steady at 90 degrees (a right angle). The rubber tubing is pulled up by hand pressure and held for 5 seconds. Sets of 20 are performed daily.

Peroneus Tendon Toning
The rubber tubing is placed around the outside of each foot, next to the little toes. The ankle is held steady at 90 degrees (a right angle). The legs are moved apart 2 to 3″ while holding the ankle firm for 5 seconds. Sets of 20 are performed daily.

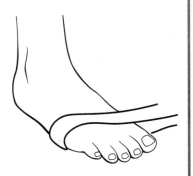

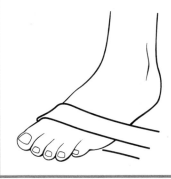

Posterior Tibialis Toning
The rubber tubing is placed around the inside of the foot next to the great toe and secured to a fixed object. The ankle is held stready at a 90-degree angle as the leg is pulled in toward the other. Sets of 20 (each held for 5 seconds) are performed daily.

and out) is toned individually. As the stability of the ankle improves, the ankle braces can be gradually withdrawn.

Activities Limitations.   These activities place too much tension across the supporting ligaments and tendons of the ankle:

Running and jogging

Playing the stop-and-go sports (racketball, tennis, basketball)

Doing Jazzercize

Jumping on a trampoline

Using a stair-stepper

Stair climbing with the ball of the foot

Using pedals repetitively (a clutch, heavy equipment, etc.)

section IV

Supports, Braces, and Casts

chapter 14

The Most Commonly Used Supports, Braces, and Casts

■ NECK

Soft Cervical Collar

Use: Cervical strain, whiplash, fibromyalgia, tension headaches

Advantages: Inexpensive, easy to put on, reasonably comfortable

Disadvantage: Doesn't restrict neck motion sufficiently

Cost: $6–7

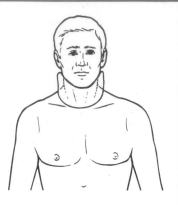

Philadelphia Collar

Use: Neck trauma transport, herniated disk, postoperative recovery

Advantages: Much improved restriction of neck motion, some vertical stretch

Disadvantages: Cost, uncomfortable, slightly more difficult to put on

Cost: Soft, $35–40; hard, $60–65

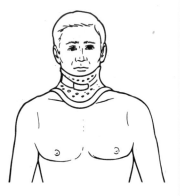

Water Bag Cervical Traction

Use: Cervical radiculopathy, cervical strain, whiplash, fibromyalgia

Cost: $40–45

Pulsating Water Massager/Electric Hand Massager

Use: Cervical strain, tension headaches

Cost: $35–45

▌ SHOULDER

Simple Shoulder Sling

Use: Acute bursitis, acute tendinitis, glenohumeral dislocation, acromioclavicular separation

Fractures: Humerus, clavicle, radial head; postoperative recovery

Advantages: Inexpensive, easy to put on, can be made at home

Disadvantages: Insufficient immobilization, can lead to frozen shoulder

Cost: $5–10

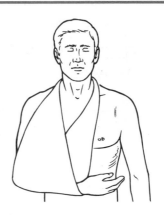

Abduction Pillow Shoulder Immobilizer

Use: Rotator cuff tendon tear, recovery from rotator cuff surgery

Advantage: Excellent immobilization in a position of abduction

Disadvantages: Hard to put on, can lead to frozen shoulder, expensive

Cost: $40–65

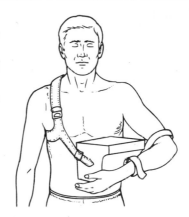

Sling and Swathe Bandage

Use: Glenohumeral dislocation, severe acromioclavicular separation

Fracture: Upper humerus

Advantages: Better control of motion and pain, inexpensive

Disadvantages: Requires a technician, can't be removed easily by the patient

Cost: $4–5

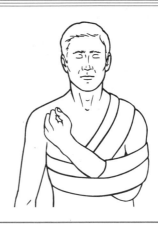

■ SHOULDER *(Continued)*

Shoulder Immobilizer

Use: Acromioclavicular separation, glenohumeral dislocation

Fracture: Humeral neck

Advantages: Easy to put on, relatively inexpensive, much less bulky, can be worn under clothing

Disadvantage: Frozen shoulder in a susceptible patient

Cost: Universal, $19–22; Velcro, $31–33

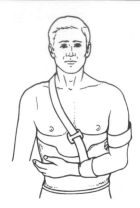

Figure-of-Eight Strap

Use: Acromioclavicular separation, dislocation

Fracture: Clavicle

Advantages: Inexpensive, easy to apply, can be worn under clothing

Disadvantage: Axillary irritation

Cost: $11–15

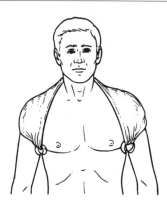

Hanging Cast

Use: No medical orthopedic indications

Fractures: Humeral surgical neck, humeral shaft

Advantage: Provides downward traction on the fractured elements

Disadvantages: Heavy and bulky compared to a simple sling, more expensive, uncomfortable, requires a technician

Cost: $50–100

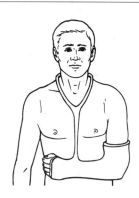

ELBOW

Tennis Elbow Band

Use: Lateral epicondylitis, extensor carpi radialis strain, brachioradialis strain

Advantages: Decreases the tension coming back to the tendon, inexpensive, easy to put on, not very restrictive

Disadvantages: Does not decrease the aggravation resulting from wrist use, probably works only for mild cases

Cost: $10–18

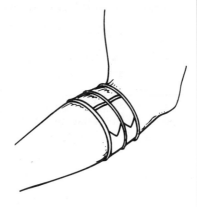

Neoprene Pull-on Elbow Brace

Use: Olecranon bursitis, arthritis of the elbow, poorly healing olecranon process fracture, cubital tunnel

Advantages: Inexpensive, easy to put on, can be worn under clothing

Disadvantage: None

Cost: $8–18

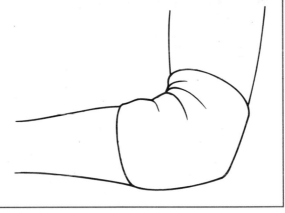

WRIST

Simple Velcro Wrist Support

Use: Sprained wrist, weightlifting support

Fracture: Carpal bones

Advantages: Inexpensive, lightweight, easy to put on

Disadvantage: Very little wrist support or restriction in wrist motion

Cost: $9–10, up to $25

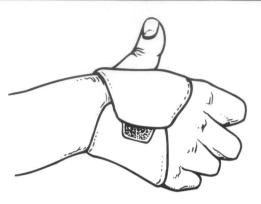

Velcro Wrist Splint with Metal Stay

Use: Lateral and medial epicondylitis, carpal tunnel syndrome, severe wrist sprains, radiocarpal arthritis, dorsal ganglion

Advantages: Good restriction of wrist motion, relatively inexpensive, lightweight, easy to put on

Disadvantages: Can cause pressure over the thumb and a temporary numbness of the local cutaneous nerve, may not restrict wrist motion sufficiently for specific conditions

Cost: $22–35

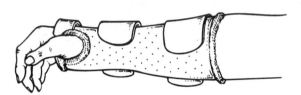

Short-Arm Cast with or without Thumb Spica

Use: Lateral and medial epicondylitis, metacarpal subluxation

Fractures: Colles, navicular, miscellaneous forearm

Advantages: Best support and restriction of the wrist, cannot be removed

Disadvantages: Bulky, heavy, susceptible to water damage, not universally available, requires a technician

Cost: Plaster, $25–27; fiberglass, $45–47

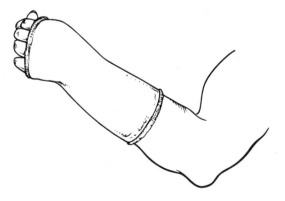

■ WRIST *(Continued)*

Radial Gutter Splint

Use: Fractures: Nondisplaced metacarpals, numbers 2 and 3, nondisplaced phalanges, numbers 1 and 2

Advantages: Lighter in weight than a short-arm cast, can be removed, more convenient

Disadvantage: Does not provide strict immobilization

Cost: Plaster, $21–23; fiberglass, $39–40

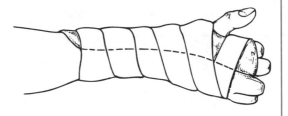

Dorsal Hood Splint

Use: De Quervain tenosynovitis, carpometacarpal arthritis

Advantages: Removable, lightweight

Disadvantages: Requires a technician, not as durable as the Velcro splints

Cost: Plaster, $15–16; fiberglass, $28–30

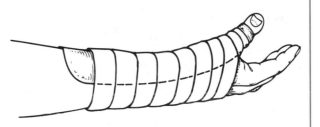

Ulnar Gutter Splint

Use: Ulnar collateral ligament strain, triangular cartilage injuries

Fractures: Boxer, nondisplaced phalanges, numbers 4 and 5

Advantages: Removable, lightweight

Disadvantages: Requires a technician, not as durable as the Velcro splints

Cost: Plaster, $21–23; fiberglass, $39–40

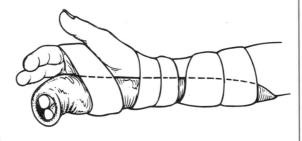

■ WRIST *(Continued)*

Long-Arm Cast with or without Thumb Spica

Use: Fractures: Navicular, complicated Colles, nondisplaced radius and ulnar shaft

Advantage: Securely holds the forearm and wrist in a fixed position

Disadvantages: Cumbersome, requires a technician, expensive

Cost: Plaster, $33–37; fiberglass, $61–68

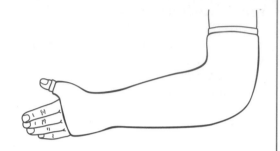

Posterior Splint

Use: Severe lateral epicondylitis, elbow dislocation

Advantages: Removable, relatively lightweight

Disadvantages: Requires a technician, may not restrict motion sufficiently

Cost: $40–44

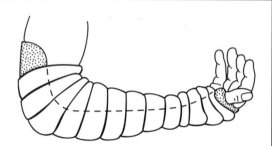

Sugar-Tong Splint

Use: Fractures: Colles, distal radius (Note: This is temporary splint only!)

Advantages: Allows swelling in the first few days, easy to recheck the fracture

Disadvantages: Insufficient immobilization compared to a short-arm cast, expensive to put on two casts

Cost: Plaster, $35–37; fiberglass, $65–67

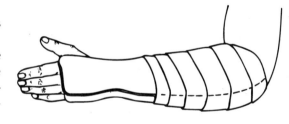

WRIST *(Continued)*

Padded Shell Velcro Thumb Splint or Velcro Thumb Spica Splint

Use: Carpometacarpal arthritis, de Quervain tenosynovitis, gamekeeper's thumb

Advantages: Lightweight, comfortable, relatively inexpensive

Disadvantage: May not sufficiently restrict motion

Cost: $26–28

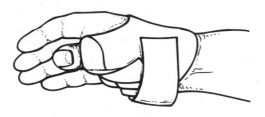

Thermoplastic Molded Thumb Splint

Use: Carpometacarpal arthritis, gamekeeper's thumb

Advantages: Custom-fitted, excellent support and immobilization

Disadvantages: Requires a technician, may be overly limiting to the patient, relatively inexpensive

Cost: $25–26

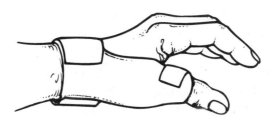

Taping for Osteoarthritis of the Thumb

Use: Carpometacarpal arthritis, gamekeeper's thumb

Advantages: Very inexpensive, permits some use without much aggravation, can be applied by the patient whenever needed

Disadvantages: Doesn't last, must be reapplied, easily soiled

Cost: $1–2

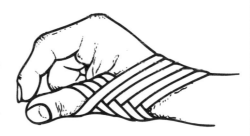

WRIST (Continued)

Thumb-Spica Cast

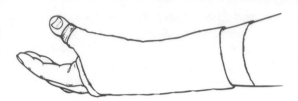

Use: Carpometacarpal arthritis, de Quervain tenosynovitis, gamekeeper's thumb

Fractures: Navicular, trapezial, metacarpal, number 1

Advantages: Best immobilization for the thumb, cannot be removed by the patient

Disadvantages: Bulky and heavy, cannot be wet, requires a technician, expensive

Cost: Plaster, $60–66; fiberglass, $109–121

Chinese Finger-Trap Traction

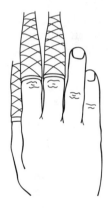

Use: Fractures: Colles, proximal phalanges (finger or toe)

Advantage: Gradual, even distribution of tensions

Disadvantage: Skin irritation

Cost: $25 (reusable)

■ HAND

Buddy-taping

Use: Simple finger sprains, trigger finger osteoarthritis of the finger joints, de Quervain tenosynovitis

Fractures: Nondisplaced phalanges, tendon avulsion fractures, tuft, distal interphalangeal dislocation

Advantages: Simple, inexpensive, can be applied by the patient, reasonable immobilization

Disadvantages: None

Cost: $1–2

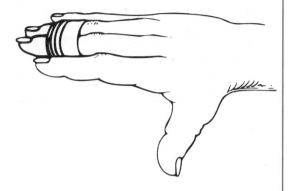

Tube Splints

Use: Simple finger sprains

Fractures: Nondisplaced phalangeal

Advantages: Simple to put on, comfortable

Disadvantages: Expensive, may not sufficiently restrict motion

Cost: $15–16

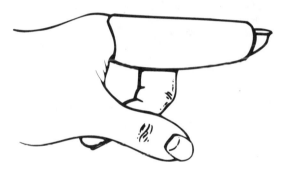

Stack Splints

Use: Mallet finger

Fractures: tuft

Advantages: Inexpensive, easy to put on

Disadvantages: None

Cost: $3–4

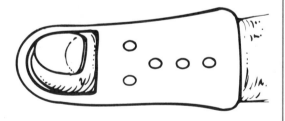

■ HAND *(Continued)*

Dorsal Splint

Use: Mallet finger, minor finger sprains, proximal interphalangeal dislocation, mallet thumb

Advantages: Easy to put on, inexpensive

Disadvantages: None

Cost: $2–3

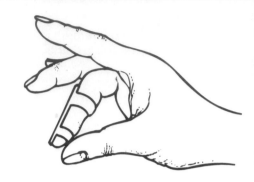

Metal Finger Splint

Use: Severe PIP or distal interphalangeal sprains

Fractures: Tuft

Advantages: Better immobilization of the PIP joint, inexpensive

Disadvantages: Difficult to keep on, may irritate the palm

Cost: $3–4

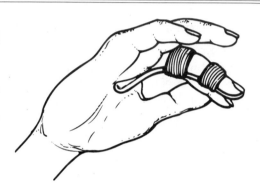

PIP Joint Splint in Extension

Use: Acute Boutonnière injury

Advantages: Simple, inexpensive

Disadvantages: Finger stiffness, range-of-motion exercises are not performed concurrently

Cost: $2–3

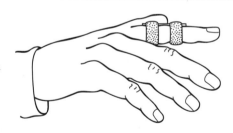

■ LUMBOSACRAL REGION

Neoprene Waist Wrap

Use: Uncomplicated lumbosacral (LS) strain, facet syndrome, weightlifting

Advantages: Easy to put on, inexpensive, comfortable, can easily be worn under clothing, easily adjusted

Disadvantages: Insufficient support and immobilization

Cost: $12–25

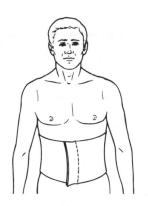

Velcro LS Corset

Use: LS strain, uncomplicated LS compression fracture, osteoarthritis, anklylosing spondylitis, recovery phase of LS radiculopathy, facet syndrome, prevention

Advantages: Easily put on, comfortable, relatively inexpensive, adjustable

Disadvantages: Insufficient support and immobilization

Cost: $15–25

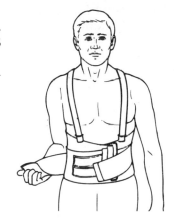

Elastic Sacroiliac Belt

Use: Sacroiliitis, iliolumbar syndrome, osteitis pubis, recovery phase of pelvic fracture

Advantages: Easy to put on, inexpensive, can be worn under clothing, easily adjusted

Disadvantages: Difficult to keep on if overweight, limited usefulness, variable patient response

Cost: $12–14

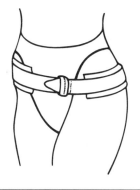

■ LUMBOSACRAL REGION *(Continued)*

LS Elastic Binder with Heated Plastic Shield

Use: Chronic low back pain, LS compression fracture, LS radiculopathy (healing phase)

Advantages: More support, maintains the LS spine in extension, more limitation of flexion

Disadvantages: Expensive, requires a technician to form the shield, not as comfortable

Cost: $125–140

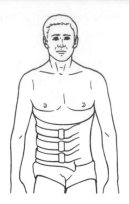

Three-point Extension Brace (Jewitt)

Use: Compression fractures, kyphosis from any cause

Advantages: Offers the greatest restriction of all braces, best control of movement

Disadvantages: Expensive, bulky and obtrusive, uncomfortable, not well tolerated, must be readjusted by a professional

Cost: $250–300

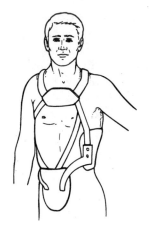

■ KNEE

Ace Wrap

Use: Any minor knee problem, rib fractures, hamstring pull, gastrocnemius injury
    Cost: $3–5

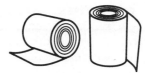

Neoprene Pull-on Knee Brace

Use: Osteoarthritis, prepatellar bursitis, first-degree medial collateral ligament or lateral collateral ligament strain, Osgood-Schlatter disease, rheumatoid arthritis, bland knee effusions
    Advantages: Easy to put on, inexpensive, simple
    Disadvantages: Very little support, slips, hard to fit on obese patients, may restrict venous flow
    Cost: Simple, $7–8, patellar cutout, $16–17

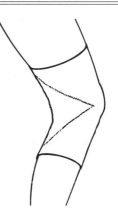

Velcro Knee Pads

Use: Prepatellar bursitis, infrapatellar bursitis, patellofemoral syndrome and osteoarthritis
    Advantages: Plastic metal cup anterior is very protective, inexpensive, easy to put on
    Disadvantages: May restrict venous blood flow
    Cost: $15–20

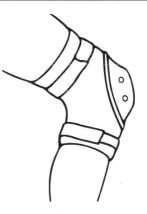

Patellar Strap

Use: Patellofemoral syndrome, patellar tendinitis, patellofemoral osteoarthritis, patellar subluxation, patellar dislocation
    Advantages: Simple, inexpensive, easy to put on and adjust
    Disadvantages: May not provide enough correction of the abnormal patellofemoral tracking, may restrict venous blood flow
    Cost: $15–16

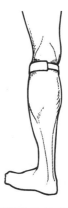

▮ KNEE *(Continued)*

Velcro Patellar Restraining Immobilizer

Use: Patellofemoral syndrome, patellar subluxation, patellar dislocation, patellofemoral ostetoarthritis, first-degree MCL or LCL strains, medial compartment osteoarthritis

Advantages: Improved patellofemoral tracking, easy to put on, patient acceptance

Disadvantages: Moderately expensive, hard to fit on obese patients

Cost: $35–60

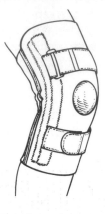

Velcro Straight Leg Brace

Use: Acute knee injury, second- or third-degree MCL or LCL strains, patellar tendinitis, medical management of a meniscus tear

Advantages: Excellent protection and immobilization of the knee, easily put on

Disadvantages: Relatively expensive, bulky, cannot wear under clothing, affects normal walking gait

Cost: 18 inch, $36–38
      24 inch, $44–46

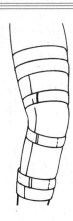

Metal-Hinged Braces (McDavid Knee Guard, Lenox-Hill Derotational Brace, Don Joy Rehabilitation Brace)

Use: Ligament instability (especially the ACL), postoperative ACL repair, third-degree MCL or LCL instability, osteoarthritis with angulation, hyperextension laxity

Advantages: Excellent and adjustable control of the knee motion and immobilization, better varus/vagus protection

Disadvantages: Very expensive, custom-made, not readily available

Cost: $800–900

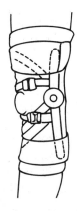

■ KNEE *(Continued)*

Long leg Cast

Use: Fractures: patellar, uncomplicated tibial plateau, minimally displaced tibial/fibular shaft, MCL or LCL avulsion, non-displaced osteochondritis

Advantage: Excellent protection and immobilization of the knee

Disadvantages: Relatively expensive, bulky, affects normal walking gait

Cost: Cylinder, $42–50, thigh to ankle, $60–70

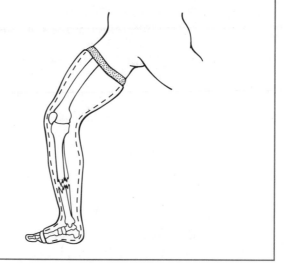

◼ ANKLE

Neoprene Pull-on Ankle Brace

Use: Minor sprains, minor degrees of pronation, mild osteoarthritis

Advantages: Simple, inexpensive, relatively easy to put on

Disadvantages: Hard to wear in a shoe, not very supportive

Cost: $7–8

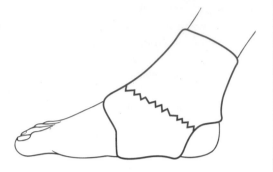

New Skin/Moleskin

Use: Achilles tendinitis, pre-Achilles bursitis, bursitis over bunion, dorsal bunion, blisters, abrasions

Advantages: Easy to apply, inexpensive, can be custom cut to shape and size

Disadvantages: None

Cost: $2–3

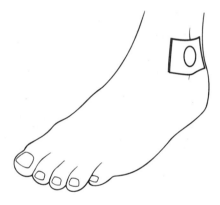

Velcro Ankle Brace

Use: Recurrent ankle sprain, osteoarthritis of the ankle, moderate pronation, posterior tibialis tenosynovitis, peroneus tenosynovitis, tarsal tunnel

Advantages: Easy to put on, relatively inexpensive, better support than a neoprene pull-on

Disadvantage: Does not provide adequate support for some conditions

Cost: $30–52

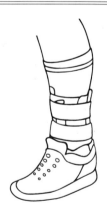

ANKLE *(Continued)*

Rocker-bottom Plastic Ankle Immobilizer

Use: Achilles tendinitis, severe ankle sprain, posterior tibialis tenosynovitis, peroneus tenosynovitis, severe plantar fasciitis, stress fracture of the foot

Advantages: Excellent support and restriction of the ankle, removable, comfortable

Disadvantages: Expensive, bulky, interferes with driving a car

Cost: $55–130 (variable depending on vendor)

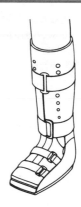

Short-leg Walking Cast

Use: Achilles tendinitis, severe ankle sprain, plantar fasciitis, severe flare of ankle arthritis

Fractures: Tibial stress, nondisplaced bimalleolar, nondisplaced fibular, avulsion of the lateral malleolus, calcaneal stress, extra-articular calcaneal, posterior process and lateral process of the talus, navicular, avulsion or nondisplaced fracture of the talus, avulsion of the base of the fifth MT, nondisplaced fracture of MT 1–4, Jones fracture of the fifth MT, march, sesamoid, great toe

Advantages: Excellent immobilization, the patient cannot remove it

Disadvantages: Expensive, makes driving unsafe, bulky, may throw off walking gait, cannot be wet, requires a technician

Cost: Plaster, $51–54; fiberglass, $94–100

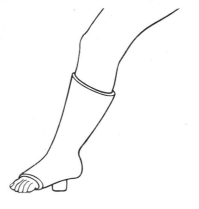

■ ANKLE *(Continued)*

Unna Boot

Use: Venous stasis ulcer, moderate ankle sprain, poorly healing wounds

Fractures: Minimally displaced fibular

Advantages: Lightweight, requires a technician

Disadvantages: Does not sufficiently immobilize or protect the ankle, cannot be wet

Cost: $21–22 (vs. athletic tape, $4–5)

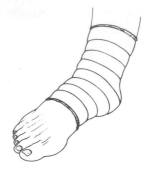

Footdrop Night Splint, Ready-made Ankle-foot Orthosis (AFO), Custom-made Ankle-foot Orthosis

Use: Stroke, Charcot-Marie-Tooth disease, polio or postpolio, any cause of footdrop, plantar fasciitis

Advantages: Protects against flexion contractures, improves gait, prevents falls

Disadvantage: Mild skin irritation

Cost: $15–30 (over-the-counter)
$40–65 (custom-made)

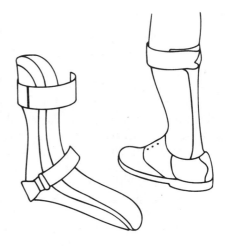

Jones Dressing with or without Posterior Splint Reinforcement

Use: Fractures: Ankle, calcaneal navicular, Jones, metatarsal

Advantages: Allows expansion for acute swelling and reinspection of the fracture, lighter in weight than a fixed cast

Disadvantage: Not rigid enough to hold a reduction

Cost: $40–50

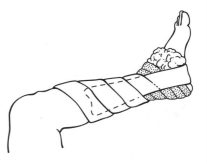

■ FOOT

Heel Cushions

Use: Heel pad syndrome, plantar fasciitis/spur, calcaneal stress fracture, ankle arthritis

Advantages: Inexpensive, effective cushioning of the heel, transferable from shoe to shoe, doesn't wear out

Disadvantage: Won't correct an arch problem or alignment problem of the ankle

Cost: $3–5

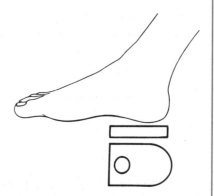

Heel Cups

Use: Heel pad syndrome, plantar fasciitis/spur, calcaneal stress fracture, severe epiphysitis, hip or knee osteoarthritis

Advantages: Inexpensive, effective cushioning of the heel, transferable from shoe to shoe

Disadvantage: Won't correct an arch problem or alignment problem of the ankle

Cost: $5–8

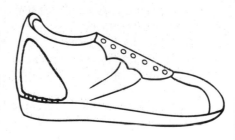

Padded Insoles (Spenco or Sorbathane)

Use: Heel pad syndrome, hammer toes, calluses, metatarsalgia, rheumatoid disease of the MTPs, Morton neuroma, ankle, knee, or hip osteoarthritis, healing phase of stress fractures of the foot

Advantages: Excellent cushioning of the entire foot, inexpensive, transferable from shoe to shoe

Disadvantage: Do not have arch supports

Cost: $12–25

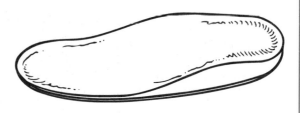

■ FOOT *(Continued)*

Padded Insoles with Arch Supports

Use: Plantar fasciitis, pes cavus, pes planus, pronated ankles, tarsal tunnel

Advantages: Soft padding plus arch support, relatively inexpensive, transferable from shoe to shoe

Disadvantage: Not enough arch support to correct moderate to severe arch abnormalities

Cost: $18–25

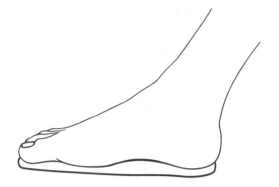

Plastic Orthotic Arch Supports (over-the-counter or custom-made)

Use: Persistent plantar fasciitis, pes cavus, pes planus, ankle pronation, tarsal tunnel

Advantage: Can correct any degree of arch abnormality

Disadvantages: Expensive, must be custom-made, time delay to obtain, hard surface without any padding

Cost: $25–28 (over-the-counter)
       $75–100 (custom-made)

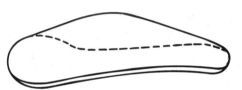

Bunion Shields

Use: Bunions

Advantages: Provides protection to the soft tissues and the joint, inexpensive

Disadvantage: Hard to fit into shoes

Cost: $5–15

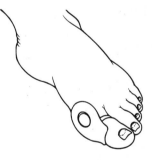

▌ FOOT *(Continued)*

Metatarsal Bar

Use: Fractures: Nondisplaced phalangeal, nondisplaced metatarsal, stress fracture of the metatarsal

Advantage: Reduced pressure over the forefoot

Disadvantages: Shoes have to be altered, may throw off normal walking gait, can be expensive if many shoes are adjusted

Cost: $20–25

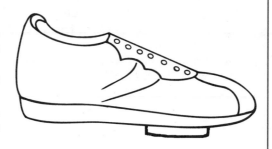

Hammer Toe Crests

Use: Hammer toes

Advantages: Easy to put on, inexpensive

Disadvantage: Mildly uncomfortable

Cost: $12–14

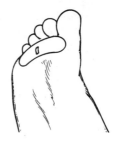

Felt Rings

Use: Bunion of the first MTP, dorsal bunion, corns, calluses, hammer toes, pre-Achilles bursitis

Advantages: Easy to apply, inexpensive

Disadvantage: Skin rash from the adhesive (rare)

Cost: $2–3

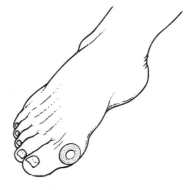

■ FOOT *(Continued)*

Toe Spacers, Cotton or Plastic
  Use: Morton neuroma, interdigital soft corns, bunions, any toe deformity
  Advantages: Easy to apply, inexpensive
  Disadvantages: None
  Cost: Cotton, $1–2; rubber, $2–3

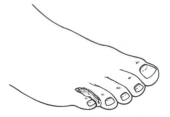

Buddy-taping of the Toes
  Use: Any toe deformity, hammer toes, turf toe, fractures: phalanges numbers 2–5
  Advantages: Easy to apply, inexpensive
  Disadvantages: None
  Cost: $1–2

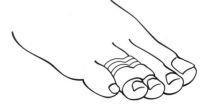

FRACTURES, MEDICATIONS, LAB VALUES

FRACTURES THAT REQUIRE REFERRAL TO A SURGICAL ORTHOPEDIST

Fracture/Dislocation	Reason for Orthopedic Referral
All compound fractures	Risk of infection and soft-tissue injury
Nearly all comminuted fractures	Unstable; risk of nonunion
Most intra-articular fractures	Risk of arthritis and poor joint function
Most spiral shaft fractures	Unstable; risk of shortening
Most displaced fractures	Unstable; risk of nonunion

SHOULDER AND UPPER ARM

Clavicle	
Associated with rib fracture	Risk of lung or great vessel damage
Distal third associated with displacement	Risk of nonunion
Humerus	
Transverse shaft fusion	Risk of nonunion
Neck fracture with shoulder dislocation	Unstable; risk of arthritis
Fragment displacement > 1 cm or angulation > 45 degrees	Unstable
Supracondylar fracture with displacement	Risk of arthritis, brachial artery or median nerve injury

ELBOW AND FOREARM

Displaced radial head fracture	Unstable
Displaced fracture of the radius or ulna	Unstable; risk of compartment syndrome

WRIST

Displaced or intra-articular distal radius fracture	Unstable; risk of arthritis
Radius foreshortened by 5 mm or angulation > 20 degrees	Risk of arthritis
Navicular fracture	Risk of avascular necrosis or nonunion
Perilunate dislocation	Referral for primary repair or fusion

THUMB

Gamekeeper's thumb, complete tear	Risk of poor function
Intra-articular metacarpal fracture of the thumb—Bennett fracture and Rolando fracture	Unstable; risk of arthritis
Dorsal dislocation of the MP joint of the thumb	Single attempt at closed reduction; Sx referral if unsuccessful
Transverse fracture at the base or neck, spiral oblique, comminuted, and condylar fracture (intra-articular)	Unstable; risk of poor function and abnormal alignment

HAND

Metacarpal fracture (except the fifth)	Unstable
Boxer's fracture of the fifth MC with angulation > 40 degrees	Unstable; referral for pin fixation
Volar dislocation of the MCP joints with avulsion fragment > 2 to 3 mm	Unstable; risk of arthritis
Volar subluxation of the DIP greater than 2 to 3 mm displacement, or involvement of > 30% of the articular surface	Referral for primary repair
Rupture of the flexor digitorum profundus tendon	Referral for primary repair

PELVIS AND HIP JOINT

Pelvic/acetabular fracture	Multiple injuries; unstable; traction
Hip fracture	Unstable; internal fixation
Fracture of the femur	Unstable; traction; internal fixation

KNEE

Supracondylar fracture	Unstable; internal fixation
Tibial plateau depressed > 6 to 8 mm	Unstable; risk of arthritis; internal fixation
Rim fracture > 10 degrees	Internal fixation
Bicondylar fracture	Skeletal traction; cast brace; internal fixation

Continued on following page

FRACTURES THAT REQUIRE REFERRAL TO A SURGICAL ORTHOPEDIST
(Continued)

Fracture/Dislocation	Reason for Orthopedic Referral
KNEE	
Tibial spines	Molded long-leg cast for 4 to 6 weeks
Subcondylar fracture	Molded long-leg cast for 4 to 6 weeks
Patellar, displaced or comminuted	Cerclage or patellectomy
Osteochondritis dissecans, symptomatic with locking	Arthroscopy
Tibial and fibular fracture	Unstable; internal fixation
ANKLE	
Unstable bimalleolar fracture	Risk of arthritis; internal fixation
Trimalleolar fracture	Risk of arthritis; internal fixation
Fracture at or above the syndesmosis	Unstable; risk of arthritis
Displaced ankle fragments	Unstable; risk of arthritis
CALCANEUS	
Intra-articular fracture	Risk of arthritis
Displaced posterior process fracture	Restore the integrity of the Achilles tendon
Nonunion of the anterior process	Internal fixation
TALUS	
Displaced neck fracture	Risk of avascular necrosis
NAVICULAR	
All displaced fractures	Unstable
FOOT	
Neuropathic fracture	Risk of nonunion or malunion
Transverse fifth metatarsal fracture	Risk of nonunion or malunion
Displaced or comminuted proximal phalangeal fracture	Risk of nonunion or malunion

NONSTEROIDAL ANTI-INFLAMMATORY DRUGS

Generic	Trade	Dose (Daily Maximum)	Cost per 100 (in Dollars)
SALICYLATE			
Acetylsalicylic acid*	Anacin, Ascriptin, Bufferin, Ecotrin	325, 500 (5–6 g)	4–5
Choline magnesium	Trilisate	0.5, 0.75 (1 g, 3 g)	77–80
Diflunisal	Dolobid	50, 500 (1500)	95–117
Salsalate*	Disalcid	500, 750 (3000)	16–22
PROPRIONIC ACIDS			
Flurbiprofen	Ansaid	50, 100 (300)	83–124
Ibuprofen*	Advil, Motrin, Nuprin, Rufen	200, 400, 600, 800 (3000)	5–18
Ketoprofen	Orudis	25, 50, 75 (300)	90–120
Naproxen	Naprosyn	250, 375, 500 (1500)	62–122
Naproxen sodium	Anaprox	275, 550 (1650)	81–121
ACETIC ACIDS			
Diclofenac sodium	Voltaren	25, 50, 75 (200)	54–116
Indomethacin*	Indocin	25, 50, 75SR (200)	20–32
Nabumetone	Relafen	500, 750 (2000)	99–130
Sulindac*	Clinoril	150, 200 (400)	82–96
Tolmetin sodium	Tolectin	200, 400 (1800)	22–61
OXICAM			
Piroxicam	Feldene	10, 20 (20)	100–214
FENAMATES			
Meclofenamate sodium	Meclomen	50, 100 (400)	24–44
Mefenamic acid	Ponstel	250 (500)	91–94

Continued on opposite page

NONSTEROIDAL ANTI-INFLAMMATORY DRUGS *(Continued)*

Generic	Trade	Dose (Daily Maximum)	Cost per 100 (in Dollars)
PYRANOCARBOXYLIC ACID			
Etodolac	Lodine	200, 300 (1200)	99–110
PYRROLOPYRROLE			
Ketorolac tromethamine	Toradol	15, 30, 60 (120–150)	117–120
PYRAZOLONE			
Phenylbutazone	Butazolidin	100 (400)	27–30

*Available in generic form

CORTICOSTEROIDS

Generic	Trade	Strength (in mg/ml)	Equivalent mg of Hydrocortisone
SHORT-ACTING PREPARATIONS (SOLUBLE)			
Hydrocortisone sodium phosphate (H)	Hydrocortone Phosphate	25, 50	25, 50
Prednisolone sodium phosphate	Hydeltrasol (H20)	20	80
LONG-ACTING PREPARATIONS (DEPOT/TIME-RELEASE)			
Triamcinolone acetonide	Kenalog-40 (K40)	40	200
Triamcinolone hexacetonide	Aristospan Intra-articular (A20)	20	100
Methylprednisolone acetate	Depo-Medrol (D80)	20, 40, 80	100–300
Dexamethasone sodium phosphate	Decadron Phosphate (Dex8)	4, 8	100, 200
Prednisolone tebutate	Hydeltra-T.B.A (HTBA)	20	80
COMBINATION PREPARATIONS (BOTH SOLUBLE AND DEPOT)			
Betamethasone sodium phosphate plus betamethasone acetate	Celestone Soluspan (C6)	6	150

CALCIUM SUPPLEMENTATION

	Amount	Calcium Content (in mg)	Yearly Cost (in dollars)
FOOD			
Milk (nonfat)	8 oz	290–300	200
Yogurt	8 oz	240–400	250
Cheese slice	8 oz	160–260	260
Cottage cheese	4 oz	80–100	960
Broccoli	8 oz	160–180	2000
Tofu	4 oz	145–155	1500
Salmon, canned	3 oz	170–200	3700
SUPPLEMENTS			
Calcium carbonate			
Oyster shell (generic)	625, 1250, 1500 mg	250, 500, 600	40
Os-Cal	625, 1250 mg	250, 500	108
Os-Cal + D	625, 1250 mg	300	107
Tum-Ex	750 mg	220	55
Calcium-rich Rolaids	550 mg	600	53
Caltrate	1500 mg	600	108
Caltrate + D (125 IU)	1500 mg	315	108

Continued on following page

CALCIUM SUPPLEMENTATION (Continued)

	Amount	Calcium Content (in mg)	Yearly Cost (in dollars)
SUPPLEMENTS			
Calcium phosphate			
Posture	1565 mg	600	115
Posture D (125 IU)	1565 mg	600	115
Calcium lactate	650 mg	85	350
Calcium gluconate	975 mg	90	522
Calcium citrate			
Citracal 950	950 mg	200	162
Citracal 1500 + D (200 IU)	1500 mg	315	162

LAB TESTS IN RHEUMATOLOGY

Rheumatoid Factor

The most significant laboratory abnormality in rheumatoid arthritis (RA)!

Antibodies formed to the Fc portion of IgG.

It may take 6 months to become positive: it is insensitive as a screening test!

Between 75 and 80% of adults with RA have significant titers, i.e., greater than 1:160; 20 to 25% are seronegative; only 20% of children with juvenile RA are seropositive; seropositivity correlates with HLA-DR4 haplotype.

The IgM rheumatoid factor is most common.

High titers are associated with more severe disease, active joint disease, presence of nodules, and poorer prognosis.

The IgG rheumatoid factor is associated with more severe disease.

The IgA rheumatoid factor is associated with bony erosions.

A positive RF can occur in non-RA individuals with TB, bacterial endocarditis, syphilis, pulmonary fibrosis, chronic active hepatitis, infectious hepatitis, as well as Sjögren's syndrome, systemic lupus erythematosus (SLE), progressive systemic sclerosis, and polymyositis; i.e., there are many false positives!

Crystals

Crystals are best identified using a polarizing microscope.

Monosodium urate crystals are needle-shaped and negatively birefringent and indicate gout.

Calcium pyrophosphate dihydrate crystals are polygonal-shaped and positively birefringent and indicate pseudogout.

Calcium hydroxyapatite crystals are glossy globules that stain with alizarin red S stain on light microscopy; electron microscopy is used to determine specific chemical content; calcium hydroxyapatite crystal deposition disease is indicated.

Antinuclear Antibodies

ANA

Homogeneous: reacts against deoxynucleoprotein and histone DNA; is the **most common** pattern of ANA; is the least specific for SLE (many false positives).

Rimmed or membranous: reacts against double-stranded DNA and native DNA; is uncommon; is far more specific for SLE than is homogeneous.

Speckled: reacts against extractable nuclear antigens (ENAs); is found in 30% of patients with SLE.

Nucleolar: reacts against ribonucleoprotein (RNP); is an unusual pattern; is more suggestive of PSS than of SLE.

Centromeric: reacts against topoisomerase I; is found in two thirds of patients with calcinosis Raynaud esophagus sclerodactyly telangiectasia syndrome.

DNA

Anti-DNA: reacts against double-stranded DNA; is diagnostic of SLE; correlates with disease activity in most patients.

ENA

Anti-RNP: reacts against antigen susceptible to RNase digestion; is found in 50% of patients with SLE and all patients with mixed connective tissue disease.

Anti-Sm: is also called anti-smith; the only ENA that is specific for SLE; is found in only 15–30% of SLE (low sensitivity).

Anti-Ro: is also called anti-SSA; reacts against RNA-protein antigen; is found in 25–40% of SLE patients, 70% of Sjögren's patients.

Anti-La: is also called anti-SSB; reacts against RNA-protein antigen; is found in 10–15% of SLE patients, 50% of Sjögren's.

LAB TESTS IN RHEUMATOLOGY *(Continued)*

Antinuclear Antibodies

INTERPRETATION

The testing for autoantibodies (ANA testing) should *not* be used as a screen for rheumatic disease! The ANA test should be used to confirm the clinical diagnosis of a patient with symptoms compatible with SLE!

Positive ANA: consider the clinical setting; titers less than 1:160 with few clinical criteria for SLE are probably false positives! Moderate titers over 1:320 to 1:5120 deserve further evaluation (a high titer is greater than 1:5120). Moderate or high titers deserve anti-DNA and anti-ENA testing for confirmation of SLE or other rheumatic conditions.

Positive ANA from drugs: often a homogeneous pattern; caused by procainamide, hydralazine, and isoniazid.

Positive ANAs and diseases: common in patients over age 50 with chronic inflammatory conditions such as (1) chronic active hepatitis, (2) chronic pulmonary fibrosis, (3) chronic infections, and (4) malignancy, particularly lymphoma. Usually the titers are below 1:640.

Positive ANA with age: 5–10% of 50-year-olds have positive ANAs; 20% of 70-year-olds have positive ANAs.

Clinical Criteria for SLE

Malar rash; discoid rash; photosensitivity; oral ulcers; arthritis; serositis; renal disease of proteinuria and/or cellular casts; neurologic disorders of seizures or psychosis; hematologic disorders of hemolytic anemia, leukopenia, lymphopenia, or thrombocytopenia; positive LE prep, anti-DNA, anti-SM, or false positive VDRL, and/or positive ANA.

SYNOVIAL FLUID ANALYSIS

	Normal Synovial Fluid	Noninflammatory Fluid (Group I)	Inflammatory Fluid (Group II)	Infectious Fluid (Group III)
APPEARANCE	Clear	Clear or slightly turbid, bloody	Turbid	Very turbid
COLOR	Colorless or slightly yellow	Yellow	Yellow-white	White-yellow
VISCOSITY	Normal	Decreased	Decreased	Decreased
TOTAL WBC PER mm^3	> 200	<2500	2500–25,000	> 50,000
DIFFERENTIAL % POLYS	7%	13–20%	50–70%	90%
BLOOD VS. FLUID GLUCOSE DIFFERENCE (mg/dL)	0	5	10–30	70–90
CLINICAL EXAMPLES		Osteoarthritis Patellofemoral syndrome Mechanical derangement SLE Hyperparathyroidism	Rheumatoid arthritis Pseudogout Gout Reiter GC Rheumatic fever TB SLE	Septic arthritis TB

■ REFERENCES

General

Anderson BC. *Stretching*. Bolinas, California: Shelter Publications, 1980.
Cyriax J. *Textbook of Orthopedic Medicine*, 8th ed. London: Baillière Tindall, 1982.
Gray RG, Tenebaum J, Gottlieb NL. Local corticosteroid injection treatment in rheumatic disorders. Semin Arthritis Rheumatol 10:231–253, 1981.
Hill JJ, Trapp RG, Colliver JA. Survey on the use of corticosteroid injections by orthopedists. Contemp Orthop 18:39–45, 1989.
Hollander JL, Brown EM, Jessar RA, Brown CY. Hydrocortisone and cortisone injection into arthritic joints: Comparative effects of and use of hydrocortisone as a local antiarthritic agent. JAMA 147:1629–1631, 1951.
Hoppenfeld S. Physical examination of the spine and extremities. New York: Appleton-Century-Crofts, 1976.
Lapidus PW, Guidotti FP. Local injections of hydrocortisone in 495 orthopedic patients. Industr Med Surg 26:234–244, 1957.
Rockwood CA, Green DP, Bucholz RW. *Fractures*, 3rd ed. Philadelphia: JB Lippincott, 1991.
Scott DB. *Techniques of Regional Anesthesia*. Norwalk, Connecticut: Appleton and Lange, 1989.
Simon RR, Koenigsknecht SJ, Stevens C. *Emergency Orthopedics*, 2nd ed. East Norwalk, Connecticut: Appleton and Lange, 1987.
Sivananda Yoga Vedanta Center. *Yoga Mind and Body*. New York: Dorling Kindersley Publishing, 1996.

Neck

Dillin W, Booth R, et al. Cervical radiculopathy: A review. Spine 11:988–991, 1986.
Frost FA, Jessen B, Siggaard-Andersen J. A control, double-blind comparison of mepivacaine injection versus saline injection for myofascial pain. Lancet 1:499–500, 1980.
Goldenberg DL, Felson DT, Dinerman H. A randomized controlled trial of amitriptyline and Naprosyn in the treatment of patients with fibromyalgia. Arthritis Rheumatol 29:1371–1377, 1986.
Honet JC, Puri K. Cervical radiculitis: Treatment and results in 82 patients. Arch Phys Med Rehabil 57:12–16, 1976.
Kelly TR. Thoracic outlet syndrome: Current concepts of treatment. Ann Surg 190:657–662, 1979.
Radanov BP, Sturzennegger M, Stefano GD. Long-term outcome after whiplash injury. Medicine 74:281–297, 1995.
Saal JS, Saal JA, Yurth EF. Nonoperative management of herniated cervical intervertebral disc with radiculopathy. Spine 21:1877–1883, 1996.
Tsairis P, Dyck PJ, Mulder DW. Natural history of brachial plexus neuropathy: Report on 99 patients. Arch Neurol 27:109–117, 1972.

Temporomandibular Joint

Toller P. Use and misuse of intra-articular corticosteroids in treatment of temporomandibular joint pain. Proc R Soc Med 70:461–463, 1977.

Shoulder

Anderson BC, Kaye S. Shoulder pain: Differential diagnosis. West J Med 138:268, 1983.
Codman EA. *The Shoulder*. Boston: Thomas Todd, 1934.
Fiddian NJ, King RJ. The winged scapula. Clin Orthop 185:228–236, 1984.

Impingement Syndrome

Brox JI, et al. Arthroscopic surgery compared with supervised exercises in patients with rotator cuff disease (stage II impingement syndrome). Br Med J 307:899–903, 1993.

Lozman PR, Hechtman KS, Uribe JW. Combined arthroscopic management of impingement syndrome and acromioclavicular joint arthritis. J South Orthop Assoc 4:177–181, 1995.

Neer CS II. Anterior acromioplasty for the chronic impingement syndrome in the shoulder: A preliminary report. J Bone Joint Surg. 54A:41–50, 1972.

Neer CS. Anterior acromioplasty for the chronic impingement syndrome of the shoulder. J Bone Joint Surg 73A:707–715, 1991.

Rotator Cuff Tendinitis/Bursitis

Chard MD, Sattelle MD, Hazleman BL. The long-term outcome of rotator cuff tendonitis: A review study. Br J Rheumatol 27:385–389, 1988.

Crisp EJ, Kendall PH. Treatment of periarthritis of the shoulder with hydrocortisone. Br Med J 1:1500–1501, 1955.

Ellis RM, Hollingworth GR, MacCollum MS. Comparison of injection techniques for shoulder pain: Results of a double-blind, randomized study. BMJ 287:1339–1341, 1983.

Fearnley M, Vadasz I. Factors influencing the response of lesions of the rotator cuff of the shoulder to local steroid injection. Ann Phys Med 10:53–63, 1969.

Petri M, Dobrow R, Neiman R, Whiting-O'Keefe Q, Seaman WE. Randomized, double-blind placebo-controlled study of the treatment of the painful shoulder. Arthritis Rheumatol 30:1040–1045, 1987.

Valtonen EJ. Double-acting betamethasone (Celestone Chronodose) in the treatment of supraspinatus tendonitis. J Intern Med 6:463–467, 1978.

White RH, Paull DM, Fleming KW. Rotator cuff tendonitis: Comparison of subacromial injection of a long-acting corticosteroid versus oral indomethacin therapy. J Rheumatol 13:608–613, 1986.

Rotator Cuff Tendon Rupture

Ahovuo J, Paavolainen P, Slatis P. The diagnostic value of arthrography and plain radiography in rotator cuff tears. Acta Orthop Scand 55:220–223, 1984.

Codman EA, Akerson IV. The pathology associated with rupture of the supraspinatus tendon. Ann Surg 93:348–359, 1931.

Darlington LG, Coomes EN. The effects of local steroid injection for supraspinatus tears. Rheumatol Rehabil 16:172–179, 1977.

Samilson RL, Binder WF. Symptomatic full-thickness tears of the rotator cuff. Orthop Clin North Am 6:449–466, 1975.

Watson M. Major ruptures of the rotator cuff: The results of surgical repair in 89 patients. J Bone Joint Surg Br 67:618–624, 1985.

Biceps Tendinitis/Tear

Mariani EM, Cofield RH, Askew LJ, Li GP, Chao EY. Rupture of the tendon of the long head of the biceps brachii: Surgical versus nonsurgical treatment. Clin Orthop 228:233–239, 1988.

Soto-Hall R, Stroot JH. Treatment of ruptures of the long head of the biceps brachii. Am J Orthop 2:192–193, 1960.

Frozen Shoulder

Andren L, Lundbery BJ. Treatment of rigid shoulders by joint distension during arthrography. Acta Orthop Scand 36:45–53, 1965.

Bulgren DY, Binder AI, Hazleman BL, et al. Frozen shoulder: A prospective clinical study with an evaluation of three treatment regimens. Ann Rheumatol Dis 43:353–360, 1984.

Jacobs LGH, Barton MAJ, Wallace WA, et al. Intra-articular distension and steroids in the management of capsulitis of the shoulder. Br Med J 302:1498–1501, 1991.

Rizk TE, Pinals RS. Frozen shoulder. Semin Arthritis Rheumatol 11:440–452, 1982.

Steinbocker O, Argyros TG. Frozen shoulder: Treatment by local injection of depot corticosteroids. Arch Phys Med Rehabil 55:209–212, 1974.

Weiss JJ. Arthrography-assisted intra-articular injection of steroids in treatment of adhesive capsulitis. Arch Phys Med Rehabil 59:285–287, 1978.

Acromioclavicular Disorders

Weinstein DM, McCann PD, McIlveen SJ, Flatow EL, Bigliani LU. Surgical treatment of complete acromioclavicular dislocations. Am J Sports Med 23:324–31, 1995.

Reflex Sympathetic Dystrophy

Adebajo A, Hazleman B. Shoulder pain and reflex sympathetic dystrophy. Curr Opin Rheumatol 2:270–275, 1990.

Lateral Epicondylitis

Boyd HB, McLeod AC. Tennis elbow. J Bone Joint Surg 55A:1183–1197, 1973.

Day BH, Gavindasamy N. Corticosteroid injection in the treatment of tennis elbow. Practice Med 220:459–462, 1978.

Fillion PL. Treatment of lateral epicondylitis. Am J Occup Ther 45:340–343, 1991.

Nirschl RP, Pettrone FA. Tennis elbow: The surgical treatment of lateral epicondylitis. J Bone Joint Surg Am 61:832–839, 1979.

Potter HG, Hannafin JA, Morsessel RM, DiCarlo EF, O'Brien SJ, Altchek DW. Lateral epicondylitis: Correlation with MR imaging, surgical and histopathologic findings. Radiology 196:43–46, 1995.

Olecranon Bursitis

Hassell AB, Fowler PD, Dawes PT. Intra-bursal tetracycline in the treatment of olecranon bursitis in patients with rheumatoid arthritis. Br J Rheumatol 33:859–860, 1994.

Knight JM, Thomas JC, Maurer RC. Treatment of septic olecranon and prepatellar bursitis with percutaneous placement of a suction-irrigation system: A report of 12 cases. Clin Orthop 206:90–93, 1986.

Smith DL, McAfee JH, Lucas LM, et al. Treatment of nonseptic olecranon bursitis: A controlled blinded prospective trial. Arch Intern Med 149:2527–2530, 1989.

Carpal Tunnel Syndrome

Ellis J. Clinical results of a cross-over treatment with pyridoxine and placebo of the carpal tunnel syndrome. Am J Clin Nutr 32:2040–2046, 1979.

Foster JB, Goodman HV. The effect of local corticosteroid injection on median nerve conduction in carpal tunnel syndrome. Ann Phys Med 6:287–294, 1962.

Gelberman RH, Aronson D, Weisman MH. Carpal-tunnel syndrome: Results of a prospective trial of steroid injection and splinting. J Bone Joint Surg Am 62:1181–1184, 1980.

Phalen GS. Carpal tunnel syndrome: 17 years of experience in diagnosis and treatment. J Bone Joint Surg 48A:211–228, 1966.

Shapiro S. Microsurgical carpal tunnel release. Neurosurgery 37:66–70, 1995.

DeQuervain's Tenosynovitis

Anderson BC, Manthey R, Brouns MC. Treatment of DeQuervain's tenosynovitis with corticosteroids. Arthritis Rheumatol 34:793–798, 1991.

Clark DD, Ricker JH, MacCollum MS. The efficacy of local steroid injection in the treatment of stenosing tenovaginitis. Plast Reconstr Surg 49:179–80, 1973.

Harvey FJ, Harvey PM, Horsly MW. DeQuervain's disease: Surgical or nonsurgical treatment. J Hand Surg 15A:83–87, 1990.

Trigger Finger

Anderson BC, Kaye S. Treatment of flexor tenosynovitis of the hand ("trigger finger") with corticosteroids. Arch Int Med 151:153–156, 1991.

Gray RG, Kiem IM, Gottlieb NL. Intratendon sheath corticosteroid treatment of rheumatoid arthritis–associated and idiopathic flexor tenosynovitis. Arthritis Rheumatol 21:92–96, 1978.

Lyu SR. Closed division of the flexor tendon sheath for trigger finger. J Bone Joint Surg 74:418–420, 1992.

Murphy D, Failla JM, Koniuch MP. Steroid versus placebo injection for trigger finger. J Hand Surg 20:628–631, 1995.

Stothard J, Kumar A. A safe percutaneous procedure for trigger finger release. J R Coll Surg 39:116–117, 1994.

Rheumatoid Arthritis

Fries JF, Spitz PW, Williams CA, et al. A toxicity for comparison of side effects among different drugs. Arthritis Rheumatol 31:121–130, 1990.

Kovarsky J. Intermediate-dose intramuscular methylprednisolone acetate in the treatment of rheumatic disease. Ann Rheumatol Dis 42:308–310, 1983.

Kushner O. Does aggressive therapy of rheumatoid arthritis affect outcome? J Rheumatol 16:1–5, 1989.

Steere AC, Bartenhagen NH, Craft JE, et al. The early clinical manifestations of Lyme disease. Ann Intern Med 99:76–82, 1983.

Weiss MM. Corticosteroids in rheumatoid arthritis. Semin Arthritis Rheumatol 19:9–21, 1989.

Zuckner J, Uddin J, Ramsey RH. Intramuscular administration of steroids in treatment of rheumatoid arthritis. Ann Rheumatol Dis 23:456–462.

Back

Basmajian JV. Acute back pain and spasm: A controlled multicenter trial of combined analgesic and antispasm agents. Spine 14:438–439, 1989.

Benzon HT. Epidural steroid injections for low back pain and lumbosacral radiculopathy. Pain 24:277–295, 1986.

Bogduk N, Cherry D. Epidural corticosteroid agents for sciatica. Med J Austral 143:402–406, 1985.

Carette S, Marcoux S, Truchon R, et al. A controlled trial of corticosteroid injection into facet joints for chronic low back pain. N Engl J Med 325:1002–1007, 1991.

Cucler JM, Bernini PA, Wiesel SW, et al. The use of epidural steroids in the treatment of lumbar radicular pain: A prospective, randomized, double blind study. J Bone Joint Surg Am 67:63–66, 1985.

Cullen AP. Carisoprodal (soma) in acute back conditions: A double-blind, radomized, placebo-controlled study. Curr Ther Res 20:557–562, 1976.

Garvey RA, Marks MR, Wiesel SW. A prospective, randomized, double-blind evaluation of trigger-point injection therapy for low-back pain. Spine 14:962–964, 1989.

Jackson RP, Jacobs RR, Montesano PX. Facet joint injection in low back pain: A prospective statistical study. Spine 13:966–971, 1988.

Kepes ER, Duncalf D. Treatment of back ache with spinal injections of local anesthetics, spinal and systemic steroids: A review. Pain 22:33–47, 1985.

Macrai IF, Wright V. Measurement of back movement. Ann Rheumatol Dis 28:584–589, 1969.

Rollings HE, Glassman JM, Joyka JP. Management of acute musculoskeletal conditions—thoracolumbar strain or sprain: A double-blind evaluation comparing the efficacy and safety of carisoprodol with cyclobenzaprine hydrochloride. Curr Ther Res 34:917–928, 1983.

Westbrook L, Cicala RJ, Wright H. Effectiveness of alprazolam in the treatment of chronic pain: Results of a preliminary study. Clin J Pain 6:32–36, 1990.

Sacroiliac Disease

Arneet F. Seronegative spondyloarthropathies. Bull Rheumatol Dis 37:1–12, 1987.

Burgox-Vargax R, Pineda C. New clinical and radiographic features of the seronegative spondyloarthropathies. Curr Opinion Rheumatol 562–574, 1991.

Trochanteric Bursitis/Piriformis Syndrome

Barton PM. Piriformis syndrome: A rational approach to management. Pain 47:345–352, 1991.

Brooker AF Jr. The surgical approach to refractory trochanteric bursitis. Johns Hopkins Med J 145:98–100, 1979.

Ege-Rasmussen KJ, Fano N. Trochanteric bursitis: Treatment by corticosteroid injection. Scand J Rheumatol 14:417–420, 1985.

Fishman LM, Zyber PA. Electrophysiologic evidence of piriformis syndrome. Arch Phys Med Rehabil 73:359–364, 1992.

Rothenberg RJ. Rheumatic disease aspects of leg length inequality. Semin Arthritis Rheumatol 17:196–205, 1988.

Avascular Necrosis of the Hip

Ficat RP. Idiopathic bone necrosis of the fermoral heal: Early diagnosis and treatment. J Bone Joint Surg 67:3–9, 1985.

Mitchesl DG, Rao VM, Dalinka MK, et al. Femoral head avascular necrosis: Correlation of MR imaging, radiographic staging, radionuclide imaging, and clinical findings. Radiology 162:709–715, 1987.

Zizic TM, Marcoux C, Hungerford DS, et al. Corticosteroid therapy associated with ischemic necrosis of bone in systemic lupus erythematosus. Am J Med 79:586–604, 1985.

Patellofemoral Syndrome

Insall J. Current concepts review patellar pain. J Bone Joint Surg 64A:147, 1982.

Osteoarthritis of the Knee

Balch HW, Gibson JM, Eighorbarev AF, Bain LS, Lynch, MP. Repeated corticosteroid injections into knee joints. Rheumatol Rehabil 19:62–66, 1970.

Friedman DM, Moore ME. The efficacy of intra-articular steroids in osteoarthritis: A double-blind study. J Rheumatol 7:850–855, 1980.

Hollander JL. Intra-articular hydrocortisone in arthritis and allied conditions: A summary of two years' clinical experience J Bone Joint Surg 35:983–990, 1953.

Kehr MJ. Comparison of intra-articular cortisone analogues in osteoarthritis of the knee. Ann Rheumatol Dis 18:325–328, 1959.

Miller JH, White J, Norton TH. The value of intra-articular injections in osteoarthritis of the knee. J Bone Joint Surg 40B:636–643, 1958.

Nakhostine M, Friedrich NF, Muller W, Kentsch A. A special high tibial osteotomy technique for treatment of unicompartmental osteoarthritis of the knee. Orthopedics 16:1255–1258, 1993.

Septic Arthritis

Blackburn WD, Alarcon GS. Prosthetic joint infections: A role for prophylaxis. Arthritis Rheumatol 34:110, 1991.

Gardner GR, Weisman MH. Pyarthrosis in patients with rheumatoid arthritis: A report of 13 years and a review of the literature from the past 40 years. Am J Med 88:503–510, 1990.

VonEssen R. Bacterial infections following intra-articular injection. Scand J Rheumatol 10:7–13, 1989.

Anserinus Bursitis

Forbes JR, Helms CA, Janzen DL. Acute pes anserinus bursitis: MR imaging. Radiology 194:525–527, 1995.

Prepatellar Bursitis

Knight JM, Thomas JC, Maurer RC. Treatment of septic olecranon and prepatellar bursitis with percutaneous placement of a suction-irrigation system: A report of 12 cases. Clin Orthop 206:90–93, 1986.

McAfee JH, Smith DL. Olecranon and prepatellar bursitis. Diagnosis and treatment. West J Med 149:607–610, 1988.

Iliotibial Band Syndrome

Barber FA, Sutker AN. Iliotibial band syndrome. Sports Med 14:144–148, 1992.

Puniello MS. Iliotibial band tightness and medial patellar glide in patients with patellofemoral syndrome. J Orthop Sports Phys Ther 17:144–148, 1993.

Meniscal Tears

Fischer SP, Fox JM, DelPizzo W, et al. Accuracy of diagnosis from MRI of the knee: A multicenter analysis of one thousand and fourteen patients. J Bone Joint Surg 73A:2–10, 1991.

Achilles Tendonitis/Rupture

Fox JM, Blazina ME, Jobe FW, et al. Degeneration and rupture of the Achilles tendon. Clin Orthop 107:221–224, 1975.

Gilcreest EL. Ruptures and tears of muscles and tendons of the lower extremity. JAMA 100:153–160, 1933.

Melmed SP. Spontaneous bilateral rupture of the calcaneal tendon during steroid therapy. J Bone Joint Surg 47B:104–105, 1965.

Ankle Injury

Cetti R. Conservative treatment of injury to the fibular ligaments of the ankle. Br J Sports Med 16:47–52, 1982.

Konradsen L, Holmer P, Sondergaard L. Early mobilizing treatment for grade III ankle ligament injuries. Foot Ankle Int 12:69–73, 1991.

Moller-larsen F, Withelund JO, Jurik AG, de Cavalho A, Lucht V. Comparison of three different treatments for ruptured lateral ankle ligaments. Acta Orthop Scand 59:564–566, 1988.

Niedermann B, Andersen A, Andersen SB, Funder V, et al. Ruptures of the lateral ligaments of the ankle: Operation or plaster cast? Acta Orthop Scand 52:579–587, 1981.

Plantar Fasciitis

Barrett SL, Day SV. Endoscopic plantar fasciotomy for chronic plantar fasciitis/heel spur syndrome: Surgical technique—early clinical results. J Foot Surg 30:568–570, 1991.

Blockey NJ. The painful heel: A controlled trial of the value of hydrocortisone. Br Med J 1:1277–1278, 1956.

Daly PJ, Kitaoka HB, Chao EY. Plantar fasciotomy for intractable plantar fasciitis. Foot Ankle Int 13:188–195, 1992.

Gould EA. Three generations of exotoses of heel inherited from father to son. J Heredity 33:228, 1942.

Lapidus PW, Guidotti FP. Painful heel: Report of 323 patients with 364 painful heels. Clin Orthop 39:178–186, 1959.

Newell SG, Miller SJ. Conservative treatment of plantar fascial strain. Physician Sports Med 5:68–73, 1977.

Wolgin M, Dook D, Graham C, Mauldin D. Conservative treatment of plantar heel pain: Long-term follow-up. Foot Ankle Int 15:97–102, 1994.

Tarsal Tunnel Syndrome

McGuigan L, Burke D, Fleming A. Tarsal tunnel syndrome and peripheral neuropathy in rheumatoid arthritis. Ann Rheumatol Dis 42:128–131, 1983.

Gout

Grahame R, Scott JT. Clinical survey of 354 patients with gout. Ann Rheumatol Dis 29:461–470, 1970.

Side Effects

Bedi SS, Ellis W. Spontaneous rupture of the calcaneal tendon in rheumatoid arthritis after steroid injection. Ann Rheumatol Dis 29:494–495, 1970.

Halpern AA, Horowitz BG, Nagel DA. Tendon ruptures associated with corticosteroid therapy. West J Med 127:378–382, 1977.

Hedner P, Persson G. Suppression of the hypothalamic-pituitary-adrenal axis after a single intramuscular injection of methylprednisolone acetate. Ann of Allerg 47:176–179, 1981.

Hollander JL, Jessar RA, Brown EM. Intra-synovial corticosteroid therapy: A decade of use. Bull Rheumatol Dis 11:239–240, 1961.

Ismail AM, Balakrishnan R, Rajakumar MK. Rupture of patellar ligament after steroid infiltration: Report of a case. J Bone Joint Surg 51B:503–505, 1969.

Kendall, PH. Untoward effects following local hydrocortisone injection. Ann Phys Med 4:170–175, 1961.

Kleinman M, Gross AE. Achilles tendon rupture following steroid injection. J Bone Joint Surg 65A:1345–1347, 1983.

Roseff R, Canoso JJ. Femoral osteonecrosis following several hundred soft tissue corticosteroid infiltrations. Am J Med 77:1119–1120, 1984.

Rostron PKM, Calver RF. Subcutaneous atrophy following methylprednisolone injection in Osgood-Schlatter epiphysitis. J Bone Joint Surg 61A:627–628, 1979.

Laboratory Testing

Barland P, Lipstein E. Selection and use of laboratory tests in the rheumatic diseases. Am J Med 100:16S–23S, 1996.

Cohen PL. What antinuclear antibodies can tell you. J Musculoskeletal Med April 10:37–46, 1993.

Sox HC, Liang MH. The erythrocyte sedimentation rate: Guidelines for rational use. Ann Intern Med 104:515–523, 1986.

White RH, Robbins DL. Clinical significance and interpretation of antinuclear antibodies. West J Med 147:210, 1987.

Young B, Gleeson M, Cripps AW. C-reactive protein: A critical review. Pathology 23:2417–2420, 1992.

Synovial Fluid Analysis

Cohen AS, Brandt KD, Krey PR. Synovial fluid. In Cohen AS ed. *Laboratory Diagnostic Procedures in the Rheumatoid Diseases*, 2nd ed. Boston: Little, Brown, 1–62, 1975.

Goldenberg DL, Reed JI. Bacterial arthritis. N Engl J Med 312:764–771, 1985.

James MJ, Cleland LG, Rofe AM, Leslie AL. Intra-articular pressure and the relationship between synovial perfusion and metabolic demand. J Rheumatol 17:521–527, 1990.

Krey PR, Bailen DA. Synovial fluid leukocytosis: A study of extremes. Am J Med 67:436–442, 1979.

Ropes MW, Bauer W. *Synovial Changes in Joint Disease*. Cambridge: Harvard University Press, 1953.

Note: Page numbers in *italics* refer to illustrations; page numbers followed by t refer to tables.

Accessory bones, of feet, 240, *241*
Achilles tendinitis, 176–179
    exercises for, 178
    injection for, *177,* 179–180
    physical therapy for, 178
Achilles tendon, exercises for, 279
Acromioclavicular strain-osteoarthritis, 31–34
    exercises for, 33
    injection for, *32*
    physical therapy for, 33
Acromioplasty, for impingement syndrome, 17
    for rotator cuff tendinitis, 22
Adhesive capsulitis, 27
Adventitial bursitis, 197–199
    exercises for, 199
    injection for, *197,* 199
    physical therapy for, 199
Anesthetic block, for Morton neuroma, 207
Ankle, 169–193, 277–280
    anatomy of, 277–278
    arthrocentesis of, *174*
    effusion of, 173–175
        exercises for, 175
        injection for, *174,* 175–176
        physical therapy for, 175
    exercises for, 277–280
    fractures of, 236–237, *237*
    physical therapy for, 277–280
    sprains of, 170–172
        exercises for, 172
        injection for, *170,* 172–173
        physical therapy for, 172
        severe, fractures accompanying, 237–238
    supports, braces and casts for, 300–302
Ankylosing spondylitis, 120
Anserine bursitis, 155–158
    exercises for, 157
    injection for, *155,* 157–158
    physical therapy for, 157
Anti-inflammatory drugs, nonsteroidal, 308–309
Antinuclear antibodies, laboratory tests for, 310–311

Apley scratch test, for glenohumeral osteoarthritis, 43
Arthritis, 18, 120
    exercises for, 272
    of carpometacarpal joint, 69–72
    of metacarpophalangeal joint, 93–96
    of radiocarpal joint, 78–81
    of sternoclavicular joint, 107
    patellofemoral, 140
    posttraumatic monoarticular, 78
    rheumatoid. See *Rheumatoid arthritis.*
    septic, 78, 93
Arthrocentesis, for anserine bursitis, 156
    of ankle, *174*
    of metacarpophalangeal joint, *94*
    of radiocarpal joint, *78*
Arthrodesis, for gamekeeper's thumb, 74
Arthrogram, for rotator cuff tendinitis, 20
    for rotator cuff tendon tears, 29
Arthrography, for Baker cyst, 159
    for impingement syndrome, 15
    for rotator cuff tendon tears, 29
Arthroplasty, for carpometacarpal osteoarthritis, 72
    for rheumatoid arthritis, 102
Arthroscopic dilation, of glenohumeral joint, 26
Arthroscopy, for knee effusion, 147
    for osteoarthritis of knee, 152
    for radiohumeral joint arthrocentesis, 63
Aspiration, of dorsal ganglion, *82,* 83
    of tibiotalar joint, 173
    of wrist, 78

Avascular necrosis, of hip, 230–231, *231*

Back, 111–124, 264–269
    anatomy of, 264–265
    exercises for, 265–269
    lumbosacral strain of, 112–115
    massage for, 264–265
    physical therapy for, 264–269
    sacroiliac strain of, 119–124
    sciatica of, 116–118
    traction for, 267
Baker cyst, 143, 158–161
    exercises for, 160
    injection for, *159,* 160–161
    physical therapy for, 160
Bible cyst, 81
Biceps tendinitis, 34–38
    exercises for, 36, 37, 38
    injection for, 37–38
    physical therapy for, 36–37
Bone scans, for gluteus medius bursitis, 131
    for trochanteric bursitis, 127
Bouchard nodes, 97
Boutonniere injury, 225–226
Braces, for ankle, 300–302
    for elbow, 287
    for hand, 293–294
    for knee, 297–299
    for lumbosacral region, 295–296
    for neck, 284
    for shoulder, 285–286
    for wrist, 288–292
Bunion(s), 194–197
    bunionectomy, 196–197, 199
    exercises for, 196
    injection for, *194,* 196
    physical therapy for, 196
Bursectomy, 199
    for prepatellar bursitis, 155
Bursitis, adventitial, 197–199
    anserine, 155–158
    exercises for, 273
    gluteus medius, 130–133
    of hip, 273
    olecranon, 58–60

Bursitis (*Continued*)
  pre-Achilles, 180–183
  prepatellar, 152–155
  retrocalcaneal, 183–185
  subscapular, 38–41
  trochanteric, 126–129

Calcaneus, fractures of, 238
Calcium supplementation,
  309–310
Capsulitis, adhesive, 27
Carpal tunnel syndrome, 74–78
  exercises for, 77
  injection for, 75, 77–78
  physical therapy for, 77
Carpometacarpal joint arthritis,
  69–72
  exercises for, 71
  injection for, 69, 71–72
  kenalog–40 for, 72t
  physical therapy for, 71
Casts, for ankle, 300–302
  for hand, 293–294
  for knee, 297–299
  for shoulder, 285–286
  for wrist, 288–292
Cervical. See also *Neck.*
Cervical arthritis, 7
Cervical radiculopathy, 7–11, *8*
  injection for, 10
  physical therapy for, 10
  prescription for, 9
Cervical strain, 4–7
  exercises for, 6
  injection for, 6–7
  physical therapy for, 6
  prescription for, 5
  range of motion for, 5
  trigger points for, *4*, 5
Cervical traction, for cervical
  radiculopathy, 9
Charcot fracture, 240
Chest, 104–119
Chiropractic manipulation, 265
Chondromalacia patella, 140
Clavicle, fractures of, 217–218,
  218
  resection of, for acromioclavi-
    cular strain osteoarthritis,
    34
Codman weighted pendulum
  exercises, for impingement
  syndrome, 17
Collateral ligament, medial,
  strained, *161*, 161–164
  ulnar, injuries of, 72
Colles fracture, radial, 220–221,
  221
Compression fractures, of spine,
  227, 227–228
  of vertebral body, *227*, 227–228
Computed tomography (CT), for
  gluteus medius bursitis, 131
  for lumbosacral strain, 113
  for sciatica, 118
  for trochanteric bursitis, 127
Corticosteroids, 309
Costochondritis, 104–106
Crystals, laboratory tests for, 310
CT. See *Computed tomography
    (CT).*
CT arthrography, for shoulder
  multidirectional instability,
  46

Cyst(s), Baker, 143, 158–161
  bible, 81
  synovial, volar, 81
  tendon, *89*, 89–91
  wrist, 81

D80, for trigger finger, 87t
De Quervain tenosynovitis,
  66–69
  depo-medrol for, 69t
  exercises for, 68
  injection for, *66*, 68
  physical therapy for, 67–68
Deep trochanteric bursitis. See
  Gluteus medius bursitis.
Depo-medrol, for de Quervain
  tenosynovitis, 69t
  for rotator cuff tendinitis, 21t
Diathermy, 265
Disk, herniated, *116*, 116–117
Diskectomy, 10
Dislocation, metacarpophalangeal, 223, 224
  of elbow, without concomitant
    fractures, 219
  of PIP joint, 226
  of thumb, 223–224
Dorsal ganglion, 81–84
  aspiration of, *82*, 83
  exercises for, 83
  injection of, *82*, 83–84
  physical therapy for, 83
Dupuytren's contracture, 91–93
  exercises for, 93
  injection for, *82*, 93
  physical therapy for, 93

Effusion, of knee, 143–146
Elbow, 50–63, 260–261
  anatomy of, 260
  dislocation of, without con-
    comitant fractures, 219
  exercises for, 261
  physical therapy for, 261
  radiohumeral joint arthrocen-
    tesis involving, 60–63
  supports and braces for, 287
EMGs, for cervical
  radiculopathy, 11
  for cervical strain, 5
Epicondylitis, lateral, *50*, 51–53
  medial, *54*, 54–58
Exercises, for Achilles tendinitis,
  178
  for Achilles tendon, 279
  for acromioclavicular (AC)
    joint, 33
  for adventitial bursitis, 199
  for ankle, 277–280
  for ankle effusion, 175
  for ankle sprain, 172
  for anserine bursitis, 157
  for arthritis, 272
  for back, 265–269
  for Baker cyst, 160
  for biceps tendinitis, 36, 37, 38
  for bunions, 196
  for bursitis, 273
  for carpal tunnel syndrome, 77
  for carpometacarpal osteoar-
    thritis, 71

Exercises (*Continued*)
  for cervical radiculopathy, 10
  for cervical strain, 6
  for de Quervain tenosynovitis,
    68
  for dorsal ganglion, 83
  for Dupuytren's contracture,
    93
  for elbow, 261
  for frozen shoulder, 25–26
  for gamekeeper's thumb, 74
  for glenohumeral osteoarthri-
    tis, 43, 44
  for gluteus medius bursitis,
    132
  for hammer toes, 204
  for hand, 263
  for hip, 270
  for impingement syndrome,
    15–16
  for knee, 275–277
  for knee effusion, 145–146
  for lateral epicondylitis, 51, 52
  for lumbosacral strain, 115
  for medial collateral ligament
    strain, 163–164
  for medial epicondylitis, 55, 56
  for meniscal tear, 167
  for neck, 252
  for olecranon bursitis, 59, 60
  for osteoarthritis, of hand, 98
    of hip, 135–136
    of knee, 151–152
  for patellofemoral diseases,
    142
  for plantar fasciitis, 190–191
  for posterior tibialis tenosyno-
    vitis, 188
  for pre-Achilles bursitis, 182
  for radiocarpal joint arthritis,
    80
  for radiohumeral joint arthro-
    centesis, 62, 63
  for rheumatoid arthritis, 101
  for rotator cuff tendinitis,
    19–20
  for rotator cuff tendon tears,
    29–30
  for rotator cuff tendons, 257
  for sacroiliac strain, 123–124
  for shoulder, 255–259
  for shoulder multidirectional
    instability, 45, 46, 47
  for sternoclavicular joint, 108–
    109
  for subscapular bursitis, 40, 41
  for tennis elbow, 262
  for trigger finger, 87
  for trochanteric bursitis, 128
  for wrist, 263
Extensor tendon, of finger,
  rupture of, 226
  of thumb, rupture of, 227

Fasciectomy, 93
Fasciitis, plantar, *188*, 188–192
Feet, accessory bones of, 240, *241*
Femoral condyle(s), medial,
  osteochondritis dissecans of,
  234
Femur, fractures of, 230
  with metastatic disease, 230
Fibromyalgia, 4, 6

Fibrositis, 4
Fibula, fractures of, 235–236
Fibulocalcaneal ligament,
    injection for, *170*
Finger, rupture of, 226–227
    trigger, *86,* 86–88, 87t
Flexor digitorum profundus
    tendon, rupture of, 227
Foot, 193–208
    bunions of, 194–197
    gout in, 199–202
    Morton neuroma of, 205–208
    supports for, 303–306
Foraminal encroachment, 7, 10
Foraminotomy, 10
Fracture(s), 212–243
    accompanying severe ankle
        sprain, 237–238
    ankle, 236–237, *237*
    calcaneal, 238
    Charcot, 240
    clavicular, 217–218, *218*
    Colles, radial, 220–221, *221*
    common, 212, 212t
    compression, of vertebral
        body, *227,* 227–228
    femoral, 230
        with metastatic disease, 230
    fibular, 235–236
    great toe, 243
    hip, 230
    humeral, 216–217, *217,* 219
    intercondylar, humeral, 219
    knee, 233
    mallet, 226
    march, of metatarsals, 241–242,
        242
    metacarpal, 223–224
    metatarsal, 240–241, 242
    midtarsal, 240
    navicular, 221–223, *222*
    neuropathic, 240
    nonoperative management of,
        213–216
    occult, of hip, *232,* 232–233
    operative management of, 213,
        307–308
    patellar, 233–234
    pelvic, 229–230
    phalangeal, 225, 226
    radial, distal, 220–221, *221*
        nondisplaced, 220
    rib, 228–229, *229*
    sesamoid, 243
    supracondylar, humeral, 219
    talar, 238
    tibial, 234, 235
        with metastatic disease, 230
    toe, 243
    ulnar, nondisplaced, 220
Frozen shoulder, 23–27
    exercises for, 25–26, 258
    injection for, 26
    physical therapy for, 25–26

Gamekeeper's thumb, 72–74,
    224, 224–225
    exercises for, 74
    injection for, *73,* 74
    physical therapy for, 74
Gastrocnemius muscle, tear of,
    236, 236
Gluteus medius bursitis, 130–133

Gluteus medius bursitis
    (Continued)
    exercises for, 132
    injection for, *130,* 132–133
    physical therapy for, 132
Golfer's elbow, 54–58
Gout, 197, 199–202
    injection for, *200,* 202
    physical therapy for, 202
Great toe, bunions of, 194–197
    fractures of, 243
    gout in, 199–202
    strain of, 242–243

Hammer toes, 202–205
    exercises for, 204
    injection for, *203,* 204–205
    physical therapy for, 204
Hand, 86–102
    Dupuytren's contracture of,
        91–93
    exercises for, 263
    osteoarthritis of, 96–98
    physical therapy for, 263
    rheumatoid arthritis of, 98–102
    supports, braces and casts for,
        293–294
    tendon cyst of, 89–91
    trigger finger of, 86–88
Heat and massage, for cervical
    radiculopathy, 10
    for cervical strain, 6
    for rheumatoid arthritis, 101
Heberden nodes, 97
Heel, traumatic irritation of, *239,*
    239–240
Heel pad syndrome, *239,*
    239–240
Herniated disk, *116,* 116–117
Herniated nucleus pulposus, 7
Hip, 125–138, 270–272
    anatomy of, *269,* 270
    avascular necrosis of, 230–231,
        231
    bursitis of, 126–133, 273
    exercises for, 270–272
    fractures of, 230
        occult, *232,* 232–233
    meralgia paresthetica of, 136–
        138
    osteoarthritis of, 133–135, *134*
    physical therapy for, 270–272
    prosthesis of, *134*
Housemaid's knee, 152
Humerus, fractures of, 216–217,
    217, 219
Hypaque 60 subacromial
    bursography, results of, *31*

Ice application, for biceps
    tendinitis, 36, 37
    for glenohumeral osteoarthri
        tis, 44
    for impingement syndrome, 15
    for lateral epicondylitis, 52
    for medial epicondylitis, 55, 56
    for rheumatoid arthritis, 101
    for shoulder multidirectional
        instability, 47
Impingement syndrome, 14–17
    exercises for, 15–16

Impingement syndrome
    (Continued)
    injection for, 17
    physical therapy for, 16
    range of motion for, 15
Infraspinatus tendons, 17
Injection, for ankle effusion,
    174, 175–176
    for Achilles tendinitis, *177,*
        179–180
    for acromioclavicular (AC)
        joint, 34
    for adventitial bursitis, *197,*
        199
    for ankle sprain, *170,* 172–173
    for anserine bursitis, *155,* 157–
        158
    for Baker cyst, *159,* 160–161
    for biceps tendinitis, 37–38
    for bunions, *194,* 196
    for carpal tunnel syndrome,
        75, 77–78
    for carpometacarpal osteoar-
        thritis, *69,* 71–72
    for cervical strain, 6–7
    for De Quervain tenosynovitis,
        66, 68
    for Dupuytren's contracture,
        82, 93
    for frozen shoulder, 26
    for gamekeeper's thumb, *73,*
        74
    for glenohumeral osteoarthri-
        tis, 44
    for gluteus medius bursitis,
        130, 132–133
    for gout, *200,* 202
    for hammer toes, *203,* 204–205
    for impingement syndrome, 17
    for knee effusion, 146
    for lateral epicondylitis, *50,*
        52–53
    for lumbosacral strain, *112,*
        115–116
    for medial collateral ligament
        strain, *161,* 164
    for medial epicondylitis, *54,* 57
    for meralgia paresthetica, *137*
    for Morton neuroma, *206,* 206–
        208
    for olecranon bursitis, *58,*
        59–60
    for osteoarthritis of hand, *96,*
        98
    for patellofemoral diseases,
        140, 142
    for plantar fasciitis, *188,* 191
    for posterior tibialis tenosyno-
        vitis, *186,* 187–188
    for pre-Achilles bursitis, *181,*
        182–183
    for prepatellar bursitis, *153,*
        154–155
    for radiocarpal joint arthritis,
        80–81
    for radiohumeral joint arthro-
        centesis, *61,* 62–63
    for retrocalcaneal bursitis, *183,*
        183–185
    for rheumatoid arthritis, *99,*
        102
    for rotator cuff tendinitis,
        21–22
    for rotator cuff tendon tears,
        30

Injection (*Continued*)
  for sacroiliac strain, *120, 123*
  for sciatica, 119
  for shoulder multidirectional
    instability, 47
  for sternochondritis, *104, 106*
  for subscapular bursitis, 40–41
  for supratellar pouch, 147–149,
    148
  for tendon cyst, *89,* 90–91
  for trigger finger, *86,* 87–88
  for trochanteric bursitis, *126,*
    128–129
  of dorsal ganglion, *82, 82,*
    83–84
  of metacarpophalangeal joint,
    95–96
  of metatarsophalangeal joint,
    194
  of sternoclavicular joint, *107,*
    108–109
Intercondylar fractures, humeral,
  219
Interphalangeal joint, proximal,
  dislocation of, 226
Intra-articular dilation, British
  method of, for frozen
  shoulder, 27

Joint, glenohumeral, 15

Kenalog-40, for carpometacarpal
  osteoarthritis, 72t
Knee, 139–169, 273–277
  anatomy of, 273–274
  anserine bursitis of, 155–158
  Baker cyst in, 158–161
  effusion of, 143–146
    aspiration of, *143,* 146
    exercises for, 145–146
    injection for, 146
    physical therapy for, 145–
      146
  exercises for, 275–277
  fractures of, 233
  housemaid's, 152
  medial collateral ligament
    strain of, 161–164
  meniscal tear of, 165–168
  osteoarthritis of, *149,* 149–151
  patellofemoral diseases of,
    140–142
  physical therapy for, 275–277
  prepatellar bursitis of, 152–155
  supports, braces, and casts for,
    297–299
  supratellar pouch of, 147–149

Lateral epicondylitis, exercises
  for, 51, 52
  injection for, *50,* 52–53
  physical therapy for, 52
Levator scapular muscle
  irritation, 38
Lidocaine injections tests, for
  rotator cuff tendinitis, 19
Loose shoulder, 44–47
Lumbar radiculopathy, *116*
Lumbosacral region, supports
  and braces for, 295–296

Lumbosacral strain, 112–115
  exercises for, 115
  injection for, *112,* 115–116
  physical therapy for, 114–115
  traction for, 115

Magnetic resonance imaging
    (MRI), for Achilles
    tendinitis, 178
  for ankle effusion, 174
  for anserine bursitis, 156
  for cervical radiculopathy, 9,
    11
  for cervical strain, 5
  for gluteus medius bursitis,
    131
  for impingement syndrome, 15
  for lumbosacral strain, 113
  for medial collateral ligament
    strain, 162
  for meniscal tear, 166
  for osteoarthritis of hip, 135
  for osteoarthritis of knee, 150
  for radiohumeral joint arthro-
    centesis, 62
  for rotator cuff tendon tears,
    27, 29
  for sciatica, 118
  for trochanteric bursitis, 127
Mallet finger, 226–227
Mallet fractures, 226
Mallet thumb, 227
Manipulation, chiropractic, 265
  for frozen shoulder, 26
March fracture, of metatarsals,
  241–242, *242*
Massage, back, 264–265
  neck, 251
Medial collateral ligament strain,
    161–164
  exercises for, 163–164
  injection for, *161,* 164
  physical therapy for, 163–164
Medial epicondylitis, 54–58
  exercises for, 55, 56
  injection for, *54,* 57
  physical therapy for, 56
Medial femoral condyle,
    osteochondritis dissecans of,
    234
Meniscal tear, 165–168
  exercises for, 167
  medial, *166*
  physical therapy for, 167
Meniscectomy, 167
  for knee effusion, 147
Meralgia paresthetica, 136–138
  injection for, *137*
Metacarpals, fractures of,
  223–224
Metacarpophalangeal joints,
    arthritis of, 93–96
  arthrocentesis of, *94*
  complete rupture of, 72, *224,*
    224–225
  dislocation of, 223, 224
  injection for, 95–96
  physical therapy for, 95–96
Metatarsals, fracture of, 240–241,
    242
  march, 241–242, *242*
  stress, 241–242, *242*
Metatarsophalangeal joints,
    injection of, 194

Metatarsophalangeal joints
    (*Continued*)
  osteoarthritis of, 194
Microscopy, 201
Midtarsals, fractures of, 240
Milwaukee shoulder, 27, 44
Morton neuroma, 205–208
  injection for, *206,* 206–208
MRI. See *Magnetic resonance*
    imaging (MRI).
Muscle relaxer, for cervical
    radiculopathy, 9
  for cervical strain, 5, 6

Navicular fractures, 221–223, *222*
Neck, 4–11, 248–252. See also
    Cervical entries.
  anatomy of, 248, 249
  exercises for, 252
  massage for, 251
  physical therapy for, 249, 251
  strain of, 4–7
  supports and braces for, 284
  traction of, 253, 284
Neer's classification, for
    impingement syndrome, 17
Nerve conduction velocity tests,
    for carpal tunnel syndrome,
    76
Neurectomy, 208
Neuropathic fractures, 240
Nonsteroidal anti-inflammatory
    drugs, 308–309

Olecranon bursitis, 58–60
  exercises for, 59, 60
  injection for, *58,* 59–60
  physical therapy for, 59
Osteoarthritis, 41–44
  exercises for, 43, 44
  injection for, 44
  of carpometacarpal joint,
    69–72
  of hand, 96–98
    injection for, *96,* 98
  of hip, 133–135, *134*
    exercises for, 135–136
    physical therapy for, 135–
      136
  of knee, *149,* 149–151
    exercises for, 151–152
    physical therapy for, 151–
      152
  of metatarsophalangeal joint,
    194
  of wrist, 78
  physical therapy for, 44
Osteochondritis dissecans, of
    medial femoral condyle, 234

Palmar fascia, Dupuytren's
    contracture of, 91–93
Paracervical muscle, 4
Patella, fractures of, 233–234
  subluxation of, 140
Patella alta, 140
Patellofemoral arthritis, 140
Patellofemoral diseases, 140–142
  exercises for, 142

Patellofemoral diseases (Continued)
  injection for, 140, 142
  physical therapy for, 142
Pellegrini-Stieda syndrome, 162
Pelvis, fractures of, 229–230
Phalanx, Boutonniere injury of, 225–226
  fractures of, 225–226
Philadelphia collar, for cervical radiculopathy, 9
Phonophoresis, for biceps tendinitis, 37
  for lateral epicondylitis, 52
  for medial epicondylitis, 56
  for rheumatoid arthritis, 101
  for tendinitis, 261
Physical therapy, for Achilles tendinitis, 178
  for acromioclavicular (AC) joint, 33
  for adventitial bursitis, 199
  for ankle, 277–280
  for ankle effusion, 175
  for ankle sprain, 172
  for anserine bursitis, 157
  for back, 264–269
  for Baker cyst, 160
  for biceps tendinitis, 36–37
  for bunions, 196
  for carpal tunnel syndrome, 77
  for carpometacarpal osteoarthritis, 71
  for cervical radiculopathy, 10
  for cervical strain, 6
  for De Quervain tenosynovitis, 67–68
  for dorsal ganglion, 83
  for Dupuytren's contracture, 93
  for elbow, 261
  for frozen shoulder, 25–26
  for gamekeeper's thumb, 74
  for glenohumeral osteoarthritis, 44
  for gluteus medius bursitis, 132
  for gout, 202
  for hammer toes, 204
  for hand, 263
  for hip, 270–272
  for impingement syndrome, 16
  for knee, 275–277
  for knee effusion, 145–146
  for lateral epicondylitis, 52
  for lumbosacral strain, 114–115
  for medial collateral ligament strain, 163–164
  for medial epicondylitis, 56
  for meniscal tear, 167
  for metacarpophalangeal joint, 95–96
  for neck, 249, 251
  for olecranon bursitis, 59
  for osteoarthritis of hand, 98
  for osteoarthritis of hip, 135–136
  for osteoarthritis of knee, 151–152
  for patellofemoral diseases, 142
  for plantar fasciitis, 190–191
  for posterior tibialis tenosynovitis, 188
  for pre-Achilles bursitis, 182

Physical therapy (Continued)
  for prepatellar bursitis, 154
  for radiocarpal joint arthritis, 80
  for radiohumeral joint arthrocentesis, 62
  for retrocalcaneal bursitis, 184
  for rheumatoid arthritis, 101
  for rotator cuff tendinitis, 20–21
  for rotator cuff tendon tears, 30
  for sacroiliac strain, 123–124
  for sciatica, 119
  for shoulder, 255–259
  for shoulder multidirectional instability, 47
  for sternochondritis, 106
  for sternoclavicular joint, 108
  for subscapular bursitis, 40
  for trigger finger, 87
  for trochanteric bursitis, 128
  for wrist, 263
PIP (proximal interphalangeal) joint, dislocation of, 226
Piriformis syndrome. See Gluteus medius bursitis.
Plantar fasciitis, 188–192
  exercises for, 190–191
  injection for, 188, 191
  physical therapy for, 190–191
Podagra, 197
Posterior tibialis tenosynovitis, 185–188
  exercises for, 188
  injection for, 186, 187–188
  physical therapy for, 188
Posttraumatic monoarticular arthritis, 78
Pre-Achilles bursitis, 180–183
  exercises for, 182
  injection for, 181, 182–183
  physical therapy for, 182
Prepatellar bursitis, 152–155
  injection for, 153, 154–155
  physical therapy for, 154
Prosthesis, hip, 134
Proximal interphalangeal (PIP) joint, dislocation of, 226

Radiculopathy, cervical, 7–11
Radiocarpal joint arthritis, 78–81
  exercises for, 80
  injection for, 80–81
  physical therapy for, 80
  synovial fluid analysis of, 78, 79
Radiohumeral joint arthrocentesis, 60–63
  exercises for, 62, 63
  injection for, 61, 62–63
  physical therapy for, 62
Radius, fractures of, distal, 220–221, 221
  nondisplaced, 220
Reiter disease, 107, 120
Retrocalcaneal bursitis, injection for, 183, 183–185
  physical therapy for, 184
Rheumatoid arthritis, 78, 93
  exercises for, 101
  injection for, 99, 102
  of hand, 98–102

Rheumatoid arthritis (Continued)
  physical therapy for, 101
Rheumatoid factor, laboratory tests for, 310
Rhomboid muscle irritation, 38
Rib, fractures of, 228–229, 229
Rotator cuff tendinitis, 14, 17–23
  exercises for, 19–20
  injection for, 21–22
  physical therapy for, 20–21
Rotator cuff tendon, exercises for, 257
Rotator cuff tendon tears, 14, 27–32
  exercises for, 29–30
  injection for, 30
  physical therapy for, 30
  risk factors for, 31

Sacroiliac strain, 119–124
  exercises for, 123–124
  injection for, 120, 123
  physical therapy for, 123–124
Scapulothoracic syndrome, 38–41
Sciatica, 116, 116–118
  injection for, 119
  physical therapy for, 119
Septic arthritis, 78, 93
Sesamoid bone, fractures of, 243
Shoulder, 14–47, 254–259
  acromioclavicular joint of, 32–34
  anatomy of, 254
  biceps tendinitis of, 34–38
  exercises for, 255–259
  frozen, 23–27
    exercises for, 258
  impingement syndrome of, 14–17
  multidirectional instability of, 44–47
  osteoarthritis of, 41–44
  physical therapy for, 255–259
  rotator cuff tendinitis of, 17–23
  rotator cuff tendon tear of, 27–32
  subluxation of, 44–47
  subscapular bursitis of, 38–41
  supports, braces, and casts for, 285–286
Shoulder immobilizer, for acromioclavicular strain-osteoarthritis, 34
Shoulder multidirectional instability, 44–47
  exercises for, 45, 46, 47
  injection for, 47
  physical therapy for, 47
Soft cervical collar, for cervical radiculopathy, 9
  for cervical strain, 6
Spine, compression fractures of, 227, 227–228
Spurling sign, 8
Staphylococcus aureus infection, in prepatellar bursitis, 152
Sternochondritis, 104–106
Sternoclavicular joint, 107–109
  arthritis of, 107
  exercises for, 108–109
  injection of, 107, 108–109
  physical therapy for, 108
Stress fractures, metatarsal, 241–242, 242

Stress fractures (*Continued*)
  tibial, *234*, 234–235
Subacromial bursal injection, *14*, *18*
Subacromial bursography, Hypaque 60 results of, *31*
Subacromial decompression, for rotator cuff tendinitis, 22
Subscapular bursitis, 38–41
  exercises for, 40, 41
  injection for, 40–41
  physical therapy for, 40
Supports, for ankle, 300–302
  for elbow, 287
  for foot, 303–306
  for hand, 293–294
  for knee, 297–299
  for lumbosacral region, 295–296
  for neck, 284
  for shoulder, 285–286
  for wrist, 288–292
Supracondylar fractures, humeral, 219
Supraspinatus, 17
Suprapatellar pouch, 147–149
  injection for, 147–149, *148*
Synovectomy, 102
  for knee effusion, 147
Synovial cyst, volar, 81
Synovial fluid, analysis of, 311
  for ankle effusion, 174
  of tibiotalar joint, 173
  of wrist, 78, 79
  aspiration of, in knee effusion, *143*, 146
Systemic lupus erythematosus, clinical criteria for, 311

Talus, fractures of, 238
Tendinitis, Achilles, 176–180
  biceps, 34–38
  phonophoresis for, 261
  rotator cuff, 14, 17, 19–22
Tendon cyst, 89–91
  injection for, *89*, 90–91
Tendon(s). See also specific tendon, e.g., *Achilles tendon.*
  excision of, 53

Tendon(s) (*Continued*)
  lengthening of, 53
Tennis elbow, 50–54
  exercises for, 262
Tenotomy, for lateral epicondylitis, 53
TENS (transcutaneous electric nerve stimulator), 267
TheraBand, for rotator cuff tendon tears, 30
Thumb, complete rupture of, *224*, 224–225
  dislocation of, 223–224
  extra-articular metacarpal fractures of, 223
  gamekeeper's, 72–74, *224*, 224–225
  intra-articular metacarpal fractures of, 223–224
  rupture of, 227
Tibia, fractures of, 234, 235
  stress, *234*, 234–235
  with metastatic disease, 230
Tibialis tenosynovitis, posterior, 185–188, *186*
Tibiotalar joint, aspiration of, 173
  synovial fluid analysis of, 173
Tietze syndrome, 104
Toe(s), fractures of, 243
  great, bunions of, 194–197
    fractures of, 243
    gout in, 199–202
    strain of, 242–243
  Morton neuroma of, 205–208
Torticollis, 4, 6
Total knee replacement, for osteoarthritis, 152
Traction, for back, 267
  for lumbosacral strain, 115
  for neck, 253, 284
  for wrist, 292
Transcutaneous electric nerve stimulator (TENS), 267
Trapezial strain, 4
Trapezius muscle, *4*
Trigger finger, 86–88
  D80 for, 87t
  exercises for, 87
  injection for, *86*, 87–88
  physical therapy for, 87
Trigger point injection, for cervical strain, *4*, 5

Trochanteric bursitis, 126–129
  exercises for, 128
  injection for, *126*, 128–129
  physical therapy for, 128
Turf toe, 242–243

Ulna, fractures of, nondisplaced, 220
Ulnar collateral ligament, injuries of, 72
Ultrasound, for cervical radiculopathy, 10
  for cervical strain, 6
  for impingement syndrome, 15
  for rotator cuff tears, 27, 29
  for rotator cuff tendinitis, 20

Vertebral body, compression fractures of, *227*, 227–228
Vertebral osteophytes, *8*
Vertical cervical traction, for cervical radiculopathy, 10
Volar synovial cyst, 81

Whiplash, 4, 38
Wrist, 66–84
  arthritis of, 69–72, 78–81
  aspiration of, 78
  carpal tunnel syndrome of, 74–78
  de Quervain tenosynovitis of, 66–69
  dorsal ganglion of, 81–84
  exercises for, 263
  osteoarthritis of, 78
  physical therapy for, 263
  supports, braces and casts for, 288–292
  synovial fluid analysis of, 78, 79
  traction for, 292
Wrist cyst, 81
Wrist sprain, 221–223, *222*
Wry neck, 4